D1548471

SSSP

Springer
Series in
Social
Psychology

SSSP

Ray Bull
Nichola Rumsey

The Social Psychology of Facial Appearance

Springer-Verlag New York Berlin Heidelberg
London Paris Tokyo

Ray Bull
Department of Psychology
Glasgow College: A Scottish Polytechnic
Cowcaddens Road
Glasgow, G4 OBA
Scotland

Nichola Rumsey
18, The Street
Didmarton, Gloucestershire
GL9 1DS
United Kingdom

Library of Congress Cataloging-in-Publication Data
Bull, Ray.
    The Social psychology of facial appearance/by Ray Bull, Nichola
Rumsey.
    p. cm.—(Springer series in social psychology)
    Bibliography: p.
    Includes indexes.
    ISBN 0-387-96607-2
    1. Interpersonal attraction.   2. Face—Social aspects.   3. Beauty,
Personal—Social aspects.   4. Body image.   I. Rumsey, Nichola.
II. Title.   III. Series.
HM132.B83   1988
302'. 13—dc19   87-32127

Typeset by Asco Trade Typesetting Ltd., Hong Kong.
Printed and bound by R.R. Donnelley and Sons, Harrisonburg, Virginia.
Printed in the United States of America.

9 8 7 6 5 4 3 2 1

ISBN 0-387-96607-2 Springer-Verlag New York Berlin Heidelberg
ISBN 3-540-96607-2 Springer-Verlag Berlin Heidelberg New York

Everyone knows that it is better to be beautiful than to be ugly. There may be some people who would prefer to be bad than good. Some might even prefer to be poor than rich. But we take it on faith that no one prefers to be ugly. The reason for this must be that people expect good things to come to the beautiful. Folklore tells us that beautiful girls marry handsome princes and live happily ever after. Heroes are handsome and villians are ugly.

Udry and Eckland (1984)

Stereotypes about physically distinctive people may begin in the eye of the beholder, but they can often end a reality. Stereotyped expectations lead people to treat members of a physically distinctive category of people in a manner that elicits the expected behavior. Once elicited, this behavior may be internalized into the self-concept of the stereotyped group members. More specifically, since their distinctive physical appearance is likely to produce self-focused attention, these people may make self-attributions for behaviors that were in reality situationally induced, and they may thus come to expect from themselves what others have expected (and elicited) from them.

McArthur (1982)

Contents

1. **Introduction** 1

2. **The Role of Facial Appearance in Liking, Dating, and Marriage**.. 9

   The Effects of Facial Appearance on Liking 9
   The Effects of Facial Appearance on Meeting and Dating 14
   The Role of Facial Appearance in Marriage 29
   Conclusion 39

3. **The Effects of Facial Appearance in Persuasion, Politics, Employ-ment, and Advertising** 41

   Facial Appearance and Persuasion 41
   The Role of Facial Appearance in Politics 50
   The Role of Facial Appearance in Employment 62
   Facial Appearance and Advertising 75
   General Conclusion 79

4. **Facial Appearance and the Criminal Justice System** 81

   The Extent to Which People Expect a Relationship Between
      Facial Appearance and Criminality 81
   The Effects of Facial Appearance on Recognizability 85
   Is There, in Fact, a Relationship Between Facial Appearance
      and Criminality? 91
   Facial Appearance and Attributions of Responsibility 101
   The Effects of Facial Appearance on "Jurors" 104
   Overall Conclusion 120

5. **The Effects of Facial Appearance in the Educational System** 121

   The Effects of Facial Appearance on Teachers' Expectations 122

The Effects of Facial Appearance on Academic Work 134
Is There Really a Relationship Between Facial Appearance and
    Academic Performance? 140
The Effects of Teachers' Facial Appearance 147
Conclusion 149

**6. The Effects of Children's Facial Appearance on Adults and the
Effects of Facial Appearance on Children** 151

Children's Facial Appearance and Their Disciplining 151
Adults' Reactions to Infants' Facial Appearance 158
At What Age Can Children Discriminate Facial Attractiveness?. 161
At What Age Do Children Demonstrate Stereotyping Based on
    Facial Appearance? 164
Overall Conclusion 177

7. The Social Psychology of Facial Disfigurement 179

The Birth and Development of Facially Disadvantaged Children . 179
A Historical Perspective on Disfigurement and Society 185
Negative Stereotyping and Negative Attitudes Toward Dis-
    figured Persons—Do They Exist? 187
The Relationship Between Societal Values and the Demand for
    Cosmetic Surgery 191
Social Interaction Involving Disfigured Persons 193
What Are the Consequences of the Negative Reactions of Others? 198
Studies of Helping Behavior Relevant to Facially Disfigured Per-
    sons 203
The Behavior of Disfigured Persons Themselves 207
Ways of Helping Facially Disfigured Persons 212
Issues to Be Considered in Future Research 213
Summary 215

**8. How Can Psychologists Help Those Disadvantaged by Their
Facial Appearance?** 217

Attitudes Toward Facially Disfigured Persons 218
The Behavior and Attitudes of Facially Disadvantaged Persons .. 223
Techniques of Attitude Change 224
The Media—Enemies or Allies? 227
How the Media Can Help 232
The Provision of Health Services for Facially Disadvantaged Per-
    sons 237
Ways of Offering Help Directly to Facially Disadvantaged People. 247
Conclusion 267

9. **Some Final Remarks** 269

Other Studies Concerning the Social Psychological Aspects of
    Beauty 269
What Is Facial Attractiveness? 278
Individual Differences Between Perceivers 282
Context Effects in Reactions to Faces 283
Theoretical Explanations 285
Further Points for Future Research 294

References 301

Author Index 337

Subject Index 353

Chapter 1

Introduction

Several years ago Coleman (1981) reported that in 1979 one of the many international cosmetics companies had an annual sales figure of $2.38 billion, nearly 1.25 million sales representatives, and over 700 products, the majority of these being for the face. Cash and Cash (1982) noted that in 1979 U.S. consumers spent over $4 million on cosmetic products. They stated that, "Although this practice would seem to be a fascinating aspect of human behavior on the basis of its generality and resilience, social-behavioral scientists have largely ignored the phenomenon so plainly (or pleasingly) in front of their eyes."

Why should people be so concerned with their facial appearance? Many psychologists have argued (e.g., Kleck & Rubenstein, 1975) not only that facial information is usually the first that is available to the perceiver, but also that it is continuously available during social interaction. Maruyama and Miller (1981) stated that "appearance is often the first dimension upon which a stranger can be evaluated. Since people tend to see others as integrated and consistent units, rather than as collections of situation-specific behaviors, a potent and immediately evident basis for an evaluation, such as physical appearance, should intrude into and affect any overall and subsequent evaluation." Furthermore, De Jong and Kleck (1986) have suggested that the continuous availability of physical appearance information during interaction "does not depend, as does attitudinal or personality information, on complex information processing and retrieval." Although we would not necessarily agree with the latter statement, we would agree with Hatfield and Sprecher (1986) that, "Other infomation may be more meaningful but far harder to ferret out." In addition, many societies have changed, and are changing, in the sense that people are becoming increasingly mobile in terms both of employment and of home. This has resulted in an increased incidence of people coming into contact with unknown others for the first time. This provides less time for individuals to get to know those persons to whom they have to respond. Therefore, it may well be the case that they have to rely on the available, limited information such as facial appearance. Early in this century, Perrin (1921) stated in the *Journal of Experimental Psychology* that, "Just why the physical characteristics of individuals should exert so profound an influence over their associates furnishes an interesting topic of speculation." Little psychological speculation and even fewer methodologically rigorous studies of the social psychology of facial appearance took place until the 1960s. Several authors have suggested (e.g., Kleinke, 1974) that by avoiding the study of the role of facial appearance, psychologists can escape from scientifically supporting the unpalatable view that looks are really important in how a person is judged. Berscheid (1981) has argued that "our collective reluctance to acknowledge the true impact of physical appearance has affected research . . . in the past and it probably continues to affect research and practice today." Although little research was conducted until the 1970s on the social psychology of facial appearance, we cannot support the notion that since then research has ignored this topic.

In fact, as the very considerable number of studies cited in the present book attest, a vast number of studies have been conducted recently. However, most of these studies are of poor quality, and it may have been this aspect of current research to which Berscheid was referring. Certainly, as pointed out by Goldstein (1983), few competent psychologists have made facial appearance their main research focus. Instead, many have published one or two (usually rather simple) studies while their main research efforts have been directed elsewhere. Thus the literature reviewed in this book is greatly lacking in terms of systematic long-term research. Goldstein argued that in this respect the development of face-related research may be unique, and he suggested that one reason for this may be the foreseen difficulties of conducting high quality research. Berscheid (1981) suggested that the strong history in American psychology of behaviorism and the environmental approach (as contrasted to the "dismal flops" of phrenology and morphology) led many researchers away from even investigating whether facial appearance has an influence on behavior. She argued that research might have been different if society were "not so enamoured of the idea that because a person's appearance *ought* not to make a difference, it *does* not."

Notwithstanding the possibility that some able researchers have purposely avoided working on facial appearance, Berscheid (1981) claimed that

> A person's physical attractiveness level has been revealed by numerous investigations to be an extraordinarily important psychological variable, for it has accounted for a statistically significant portion of the variance in almost all situations in which it has been investigated and for almost all dependent measures which have been constructed to show its effect. This effect, in general, is such that the physically attractive are preferred to the unattractive and thus receive numerous preferential social treatments. . . . the psychological effects of physical attractiveness have been found to be pervasive in frequency, considerable in strength, and generally monolithic in nature.

We leave it to readers of our book to judge whether Berscheid's statement is a valid one with respect to facial appearance. (Our own view is that it is an overstatement.) Readers may also wish, when going through our overview of the research, to determine for themselves whether it supports the claims recently made by Hatfield and Sprecher (1986) that

> There seem to be four steps in the stereotyping process that ensures that beauty equals goodness
>
> 1. Most people feel that discriminating against the ugly is not fair, but yet . . .
> 2. Privately, most of us simply take it for granted that attractive and unattractive people are different. Most often we perceive that attractive people have the more desirable traits.
> 3. As a consequence, we *treat* good-looking versus ugly people quite differently; the good-looking get the better treatment.
> 4. How does such prejudice affect the victims of our discrimination? Over time, a sort of "self-fulfilling prophecy" occurs. The way we treat attractive versus unattractive people shapes the way they think about themselves and, as a consequence, the kind of people they become.

Similarly, McArthur (1982) suggested that stereotyped expectations lead people to treat members of physically distinctive categories in a manner that elicits the expected behavior. Once elicited, this behavior may be internalized into the self-concepts of the stereotyped people so that they come to make self-attributions for behaviors that were situationally induced. R. Jones (1982) additionally argued that "when we have categorized someone in a certain way, we are more likely to attend to and remember actual behaviors consistent with the categorization and to fill in memory gaps with attributes for which we have no evidence (but are consistent with the initial categorization). We may even remember only the categorization itself, and forget the features that prompted us to make it" (see also B. Clifford & Bull, 1978).

Hatfield and Sprecher (1986) suggested that "people generally *say* looks are not important to them, but their actions belie their statements." One reason why it may to some extent be true that most people are not fully aware of the effects of facial appearance could be, as Nisbett and Wilson (1977) suggested, that whatever effects occur may largely be the result of unconscious processing. However, a number of professional groups (e.g., dentists, surgeons, and lawyers) recently may have increased their awareness of facial issues. Lucker, Ribbens, and McNamara (1981) made the point that techniques of facial surgery are now so advanced and fairly widely available (at least to those who can pay) that the resultant opportunities to alter facial appearance require a worthwhile understanding of the possible psychological benefits of such interventions. Berscheid and Gangestad (1982) stated that "the increasing concern health practitioners are now giving to the social and psychological impact of alterations in facial form has come about through mounting evidence that an individual's facial physical attractiveness has an important impact upon his or her life."

In 1986 Berscheid noted that practitioners in a variety of professions are increasingly asking just how important is facial appearance. She noted that lawyers representing clients whose appearance has been irrevocably altered for the worse through the negligence of others often want to know how much we, the experts, think a particular decrease in attractiveness is "worth" in monetary damages. How much, they ask, should the manufacturer of a flammable nightgown be ordered to pay to the little girl whose face and body were burned beyond the remedial talents of plastic surgeons? How much should be awarded to the boy whose face was ripped beyond repair by a savage dog that escaped his owner's leash? What factors have to be taken into consideration? Will their physical unattractiveness affect their self-esteem? Will it influence their marital prospects, their job prospects? Will it influence their close relationships with their parents and siblings and peers?

Berscheid continued by pointing out that

> . . . judges and juries aren't the only ones who have to make very concrete judgements about how important physical attractiveness is. Those in the dental and medical professions make such determinations everyday. The orthodontic surgeon, for example, has to decide whether breaking a jaw in order to acheive a perfect "bite" is worth lessening the person's physical attractiveness. Again, social psychologists can take some credit for the fact that appearance is now more frequently considered by practitioners when treatments that will improve function but also will alter appearance are contemplated. But how much, they ask, is a specific increase or decrease in attractiveness level worth against a specific improvement of function?

This book overviews the published research that is available to those who wish to construct answers to these (and other) questions. However, the majority of research has been so unsystematic and so atheoretical as possibly to preclude worthwhile answers. Mere awareness of these issues is not enough; a systematically organized body of knowledge is necessary. Even then, as Wells (1983) pointed out, awareness may not guarantee society's being able to modify, should it wish to do so, the social psychological effects of facial appearance.

In deciding what to include in this book we chose, largely for space reasons, to exclude the topic of facial expression as such. Clearly there are facial expression differences both within and between faces. However, the majority of the studies cited in this book have kept facial expression constant. A determination of whether this restricts the generalization of results from such studies to real life (in the way discussed in Chapter 9) awaits the results of future research, since few studies have varied concomitantly facial expression and facial appearance factors such as attractiveness (see Mueser, Grau, Sussman, & Rosen, 1984).

In the preface to his 1978 book (with Crossman) Adams made the point that he doubted the conclusions arrived at by previous authors of research papers on the social role of facial appearance. In order to confirm his doubts he undertook a program of research on this topic that led him to conclude that "the doubting Thomas has had his head turned—looks really matter." However, having written our review of research we would not necessarily agree with Adams. Looks may well be found to matter in rather basic, ecologically invalid research, but the evidence that they have important effects in real life is as yet rather weak. That is the conclusion we shall arrive at in our final chapter. However, let us now briefly outline the contents of each chapter.

Chapter 2 examines research on the effects of facial appearance in liking, dating, and marriage. With regard to liking, early research (i.e., from around 20 years ago) found what appeared to be pronounced effects of facial attractiveness. Even those later studies that also manipulated other independent variables (e.g., attitude similarity) found facial appearance seemingly important. However, many of these studies could be criticized for having procedures that did not resemble real-life situations. Early research also claimed that facial attractiveness plays an important role in meeting and dating, but again the procedures were deficient in terms of ecological validity. More recent research has taken the trouble to examine concomitantly the effects of other factors (such as the subjects' level of facial attractiveness), but there is little consensus as to the power of these factors or the nature of their interaction with the factor of facial appearance. Some studies of real-life (as opposed to experimenter-imposed) dating have been conducted, and these tend to support the idea that facial appearance plays a central role in such settings, although the effect of facial attractiveness may not be monotonic. In Chapter 2 we begin to develop the notion (followed through in subsequent chapters) that one important (indeed, probably the crucial) effect of facial appearance is concerned not simply with some kind of direct, instantaneous effect upon the perceiver, but with how it affects the dynamics of encounters. Studies of long-term interactions/dating (as opposed to simple "one shot" studies of students' ratings of photographs) are also mentioned. Research on the role of facial appearance in marriage is reviewed, and we examine the questions of whether marriage partners are similar to each other in facial appearance and/ or whether beautiful women become involved with prestigious men. We overview research on the effects of having a facially attractive partner, and that on the relationships between facial appearance and (*a*) marital adjustment, (*b*) sexuality, and (*c*) infidelity.

In Chapter 3 we examine research on the effects of facial appearance in persuasion, politics, employment, and advertising. Twenty years ago the findings of early research suggested that a communicator's facial attractiveness led to her being more persuasive, and that this effect was mediated by liking and/or credibility. More recent and ecologically valid work has examined the ways in which a communicator's facial appearance could affect the information processing strategies employed by the recipients of a message. This provides one of the several opportunities that we have taken throughout this book to point out that the study of a topic (i.e., facial appearance) that traditionally falls within the scope of social psychology is unlikely to bear fruit unless the concomitant role of cognitive factors is also examined. In politics, as with persuasion, the history of methodologically respectable studies is short. Studies have found that political inclination can be judged fairly reliably from facial appearance. The research that has focused on the "women's movement" can be used to chart how the view that "only ugly women are feminists" has become modified over recent years. Studies of the effects of facial appearance in employment can also be used to examine recent (and ongoing) changes in facial biases, especially toward females. This research can be used to question the naive notion that the higher a person's facial attractiveness the more she (he) benefits from it. Research concerning employment also provides us with a chance to examine another notion that we mention in several chapters, that facial appearance (e.g., level of attractiveness) has a more powerful effect when the stimulus person's possession of ecologically valid factors (e.g., job-related qualifications) is low, or unknown. To the perceiver the stimulus persons often employed in advertising have unknown qualities (save when famous people are used). Unfortunately (probably for commercial reasons) few studies of the effects of facial appearance in advertising have been published. Some commentators have pointed out that the use of facially attractive models has increased considerably in the last two decades. Such usage could be based on a limited appreciation of the research reviewed earlier in this chapter, although a realization that advertising model facial appearance might influence how the related message is cognitively processed could be appropriate.

Chapter 4 focuses on the role of facial appearance in the criminal justice system. We review studies of the extent to which the general public expect there to be a relationship between facial appearance and criminality. It seems beyond doubt that people do consensually share such expectations. However, the evidence is not strong that those who commit crimes have certain types of facial appearance (e.g., abnormal). Related research fails to offer a clear conclusion concerning the nature of the relationship of facial appearance to (a) recognizability and (b) attributions of responsibility. Similarly, the nature of the effects of the facial appearance of either victims or defendants upon "jurors" is not clear, even though a very considerable number of studies have been conducted. Sadly, most of these studies have been so lacking in ecological validity as to make unjustified almost any extrapolation from them to the criminal justice system, especially since the real-life difference between (a) judgment of guilt and (b) sentencing has usually been ignored. Ecological validity may not necessarily be required if a study is conducted solely to test a psychological theory; however, many publications on this topic hardly mention such theory.

In Chapter 5 we examine research on the effects of facial appearance in the educational system (the disciplining of children is covered in Chapter 6). We review work on the effects of children's facial attractiveness on teachers' expectations of them and on the assessment of their work. Although early work (i.e., that of 15 years ago) claimed to have found significant effects, the actual size of such effects may be rather small. Later studies additionally varied other factors (e.g., academic performance), and when this is done the effects of facial appearance may well be considerably attenuated or perhaps may have a meaningful effect only when academic achievement is low. Studies of mere expectation are relatively easy to conduct; what are more difficult to achieve in the educational system (or indeed, elsewhere) are studies of behavior. There is limited evidence that facial apearance and actual academic performance are related. In Chapter 5 we examine the possibility that (as in Chapter 4) unattractiveness or facial abnormality is assumed to be associated with undesirable characteristics. Chapter 7 focuses more explicitly on this notion, and Chapter 8 examines for counselors, as does Chapter 5 for teachers, the effects of their facial appearance.

Chapter 6 reviews the literature concerning the effects of children's facial appearance on adults (save for that covered by Chapter 5). It also takes a developmental perspective by examining research on the effects of facial appearance on children of various ages. Consensus does not exist in the research on the effects of children's facial appearance on their disciplining. However, that little research that exists concerning physically abused children could be taken to imply that their facial appearance may play a role, particularly in the light of research on adults' reactions to infants' faces that suggests a relationship with caregiving behavior. This chapter also examines the age at which children may start to be influenced by the facial appearance of others. There is evidence that not only infants but also neonates may be able to discriminate facial attractiveness. However, this sould not be taken to suggest that they behave or make judgments based on facial attractiveness. Research that has examined the issue of the age at which children demonstrate stereotyping based on facial appearance similar to that shown by adults suggests that this does not occur until much later (probably in strong form between ages 6 and 9 years).

The first part of Chapter 7 is also concerned with children. This chapter overviews research on the social psychology of facial disfigurement. It begins by examining work on the birth and development of facially disadvantaged children. We then focus on studies designed to examine whether negative behavior occurs toward disfigured persons and we conclude that responses that could be taken by disfigured persons to indicate negativity, avoidance, and rejection do occur but that these may be caused more by people not being sure how to behave rather than by purposive rejection. Relevant research concerning helping behavior is reviewed, as is that on the demand for cosmetic surgery. One of the main themes of Chapter 7 is that social interactions involving facially disfigured persons may not run smoothly, this relating perhaps to problems of privacy, loneliness, and self-definition. Few studies have examined the behavior of facially disfigured persons, but it may be, because of the reciprocal nature of social interaction, that an enhanced level of social skill could greatly benefit those individuals who are facially disadvantaged.

Chapter 8 examines this suggestion in greater depth, having as its main focus the extent to which psychology can help those disadvantaged by their facial appearance. It begins by reviewing research concerning attitudes toward facially disfigured persons, and this sets the scene for our discussion of how negative attitudes might be changed. The role of the media in the establishment and modification of attitudes is highlighted, and suggestions are made for how the media could be used to reduce facial prejudice. We then turn to a discussion of the provision of health services for facially disadvantaged persons, and we argue that more than mere surgical care is necessary. Counseling could possibly be of benefit, not only from the psychological perspective but also because it may prove cost effective. At this point we examine research on the role of facial appearance in counseling and in mental health. The final part of Chapter 8 examines the notion of whether there is a relationship between facial appearance and social skill, and whether social skill training could be of benefit to facially disadvantaged persons.

Chapter 9 is entitled "Some Final Remarks." It begins by briefly mentioning studies of facial appearance that do not readily fit in with the organization of the previous chapters. We then discuss what is meant (so far as is known) by facial attractiveness and the extent to which people react similarly to faces. The possible influences of individual perceiver differences and contextual effects on reactions to faces are discussed. An overview is then presented of theoretical explanations that have been put forward to account for some of the findings mentioned in this book, and we offer the opinion that research on the social psychology of facial appearance is woefully lacking in theoretical content, the majority of the literature being atheoretical. This final chapter ends with some further suggestions for future research, an important one being that we should investigate the validity not only of the notion that "what is beautiful is therefore good" but also the more palatable notion that "what is good is therefore beautiful" (see H. Cavior & Dokecki, 1973).

Chapter 2

The Role of Facial Appearance in Liking, Dating, and Marriage

The Effects of Facial Appearance on Liking

In 1966 Walster, Aronson, Abrahams, and Rottman published one of the first studies examining the effect of facial appearance on liking and dating. (For an interesting account of this study see Berscheid's foreword to Hatfield and Sprecher's 1986 book). College students who purchased a ticket for a "computer-dance" were guaranteed a partner for the duration of the dance. (In fact the males and females were paired at random.) During the evening's intermission the students filled in a questionnaire concerning how much they liked their date and how much they wanted to date their partner again. It was found that the only predictor of this popularity was physical attractiveness, ⌐ which was assessed at the box office as each student purchased a ticket for the dance. Intelligence and social skill were found to be unrelated to liking. Brislin and Lewis (1968) conducted a very similar study and they again found a very high positive correlation between independently evaluated physical attractiveness and randomly assigned partners' desire for a future date (the latter data were gathered 2 hours after the dance had started). In addition, Brislin and Lewis found significant, although rather smaller, correlations between individuals' desire to date their partner again and their rating of their partner's (a) sociability and (b) similarity of interest to their own. (See below for further studies contrasting the effects of attitude similarity and facial attractiveness on liking.)

Subsequent studies seemed to confirm the powerful effect of facial attractiveness on liking. A. Miller (1970a), for example, found people whose facial photographs had been judged as attractive to be rated more positively on an adjective checklist, particularly females. Dion, Berscheid, and Walster (1972) found that facially attractive people were expected to be more likely to possess almost every soically desirable personality trait (e.g., warm, sensitive, kind, interesting, strong, sociable) as determined by a preliminary study.

Similar results were found by Byrne, London, and Reeves (1968), by Stroebe, Insko, Thompson, and Layton (1971), by B. Thornton and Linnstaedter (1980), and by Kupke, Hobbs, and Cheney (1979), who, instead of merely using photographs, examined females' liking for and interpersonal attraction toward males with whom they had just had a 15-minute "casual, social" con- versation. Kupke, Hobbs, and Cheney found that the females' evaluations of the male whom they had just met for the first time were significantly affected by his physical attractiveness (assessed by independent raters).

At the time of their publication these results, especially those of Walster et al. (1966), were thought of as rather surprising, so much so that H. Miller and Rivenbark (1970), for example, took the trouble to ask students to rate the importance for them of physical attractiveness in a variety of situations. They found that males and females rated it as only moderately important even for first meetings and social functions, and they suggested that their subjects were "either not fully aware or not fully honest about how important physical attractiveness really is to them." Soon, however, studies were published that, unlike those of A. Miller (1970a) and Dion et al. (1972), varied other stimulus factors along with facial appearance, as had Walster et al. (1966).

Varying Other Independent Variables

Smits and Cherhoniak (1976) asked male students to rate a stimulus female who was either high or low in facial attractiveness and whose personality was described as warm/friendly or as cold/unfriendly. Ratings of "social attrac- tiveness" were significantly affected by physical attractiveness but not by friendliness, whereas ratings of "personality" were affected by both indepen- dent variables. (The subjects' self-rated physical attractiveness had no effect.) Even as recently as 1976 Smits and Cherhoniak deemed it worth stating that, "The interesting finding is that physical appearance can affect ratings of per- sonality."

In addition to varying physical attractiveness Kleinke, Staneski, and Pipp (1975) varied the behavior of the stimulus person. Male students were asked to spend 15 minutes getting to know a female who was either physically attractive or unattractive and who spent 90% or 10% of the interaction gazing at the subjects, while on some occasions moving her chair closer. The subjects indicated that they liked more the attractive confederate and they rated her more positively on a number of bipolar adjective scales, these effects of attractiveness being much more pronounced when the confederate gazed at the subjects for only 10% of the time. The amount of confederate gaze itself had a minimal effect on these ratings. The subjects' own gaze behavior is not reported to have been affected by confederate facial attractiveness. Kleinke et al. concluded that, "The most important variable affecting males' ratings of their female partners in the present study was the females' attractiveness." However, since subjects' gaze and talking behavior seems to have been un- affected by attractiveness, previous studies' assumptions that more positive ratings would occasion in subjects more positive behavior toward attractive stimuli seem unwarranted.

McKelvie and Matthews (1976) also varied another factor alongside facial attractiveness. In their study male and female students rated their liking of photographed females whose attractiveness and favorability of character were varied. McKelvie and Matthews stated that, "Although the relationship between physical attractiveness and liking appears to be well established, it is not clear how to account for it." They suggested that on the one hand "the reinforcing properties of physically attractive people" may be what makes them more likeable. On the other hand they argued that liking may be determined by the kind of attributes a person is believed to possess. This latter, indirect explanation holds that the attractiveness effect occurs because appearance affects beliefs about the attributes people possess. By varying both facial attractiveness and favorability of the character descriptions given to the stimulus persons McKelvie and Matthews attempted to determine which of these two explanations was more appropriate. They noted that Lampel and Anderson (1968) had found personality descriptions to have no effect in terms of desirability for dating when accompanied by an unattractive photograph, but that this variable did have an affect when accompanying facially attractive photographs. McKelvie and Matthews found that degree of liking was significantly affected both by facial attractiveness and by character, with character having the stronger effect, particularly with attractive rather than unattractive faces (as found by Lampel and Anderson). Male subjects were more influenced by facial attractiveness than by character, whereas females evidenced the reverse. McKelvie and Matthews concluded that their results were inconsistent with the indirect facial attractiveness———→character———→ liking effect, especially since attractiveness "influenced the effect of character itself," and that a reward model of the effect of facial attractiveness may be more appropriate.

Zakin (1983) examined the effects of facial appearance on children's liking. (Further studies of the effects of facial appearance on children are covered in Chapters 5 and 6.) He found, somewhat to his surprise, that photographic facial attractiveness was more important than described social or athletic ability in influencing children's choice of which new, as yet unmet, classmate they would choose as a friend. No effect of facial appearance, however, was found on judgments of predicted popularity.

From the studies reviewed above it might seem that facial appearance has a strong effect on liking. However, as Wells (1983) has pointed out, such studies tend to oversimplify matters and they often have very little ecological validity. Only those by Kupke, Hobbs, and Cheney (1979) and Walster et al. (1966) involved actual behavior rather than mere expectation. (The latter found a female student's physical attractiveness to predict how often her computer-date partner subsequently asked her for a date.) In addition, early studies of the possible effects of facial appearance upon liking did not pay much attention to possibly important subject individual difference factors.

Subject Factors

In 1976 Pheterson and Horai found that it was only high scorers on a sensation-seeking scale whose liking ratings were affected by stimulus facial attractiveness. Their analysis for the effects of this individual difference subject factor revealed that low sensation seekers were uninfluenced by facial attractiveness.

Mathes and Edwards (1978) found speakers' physical attractiveness to influence whom among their group the speakers nominated to receive a small financial reward. However, this main effect was caused solely by subjects of the opposite sex from the nominated speaker. Similarly, in their second study the physical attractiveness of a photographed person said to be requesting a donation of money toward his or her lunch only had a positive effect on the stated donating intentions of subjects of the opposite sex from the requestor.

In 1979 Touhey made the point that "virtually nothing is known about individual differences in subjects' responses to persons who vary in attractiveness." He found facial attractiveness to influence liking for a member of the opposite sex and other ratings on an interpersonal judgment scale only for those male and female subjects who were high scorers on a "Macho Scale" of sexist attitudes. Furthermore, he found a similar effect of this subject factor on the amount of information recalled by subjects from the biographical account of the stimulus person that they had read some 15 minutes earlier. From his data Touhey concluded that whereas the high scorers on the macho scale were affected by facial appearance, the low scores (particularly females) were affected by the written biographical account.

Husain and Kureshi (1983) also found the effect of facial attractiveness on liking to be qualified by a subject factor, namely the subjects' self-rating of their own level of facial attractiveness. (Another noteworthy aspect of this study is that it is one of the few studies of the social effects of facial appearance that has been conducted outside the English-speaking world.) Males, irrespective of their self-rating, liked most the highly attractive photographs, as did females whose self-ratings were medium or high. However, females whose self-ratings were low liked most the medium-attractive male faces.

R. Bailey and Schreiber (1981) found that subjects liked less those persons whom they were led to believe had rated the subjects' physical attractiveness as lower than had the subjects themselves. Individuals whom the subjects believed to have rated them equal to or higher than their own self-rating were liked more.

Attitude Similarity

A subject factor that has been more extensively studied than those mentioned above is that of similarity in attitudes to the stimulus person. Byrne et al. (1968) found that both similarity of attitude and physical attractiveness had significant effects on interpersonal attraction. Byrne, Ervin, and Lamberth (1970) asked students "to spend 30 minutes together at the Student Union on a 'coke date'." The subjects' subsequent evaluation of their date on an interpersonal judgment scale was found to be affected both by attitude similarity and by physical attractiveness. In an end-of-term follow-up both factors were found to related to memory of the date's name, incidence of talking to one another since the date, and desire to date the other person in the future.

Curran and Lippold (1975) criticized Byrne et al.'s studies for randomly pairing dates with regard to physical attractiveness. They argued that if in real life members of dating couples tend to be similiar to each other in attractiveness (see later in this chapter) then random pairing could produce artifactual effects. Curran and Lippold asked students to participate in a "computer-dating service," and they found that even though members of couples were similar to each other in level of physical attractiveness, the partner's physical attractiveness had a much greater effect on interpersonal attraction than did attitude similarity. However, Curran and Lippold's study seems to lack any guarantee (as do many others) that dates were aware of their partner's attitudes.

Stroebe et al. (1971) found, in addition, that different forms of relationships (e.g., dating, marrying, liking, working) were differentially affected by physical attractiveness and similarity of attitude. For attractive females attitude similarity had a clearly significant effect, whereas it (narrowly) did not for unattractive female stimuli.

N. Cavior, Miller, and Cohen (1975) also examined whether attitude similarity would qualify the effects of stimulus physical attractiveness. Unlike most of the studies mentioned above, their study was not concerned with subjects' ratings of strangers' photographs made in rather meaningless settings. Instead they examined the judgments of teenage classmates who had been in school together for years. They found that liking/dating preference was significantly influenced, as expected, by subjects' beliefs concerning the stimulus persons' similarity in attitudes to their own. For those readers who might expect this more ecologically valid study to find a reduced effect of physical attractiveness, the finding that on opposite-sex judgments it had an even stronger effect than perceived attitude similarity may come as rather a surprise. An additional interesting finding was that subjects' ratings of their classmates' physical attractiveness and their judgments of classmates' attitude similarity to their own beliefs were positively correlated. In other words, the subjects indicated that individuals whom they considered to be physically attractive would be more likely to have attitudes similar to their own (and vice versa).

A similar finding was noted by Schoedel, Frederickson, and Knight (1975), who found their subjects to assume that attractive strangers of the opposite sex would have attitudes similar to their own. Schoedel et al. stated that it would seem reasonable to suggest that "the subject anticipates positive reinforcement from individuals who have been found to be reinforcing. Thus, if a subject receives positive reinforcement (physical attractiveness) from another person, he may expect further reinforcement and this expectation may generalize to other forms of reinforcement (attitude similarity)." Alternatively they suggested that a cognitive consistency model could account for their findings. (To what extent these "reinforcement" and "cognitive consistency" notions merit being described as models or theories is discussed in the concluding chapter.) Schoedel et al. made the worthwhile suggestions (a) that "These data imply that physically attractive individuals have an added advantage in social situations where attitudes rather than appearance are presumed to be of primary importance. . . . the attribution of similar attitudes to attractive individuals might be expected to result in their being treated preferentially, while unattractive individuals might receive negative feedback from others because they are perceived as dissimilar" in attitude, and (b) that "an attractive candidate for a political office might be expected to receive more votes because voters perceive his views as being similar to their own" (Chapter 3 examines the role of facial appearance in politics).

Mashman (1978) also found that subjects' assumed similarity between stimulus persons' attitudes and their own increased with stimulus physical attractiveness, particularly for females' assumptions about males. This sex effect was the opposite of what Mashman predicted, and to his rather weak explanations of this we might add that it may be females who, when finding a male to be physically attractive, have a stronger need to assume that his attitudes are similar to their own. Perhaps males do not consider females' attitudes to be quite so important.

No such sex of subject effect was found by Marks, Miller, and Maruyama (1981), who stated (somewhat surprisingly in view of the studies reviewed above) that "although the literature on physical attractiveness strongly suggests that people should perceive attractive strangers as being similar to themselves, it contains no direct test of enhancement of assumed similarity between self and physically attractive others." However, since Marks et al. inexplicably used only female faces as stimuli there was no opportunity to examine the effects of male attractiveness on their female (and male) subjects. Nevertheless, their subjects did evidence an effect of facial attractiveness on assumed attitude similarity.

Thus, if it is indeed the case that people assume facially attractive others to have attitudes similar to their own, then in seeking out a partner for dating or a longer lasting relationship, target physical attractiveness could be used as an easily discernible guide to attitude similarity. (The conclusion from the above, largely correlational studies, could also be that we find those known to share our attitudes to be more facially attractive.) It is to studies of the effects of facial appearance on dating that we now turn. Its effects on marriage will be covered in the subsequent section.

The Effects of Facial Appearance on Meeting and Dating

At the beginning of this chapter we briefly described the study by Walster et al. (1966) that found the main determinant of whether subjects wished to (and, in fact, did) date their partner again to be the partner's physical attractiveness. In 1871 Darwin had noted that, "In civilized life, man is largely, but by no means exclusively, influenced in the choice of his wife by external appearance." The remainder of this chapter is concerned with the effects of facial appearance on dating and marriage.

In 1971 Berscheid, Dion, Walster, and Walster found that the information provided to subjects about the possibility of someone rejecting them as a date did not have a strong effect on subjects' desire to date attractive individuals. However, unlike Walster et al. (1966), they did find evidence that subjects' own level of physical attractiveness related to the level of attractiveness desired of a date.

Curran (1973), however, pointed out that the 1966 Walster et al. study, being based on randomly organized pairings of a "computer-dance" (as was the first study of Berscheid et al. [1971]), was not that representative of most real-life dating situations. In this study student respondents to an "advertisement for a computer dating service (Psych-A-Date)" were paired not at random but with regard to their similarity in independently rate physical attractiveness. Even for these similar-in-attractiveness couples, partner's physical attractiveness was significantly related to interpersonal attraction, especially for males' ratings of their female partners. However, the attraction females— felt toward their male partners was significantly related only to *their* rating of his physical attractiveness, and not to independently evaluated physical attractiveness. These findings suggest that the females' rating of male facial attractiveness may be affected by their liking for the male, whereas this may not be the case for males' reactions to females. (Efran's [1974] finding described in Chapter 5, and that of Gross and Crofton [1977] in Chapter 6, are related to this point.) Another interesting aspect of Curran's rather ecologically invalid study was that although females' self-ratings of physical attractiveness and the independent ratings of this factor were significantly correlated, they were not so for males.

Stretch and Figley (1980) also found physical attractiveness to have a stronger significant effect on males' than on females' ratings of a (randomly chosen) potential dating partner when they did not, in fact, meet. Whether or not the potential date was ingratiating and boastful in an audiotape had no effect on the ratings.

Is It Wise to Date Attractive People?

Robertiello (1976) was concerned with the mental health consequences of the apparently very powerful effect of female physical attractiveness on males' dating choices. He cited one client as describing his stressing girlfriend as "a chronic alcoholic, . . . a castrating bitch, and a psychotic, but she was . . . extraordinarily physically attractive to him." Robertiello noted that, "Though he was a very intelligent, sophisticated man, he felt his attraction to her should override his cognitive appraisal of her and he was irresistibly fated to persist in a relationship with her."

Likely Acceptance as a Date

Huston (1973) also commented on whether males are powerfully drawn to physically attractive women irrespective of the possible outcomes. He asked male students to choose a date from a photographic array of six females. Some of the males were led to believe that the six females, having seen their picture, had indicated that they would agree to date them. The other males received no information on possible dating acceptance by the females. An effect of female physical attractiveness upon male choice was found in that highly physically attractive females were chosen more frequently than were either medium- or low-attractiveness females. This effect was particularly strong for those males who were led to believe that the attractive females had agreed to date them, but it was still present in the choices of those given no information about likely acceptance. These latter males were also asked to estimate the likelihood of the females accepting them as dates. Here again, an effect of physical attractiveness was found in that the estimated acceptance of highly attractive females was significantly lower than that concerning females of medium or low levels of attractiveness.

W. Bernstein, Stephenson, Snyder, and Wicklund (1983) noted a somewhat similar effect of physical attractiveness. They found male students to sit next to attractive females only when their "approach can occur under the guise of a motive other than desire to be with the attractive woman. This is because keeping one's true approach motive ambiguous may make direct personal rejection less likely." In this study males who believed that they were taking part in a "movie rating exercise" were offered one of two TV monitors to watch. In front of each monitor were two chairs only 3 inches apart. In front of one monitor was a female whose attractiveness had been independently rated. Half the males were informed that a different movie would be on each of the two monitors, the other half that both monitors would be showing the same movie. It was found for attractive females that significantly more males chose to sit with them in the different-movie condition than in the same-movie condition. That is, more sat next to an attractive female when they "had an excuse to do so (i.e. a movie preference)." When the females were unattractive the males avoided them regardless of movie condition. (Avoidance of those with unattractive faces is more fully discussed in Chapter 7.) W. Bernstein et al. concluded that when an excuse for affiliation was available males will approach attractive females. However, if such an excuse is not available the males' fear of rejection may prevent their approaching attractive women. They found that it was only the attractive males whose behavior seemed unaffected by possible rejection in that the males who sat with an attractive female in the same-movie condition were significantly more attractive than those who avoided females in this movie condition.

Kiesler and Baral (1970) also found an individual difference relating to fear of rejection to influence whether or not males asked an attractive female for a date. Those males whose self-esteem had been raised did so more than did those whose self-esteem had been lowered. (For more on facial appearance and self-esteem, see Chapter 8.)

In Huston's (1973) study, described previously, the males were asked to rate their own level of physical attractiveness. These self-ratings were found to have no effect on whether the males chose as a possible date a highly attractive female. They did, nevertheless, affect the males' estimates of the likelihood that a female would accept an offer of a date. Thus, although the males who judged themselves not to be physically attractive did rate the likely success of their offer of a date to an attractive female to be lower, they nevertheless chose attractive females. Whether the results of this "photographs plus stated intentions" study would generalize to actual live interactions is an open question.

Subjects' Own Level of Attractiveness

Weinberger and Cash (1982) examined for females the effects of their own physical attractiveness on dating acceptance or rejection. Female subjects briefly interacted with two males whom they believed also to be subjects in a study on dating behavior. Having interacted with the men the women rated their interest in dating each of the males and their estimation of the males' acceptance of them as a dating partner. It was found that the more physically attractive females expressed lower interest in dating the first male. However, when they were then informed that the first male had expressed a wish not to date them, it was noted that the attractive females found the decision of the second male "increasingly important." Weinberger and Cash concluded that, "The less attractive women may not have had very high generalized expectation of getting a date to begin with, so although acceptance was important to them, being rejected did not violate their expectation to the extent that it did for the more attractive women."

Shanteau and Nagy (1979) also examined the effects on females of males' acceptance of them as dating partners. In their first study the females were found to prefer as dates the more physically attractive males, but only under conditions in which they were told by the researchers that it was likely that the males would accept them as dates. In the second and third studies the females themselves provided the estimates of whether the males would be likely to accept them as dates. Under these circumstance male physical attractiveness and the females' estimates of their own acceptance were inversely related, and most date preferences were for males of intermediate attractiveness. It seems that the women took their estimates of the males' acceptance of them into account when choosing a possible dating partner, even when it was clear to the subjects that they would not, in reality, be dating any of the males.

In attempting to explain why they found probability of acceptance to have a greater effect than had previous studies, Shanteau and Nagy suggested that the powerful effect of high attractiveness in previous studies may have something to do with the fact that these studies "have generally attempted to study actual dating situations," whereas their study did not. However, to argue (as Shanteau and Nagy did) that their subjects took probability of acceptance more into account because they "did not actually expect to go out with their dating choice" seems rather perverse.

Over a quarter of Shanteau and Nagy's subjects did not in fact take probability into account. These subjects chose the most attractive males as dates. Shanteau and Nagy reported that these females tended to judge it to be equally likely that all the men would date them. However, these females were not found to be more physically attractive (by independent ratings) than those who took probability of acceptance into account when nominating a dating choice. (Unfortunately, self-ratings of facial attractiveness were not collected in this study.)

Hagiwara (1975), however, did examine the effects of female students' self-rated attractiveness on their ratings of males' desirability as a date. The lower a male's attractiveness, the less was he desired as a date, especially by the women whose self-ratings were high.

Pellegrini, Hicks, and Meyers-Winton (1980) also found self-rated attractiveness to be important. Their male subjects whose self-rated attractiveness was high endorsed the belief that "romantic love attraction" is easier "to win" for men than it is for women, whereas those male whose self-rated attractiveness was low said that it was easier for women to win. An analogous effect was found for the female subjects.

Dating Frequency

In a similar vein, Morse, Reis, Gruzen, and Wolff (1974) found a negative relationship between male subjects' heterosexual dating frequency (self-reported) and their evaluations of female and male stimulus attractiveness. These authors suggested that, "Men who refrain from dating may do so because they perceive females as too attractive to be attainable and because they see other men as so attractive (to females, presumably) as to make any contest with them for dates seem futile." The possible relationships between self-regard and facial appearance are more fully discussed in Chapter 8. However, it is worth nothing here that both Berscheid et al. (1971) and Spreadbury and Reeves (1979) found that their physically attractive subjects reported themselves as having had more dates, with more individuals, than did unattractive subjects.

Studies of Real Life

In their paper on dating behavior Krebs and Adinolfi (1975) pointed out that, "Although past studies consistently have found that physical attractiveness affects impression formation and social contact with the opposite sex, the extent to which their findings can be generalized from the experimental contexts in which they occurred to everyday life remains undetermined. Many studies failed to employ actual people as stimuli," using photographs instead, and "Other studies allowed only short-term contact between subjects in relatively artificial situations." Krebs and Adinolfi's study examined the relationship between facial attractiveness and (a) opposite sex dating and (b) same-sex social contact. In addition their study "also measured for the first time (cf. Berscheid & Walster, 1974) the personalities of the physically attractive and unattractive in order to test the validity of the traits observers attribute to them. It tested whether the physically attractive are actually more likeable, friendly, confident, sensitive and flexible [A. Miller, 1970a] than the physically unattractive."

Krebs and Adinolfi found independently rated female (but not male) facial attractiveness to be positively related to dating frequency. The subjects' scores on sociometric ratings provided by their "same-sex dormmates after two months on campus" enabled them to be described as being in a socially accepted, a socially rejected, an isolated, or a control group. It was found that the facial attractiveness of the accepted group was higher than that of the control group, which was higher than of the isolated group. Contrary to their expectation, Krebs and Adinolfi found that subjects in the rejected group had the highest facial attractiveness. One possible reason for this unexpected finding could be that the facial attractiveness ratings were found to have only a few, weak relationships with the scores the subjects obtained on a variety of personality and other measurers. *If* it is the case that facially attractive people, in fact, are not found to possess the traits that same-sex strangers attribute to them, then the resulting contrast could result in rejection. Another explanation of why the most physically attractive were rejected by their same-sex dormmates may be the jealousy caused by the positive relationship found between attractiveness and dating frequency.

Concerning rejection, Krebs and Adinolfi made the important point that

> The low incidence of dating for the physically unattractive customarily has been interpreted as rejection by the opposite sex. The present findings on social contact with the same sex suggest a possible refinement of this interpretation. In order to be actively rejected, one must be noticed; but the present data suggest that the physically unattractive tend to be ignored. It may be less that the physically unattractive make a bad impression and more that they do not make an impression at all.

This could be caused by their "failing to develop socially effective personality lifestyles." Chapter 8 in this book examines this possibility. However, it is still worth quoting here Krebs and Adinolfi's view that a possible sequence for such an effect

> . . . is as follows: early in life physical attractiveness affects social reactions, which in turn affects the development of personality. The physically attractive are admired and pursued. Because they are pursued they develop a high level of self-esteem, which mediates the development of personality dispositions oriented towards ambition and success. The physically unattractive are ignored, which forces them to withdraw from social relations; and they develop asocial, self-protective personality dispositions.

However plausible this suggestion may seem, we should note that Krebs and Adinolfi did not find strong evidence to support it. Nevertheless, theirs was a praiseworthy attempt to gather real-life, meaningful data to relate to facial appearance.

Another attempt to study the effects of physical appearance on dating in a somewhat more realistic setting than is usually the case was undertaken by Mathes (1975), who noted that the effect of physical attractiveness found in the "computer-dance" study by Walster et al. (1966) may have been so strong because only one encounter between the dating partners was studied. He suggested that, "On the first encounter the only reliable information available about a partner is his or her physical attractiveness and hence liking is based solely on it," and that with subsequent encounters further information, such as that concerning personality, becomes more available. Mathes' subjects were allocated to heterosexual pairs who were asked to "go on a series of five, 40-minute encounters, each separated by approximately one week. Couples were asked to set up their own encounters and to use each encounter to become further acquainted." After each encounter each subject rated his or her partner for liking. The subjects were either high or low in physical attractiveness and either high or low scorers on an anxiety questionnaire.

A main effect of physical attractiveness on liking was found, and an interaction with number of encounters revealed that although there was *no* effect of attractiveness for the first encounter, the liking ratings made at the end of subsequent encounters were affected by attractiveness. Subjects scoring high on the anxiety questionnaire were liked more than low scorers across all five encounters. From his findings Mathes concluded that the effect of physical attractiveness does not diminish over encounters. He also noted that in his study, because of its artificality, the subjects may have had a "lack of ego involvement. . . . Possibly their purpose in participating in the study was primarily to obtain points towards their final grades, not to become involved with someone of the opposite sex."

With this point we would strongly agree. Attempting to understand the possible effects of facial appearance on dating by getting students, for course credits, to engage in clearly ecological invalid encounters may not only be a waste of time, it may also lead to misleading conclusions about real-life behavior. It seems far better to devote energy and ingenuity to studying real-life dating and its outcomes. Alternatively, researchers could try to gain some information concerning whether their student subjects, such as those in the Krebs and Adinolfi study, do actually become "ego involved" and behave in a way commensurate with real-life dating.

Dynamics of Encounters

J. Cunningham (1976) pointed out that most psychological studies of dating had focused on individual difference factors rather than on the dynamic properties of such relationships. One study that did examine the effects of facial attractiveness on the dynamics of the "getting-acquainted" process for heterosexuals was conducted by Snyder, Tanke, and Berscheid (1977). In this study male students were asked to hold getting-acquainted telephone conversations with female students. Each male was led to believe that the female with whom he was about to converse was either attractive or unattractive (when, in fact, female attractiveness varied randomly). Raters blind to the female's supposed attractiveness listened to either the male or female part of the conversation. It was found that the men who believed their conversational partner to be facially attractive were rated from their conversations as being more sociable and outgoing than were the men who had allegedly unattractive partners. Furthermore, the females who were supposedly attractive were rated from their conversation as more sociable and outgoing even though they knew nothing about the attractiveness manipulation. Thus, not only did the facial appearance variable effect the males' conversational manner, it also caused their manner to affect the manner of the females.

In 1981 Andersen and Bem replicated the findings of Snyder et al. (1977) for the subjects who saw their alleged partner's photograph. This was the case not only for the manipulation of female attractiveness (which is what Snyder et al. varied), but also the manipulation of male attractiveness. In addition Andersen and Bem employed same-sex pairings. They found effects of facial attractiveness similar to those found by Snyder et al. in their opposite-sex encounters, but weaker effects in the same-sex encounters, particularly for males. However, it was only those subjects who scored above the mean on a sex-typing inventory who were affected by partner attractiveness.

In contrast to Synder et al.'s findings regarding the speech of the "photographed" partner, no simple main effect of attractiveness was found. Such an effect was found only for those conversing with a female who scored above the mean on sex-typing. The conversations of those who conversed with females with below average sex-typing demonstrated a reversed effect of attractiveness. That is, an attractive photograph plus conversation with a female who saw that photograph and who scored low on sex-typing led to the "photographed" person's conversation being rated as less responsive and less self-assured than when an unattractive photograph was used. Andersen and Bem noted that, "This reversal for targets interacting with androgynous women must presumably derive from some behavior on the part of androgynous women perceivers. In this regard it will be recalled that androgynous perceivers of both sexes were rated overall as no more responsive toward attractive targets than toward unattractive targets."

Andersen and Bem also asked at the end of each conversation how much the subjects now liked the former stranger with whom they had conversed. Attractiveness was found to have a significant effect on liking except upon androgynous women, even though these women had "differentiated in the conventional direction" between facially attractive and unattractive targets even more strongly than had sex-typed women when asked for their preconversation, postphotograph impression of their partners. Thus, as stated earlier in this chapter, subject individual differences may often have a qualifying or nullifying influence on the effects of facial appearance.

A null effect of physical atttractiveness was noted by Crouse and Mehrabian (1977), who found, as had Andersen and Bem for their androgynous subjects, that partner attractiveness had no effect upon subjects' "verbal affiliative behavior." Crouse and Mehrabian pointed out that most studies of the effects of attractiveness had not been concerned with live, face-to-face interactions but had merely used photographs. In their study, volunteer students were led to believe that they were taking part in a study involving listening to music. Upon arrival at the laboratory they were introduced to a "subject" of the opposite sex who was really a confederate. They were then informed that "the original machine for playing the music had broken down" and that the experimenter was going to fetch another. During the ensuing 5 minutes any conversation between the subject and the confederate was unobtrusively recorded, the confederate behaving in accordance with a prearranged, semifixed schedule. Then a few minutes of music were played and the subject rated this. Finally the subject was asked to rate the other "subject" on a 22-item questionnaire. Although the manipulation of confederate physical attractiveness had the expected significant effects for ratings of attractiveness, acceptability as a date, acceptability as a marriage partner, it had no effect on verbal affiliative behavior.

This null effect of physical attractiveness does not replicate the findings of Snyder et al. (1977). One explanation put forward by Crouse and Mehrabian for their null finding was that subjects may be affected by "target attractiveness only when they were asked to view targets in a romantic context (e.g., dating and marriage)." However, a romantic context seems to have been no more present in the study by Snyder et al. than it was in that by Crouse and Mehrabian. Nevertheless, there is one important difference between these two studies (in addition to that concerning conversation partners' behavioral variability), and this involves the subjects' beliefs about the the aims of the study. In the case of Snyder et al. the subjects were informed that the study was concerned with "getting acquainted," whereas in that of Crouse and Mehrabian they appear to have been misled. (This difference serves to highlight the point that in investigations of the effects of facial appearance, the more ecologically valid the study the greater should be the concern with ethical matters).

Studying in real life the effects of facial appearance on dating is likely to be fraught not only with ethical problems but also with methodological ones. One way in which real-life dating has been studied involves the cooperation of dating organizations.

Real-Life "Computer Dating"

Members of dating organizations are typically provided not only with information about possible partners' physical attractiveness, but also with information concerning their occupation, background, attitudes, interests, and so on. These circumstances would seem to provide a more valid test of the importance of facial appearance than do the artifical studies of so-called dating in college students. Thus, it is worthy of note that Riggio and Woll (1984) found that members of a video-dating organization who were selected more frequently as dates were the ones who were rated (independently) as the more physically attractive. In addition, these more attractive members were more likely to have their selections reciprocated by individuals whom they chose. However, being selected as a date should not be taken to suggest that facially attractive people will necessarily have more success in dating relationships.

In 1982 Folkes examined whether the importance of similarity in physical attractiveness noted in the rather artificial studies of Berscheid et al. (1971), Huston (1973), and Shanteau and Nagy (1979) would be found in real-life dating. She did not cite the finding of Harrison and Saeed (1977) that in "lonely heart" advertisements in a "nationally circulated, weekly tabloid" they had found individuals who described themselves as physically attractive to more frequently mention that possible partners should be attractive. Folkes suggested that the effect of similarity found in the studies of students could have been due to the greater homogeneity among college populations than among the general population, and to the possibility that facial appearance may be more important for college students than for other people. The subjects in Folkes' study had access, via the dating service, not only to the photographs and video recordings of possible partners but also to information about their occupation, general attitudes, interests, and background. The dating service allowed each member to choose 13 opposite-sex persons to meet. When one member expressed an interest in another, the chosen member was notified and given details of the chooser. If the chosen member reciprocated the choice both members of the dyad were given each other's surname and telephone number.

Folkes studied 67 dyads that were formed in this way. Her dependent variable was an index of progress in forming a relationship. Members of each dyad were contacted between 10 and 17 days after both individuals had been given the other's telephone numbers. They were separately asked whether any communication between them had occurred, if there had been a date, and if there had been more than one date. (No disagreement among dyads was found on these measures.) Attractiveness was independently rated using the photographs and video recordings. Folkes found that although those couples who had progressed beyond a second date were no more similar to each other in age or in occupation than were those dyads who had not progressed as far, the correlation between dating progression and attractiveness similarity was significant. The further the dyad had progressed the greater was the similarity (expect for having been on a second date, where a slight reversal of the trend occurred). Thus similarity in facial attractiveness may well not only be important for college students taking part in experiments, it may also be important in real life. (Its role in marriage will be discussed later in this chapter's section on marriage.)

Dating in Bars

One location in which real-life dating behavior may be unobtrusively observed is that of the "singles bar" where people may go to meet possible partners. Glenwick, Jason, and Elman (1978) observed between 10:30 p.m. and midnight how frequently "unattached" women in New York singles bars were approached by men. They found that there was no relationship between female physical attractiveness and the number of approaches made. Thus, in real-life interactions it may not necessarily be the case that physically attractive people receive more approaches. However, as with many field studies, the uncontrolled nature of Glenwick et al.'s study raises more questions than the study answers. One variable that might have confounded their data was the finding of Pennebaker et al. (1979) that individuals' attractiveness ratings in bars of people of the opposite sex (but not of the same sex) increased between 10:30 p.m. and midnight. Thus, whether there is a relationship between facial attractiveness and the number of approaches received may be a function of how near to closing time in a bar it may be. If the subjects in Pennebaker et al.'s study became more pleasantly aroused as the late evening progressed then this may have led to more generous opposite-sex attractiveness ratings. There certainly is evidence (see Chapter 9) that arousal influences the ratings of physical attractiveness that subjects award. However, since a replication of Pennebaker et al.'s "closing time" study by Sprecher et al. (1984) failed to find such an effect, other weaknesses of the study by Glenwick et al., such as the short observation duration of 5 minutes per stimulus, should be rectified in future studies that seek to determine whether in real-life dating situations it is the more physically attractive people who receive more dating choices.

Sexual Experience

If it is the facially attractive who receive more dating choices, why should this be? One possible explanation is related to the assumptions people make about attractive individuals. One assumption that may be made is that physically attractive people are more sexually skilled and experienced. Hatfield and Sprecher (1986) stated that, "Handsome men and beautiful women are seen as being more exciting and active sexual partners." They cited some unpublished 1983 studies by Smith, Sprecher, and De Lamater that found (a) that people's estimates of how sexually advanced and "vigorous" were various photographed individuals correlated positively with stimulus attractiveness, and (b) that people expected physically attractive couples to engaged more frequently in a variety of sexual activities.

Evidence to support the validity of these assumptions comes from studies by Kaats and Davis and from Curran and his co-workers. Kaats and Davis

(1970) found that a significantly greater proportion of physically attractive female students indicated that they were not virgins than did females independently rated as being either medium or low in attractiveness. The attractive females also reported experiencing more noncoital sexual activities.

In 1975 Curran claimed to have found among students who agreed to fill in a sexual experience questionnaire that the more physically attractive ones reported more "advanced" sexual experience. This relationship, however, was only found to be significant for independently rated male attractiveness. For females, the only significant relationship between sexual experience and their attractiveness was for their computer-date's rating of his partner's attractiveness after he had dated her (i.e., there was no significant relationship between independent ratings of females' attractiveness and their reported experiences). Why women who indicated that they were sexually experienced were subsequently rated as attractive by males who had dated them is open to speculation. Gross and Crofton (1977) (see Chapter 6) found evidence to support the notion that "What is good is beautiful"!

In other studies, however, Curran does report finding significant, although small, positive correlations between independently rated female (and male) physical attractiveness and the degree of reported sexual experience (Curran & Lippold, 1975; Curran, Neff, & Lippold, 1973).

Further evidence to support the notion that attractive people may be chosen as dates because of their greater sexuality comes from G. Wilson and Brazendale (1974), who found attractive females' preferences among risque "seaside postcards" to differ from those of unattractive females.

However, not all the evidence concerning sexuality finds a direct positive relationship with physical/facial attractiveness. Hocking, Walker, and Fink (1982) found Midwestern students to rate a female who had experienced premarital sexual intercourse as less moral when she was described as attractive than when unattractive. Furthermore, some studies concerning rape and other undersirable outcomes have found attractiveness not to be to a woman's advantage (see Chapter 4). Nevertheless, what research evidence there is does tend to support the notion that there may be a positive relationship between facial attractiveness and degree of sexual experience.

From the studies cited above it seems that facial appearance may well play a role in dating, in addition to its possible effect on liking. However, the majority of studies cited so far in this chapter been rather simple, "one-shot" studies. They have often been conducted on college students in rather artificial circumstances. Rarely have they studied ongoing, long-term interactions.

Long-Term Interactions

One study that stands out from the rest in terms of its quality is that by Reis et al. (1982), who made the point that, "The vast majority of studies of the 'what is beautiful is good' stereotype deal with first impressions of others who are not known to the subject and about whom limited information is available. In contrast, the bulk of our social contacts occur with people whom we have met previously. . . . Consequently, the effects of physical attractiveness in everyday life require further elaboration." They suggested that the social effects of facial appearance may change substantially as more information becomes available about the target person as a relationship develops. Their study was, in part, based on one by Reis, Nezlek, and Wheeler (1980) that found (a) that attractiveness correlated positively for both sexes with reported social intimacy and satisfaction, and (b) that attractive males had more and longer lasting interactions with a greater number of females than did unattractive males, although females' attractiveness bore no such relationship to their interactions with males.

Reis et al. (1982) tried not only to repeat and improve upon the 1980 study but also "to find out why attractiveness relates to social participation." They suggested that one reason might be simply that "we seek out attractive others because they are aesthetically pleasing to look at and because we have been taught that 'what is beautiful is good' and therefore desirable." On the other hand they suggested that "a more insidious and significant self-fulfilling prophecy may be occurring. Merely believing another person to be attractive may be sufficient to alter their behavior. If appearance plays an important role in how people are responded to and evaluated from infancy, a lifetime of differential treatment might well be responsible for variations in the behavior of attractive and unattractive person." Whatever the possible theoretical explanations of the social effects of facial appearance (our concluding chapter makes mention of some of the various theories and notions that have been offered), Reis et al. made the point that, "There are few studies available that directly assess the reasons why pretty people seem to have a social advantage."

In their study male and female senior students who lived on campus at a university in the Northeastern United States filled in a social interaction record for, on average, a 2-week period. This procedure required the subjects "to complete a short fixed-format entry for every interaction of 10 minutes or longer." For males significant positive correlations were found (as in 1980) between physical attractiveness (which was independently rated from photographs taken from "midthigh to over-the-head") and (a) number of females interacted with and (b) time spent with females. For male subjects significant negative correlations were found between attractiveness and time spent with males. However, for female subjects no such relationships with physical attractiveness were found (again confirming the 1980 findings). Only for interactions with groups of mixed sex were there significant (marginal) correlations for female attractiveness, and these were negative.

Closer examination of the data for males revealed that the correlation of male attractiveness with interactions with females was due more to interactions with females who were not classed as among the first-, second-, and third-best female friends than it was to interactions with the "close" female friends. That is, "attractive males expanded their interaction with females by increasing contact with less close female friends." Somewhat similarly, attractive males were found to have more interactions with "less close" male friends, but significantly fewer interactions with closer male friends.

Reis et al. (1982) also asked their subjects to rate each interaction for its intimacy, amount of self- and other-disclosure, satisfaction, and "pleasantness." For males (and somewhat for females) attractiveness correlated with rated intimacy, and with both self- and other-disclosure. However, for males it did not correlate with either satisfaction or pleasantness. For females satisfaction and pleasantness did correlate with attractiveness, the former largely for same-sex interactions and the latter for opposite- and mixed-sex interactions. With regard to their ratings concerning who initiated and influenced each interaction, attractive males reported more self-initiations than did unattractive males, whereas for females this effect was reversed.

The subjects in this study also completed a number of psychological questionnaires once the interaction record-keeping phase had been completed. The correlations described above between physical attractiveness and social interaction were investigated by partialing out from them the relationships found between the social interaction record data and (a) several questionnaire measures of social competence (such as the Dating and Assertion Questionnaire and the Social Avoidance and Distress Scale, two assertiveness scales); (b) a questionnaire measure of self-esteem; and (c) a questionnaire concerned with interpersonal rejection/trust. (Part of Chapter 8 focuses on the relationships between facial appearance and such indices.) When this was done it was found that this partialing somewhat reduced the relationships between appearance and the social interaction data, but it by no means eliminated them. From this Reis et al. concluded for males that "apparently, part of the effect of appearance on social interaction may be mediated by attractiveness-rated differences in social competence: however, an independent influence remained." For females they found that "the effects of social competence on interaction were opposite to those of attractiveness, suggesting that they operate divergently."

Overall, Reis et al. found that physical attractiveness and measures of social interaction were much more strongly (and positively) related for men than they were for women. We should note that Cash and Burns (1977) found males' physical attractiveness, but not females, to correlate positively with their self-rated "obtained reinforcement" (i.e., the frequency and enjoyability) for pleasant events in the preceding month. Reis et al. suggested that their finding "contradicts studies showing that attractiveness plays a focal role in females' popularity." However, as stated above, the majority of these studies have minimal validity (unlike that of Reis et al.), one reason for this being that they have rarely analyzed data from everyday, real-life interactions. In such interactions social dynamics as well as facial appearance are clearly likely to be important. Reis et al.'s finding that the initiation of social interaction was positively correlated with physical attractiveness for males and negatively for females may well go some way in explaining why their findings for females appeared to contradict what the findings of previous, simple studies would suggest, especially since Reis et al. found that "attractive women were not more skilled on any of the competence measures we collected."

The 1982 study by Reis et al. can be taken as suggesting that the self-fulfilling prophecy, which they hypothesized may operate in real life, seems likely to be the case for males; that is, via feedback from their social environment attractive males actually become more socially adept. The picture seems not so clear regarding females. Nevertheless, Reis et al. made the important point that "attractive persons' interactions were more qualitatively rewarding, generally across both close and less close friends. Would anyone judge these phenomena to be superficial or of limited importance? We think not. Because perceptions of beauty and their social ramifications bear heavily on these behaviors, beauty is a vital and significant variable worthy of investigation."

One aspect of life that is certainly of importance is marriage. It is to the role of facial appearance in marriage that we shall soon turn, but before we do that let us examine studies of the effects of facial appearance on the success of the long-term dating that typically precedes marriage.

Long-Term Dating

C. Hill, Rubin, and Peplau (1976) noted many steady-dating couples who were dissimilar in physical attractiveness to have "broken up" 2 years later, whereas those couples of similar attractiveness had tended to remain together. White (1980) also found that within-dating-couple similarity in physical attractiveness was predictive of courtship progress. He found "serious" daters and those who were engaged or married to be more similar to their partners in independently rated attractiveness than were casual daters. Perhaps surprisingly, couples who were "cohabitants" were not similar to each other in attractiveness. White also found 9 months later that those casually or seriously dating couples who had now broken up had been more dissimilar in attractiveness than had those who had stayed together. No such effect, however, was found among those in the engaged/married or cohabiting partnership (possibly because the sample sizes in these groups were so small at 3 and 5, respectively). Contrary to the findings of previous studies concerning people's expectations about attractive women, White found no evidence that the females who were more attractive than their partners had a greater desire to date or to have sex with other people. However, such a relationship was found for males who were dating (but not for those who were cohabiting or engaged/married).

White suggested that one possible explanation of his findings could be equity theory, but we should note that over the years this notion has been so poorly articulated that as yet it may not be possible to compare it effectively with other competing explanations. White concluded that, "Equity theorists must demonstrate that differences in attractiveness must result in tension generated by violation of the equity norm." Some data on this question were provided in the same year by Critelli and Waid (1980), who found, even though there was an overall significant positive correlation for within couple attractiveness, that "subjects who believed that their partners were the more attractive member of the dyad loved their partners more and indicated greater submission in their relationships."

If the existence of love is predictive of marriage, and if it is the facially attractive who are liked more, who have more and varied dates, and who end up being loved more, then perhaps a greater proportion of them get married.

The Role of Facial Appearance in Marriage

One of the earliest data-based studies of the relationship between facial appearance and marriage was published in 1938 by S. Holmes and Hatch. They rated in the classroom the faical beauty of several hundred female students at the University of California. A few years after their graduation information concerning whether these women had married was obtained. It was found that a greater proportion (34%) of the "beautiful" women had married than of the "good looking" (28%), "plain" (16%), or "homely" (11%).

Nida and Williams (1977) asked students to rate as a possible marriage partner an opposite-sexed stranger whose photograph they saw and whose "trait description" they read. A significant effect of facial attractiveness was found, and this rather basic study suggests, along with Holmes and Hatch's more ecologically valid data, that facial appearance and marriage may be re-lated. Why should this be? A number of suggestions have been put forward, many of which have not been empirically investigated. Two related sugges-tions that have been studied are (a) that facially attractive women marry men who are desirable as marriage partners because of their physical attractive-ness or their wealth, status, and prestige, and (b) that an individual is more positively evaluated by others the more facially attractive is his or her partner. We will now consider each of these suggestions in turn. In the final part of this section on marriage we will overview studies of the relationship between facial attractiveness and marital adjustment.

Are Marriage Partners Similar to Each Other in Facial Attractiveness?

Above we cited Nida and Williams' finding that people evaluate physically attractive others more positively as possible marriage partners. However, as Vandenberg (1972) pointed out, we should ask "to what extent such expressed preferences are predictive of actual choice." Whatever studies like that of Nida and Williams, or studies of dating, or anecdotal and personal experience may suggest, what is the actual relationship within spouses' facial attractiveness? The facially attractive may to some extent be liked and dated more, but whom do they marry?

Murstein (1972) suggested that an "exchange-market" or equity model might apply in which people are married to spouses of similar physical attractiveness to themselves. He noted that early research on dating (e.g., Brislin & Lewis, 1968; Walster et al., 1966) suggested (in rather ecologically invalid settings) that subjects all seemed to prefer a highly attractive partner, independently of their own attractiveness. However, better research on dating conducted since 1972 (which was discussed previously) has found that people often do take into account their own level of physical attractiveness. In friendships also, similarity in physical attractiveness may be a factor. Cash and Derlega (1978) found that same sex "close friends" were significantly more alike in terms of independent ratings than would be expected by chance alone.

Murstein found that photographs of members engaged or "going-steady" couples (when presented individually) were rated as more similar in physical attractiveness than would be expected by chance. A within-couples similarity effect was also found for the photographed persons' self-ratings of physical attractiveness. Murstein concluded from his data (a) that his subjects believed their partners to be similar to themselves in physical attractiveness and that this perception was accurate, and (b) that even though many possibly marriage-relevant factors were free to vary in his study "the fact that equality of physical attractiveness tends to influence marital choice even when these other variables are not controlled testifies to its ubiquitousness during the entire course of marital courtship."

Murstein's (1972) subjects were merely going steady. What of married partners? In the same year Shepherd and Ellis (1972) obtained a set of 36 negatives of wedding photographs from a local newspaper. The face of each partner was then printed separately and all 72 faces were rated by students for how "good-looking" they were. A correlation of +.39 was found between spouses' facial attractiveness. Shepherd and Ellis concluded that this significant correlation, "though not spectacular, is noteworthy." A higher correlation between spouses' attractiveness of +.73 was in the same year reported by N. Cavior and Boblett (1972), although the correlation they found for dating couples was much lower at +.19. Murstein and Christy (1976) and McKillip and Riedel (1983) also found a significant correlation, as did Price and Vandenberg (1979), even when they partialed out the age of the photographed individuals.

Price and Vandenberg pointed out that the size of the reported attractiveness correlations "fits well into the general pattern of small to moderate spouse similarity which is observed for physical traits." They cited Spuhler's (1968) work on physical traits in which he reviewed studies that had found small, significant within-couple correlations for a variety of facial features. (In this book's concluding chapter we will discuss the relationship between facial attractiveness and facial features.)

From the studies mentioned previously it would seem that support does exist for Murstein's attractiveness equity model. Terry and Macklin (1977) investigated whether people would employ this model when asked to select from females' photographs which of them were married to photographed males. Evidence for an attractiveness similarity effect was found in that the subjects reliably chose as the wife the woman most similar (of the four presented) to each male in terms of physical attractiveness. The actual correlation between spouses' attractiveness was also significant. However, since the subjects made these attractiveness ratings before performing the wife selection task they may have been predisposed to selecting wives on the basis of physical attractiveness.

R. Bailey and Price (1978) examined whether members of married couples would rate their own physical attractiveness at a level similar to the rating they allotted to their partner. No evidence was found for this, possibly because 84% of the wives and 75% of the husbands rated their spouse's attractiveness as higher than their own. Bailey and Price noted, with surprise, that only members of couples who were recently married (rather than the longer married couples) rated their spouse's attractiveness similarly to independent raters. We might suggest that Gross and Crofton's (1977) notion of "what is good becomes beautiful" may have operated here, particularly for the longer married couples. Bailey and Price concluded that, "The results suggest the perceived attractiveness similarity between self and spouse was relatively unimportant as far as the maintenance of a marriage relationship was concerned." We shall examine this suggestion more fully later in this chapter.

Although R. Bailey and Price (1978) did not find that members of a couple rated their spouse as similar in physical attractiveness to themselves, in 1984 R. Bailey and Kelly reported such effects for "going-steady" and engaged couples, and they concluded that, "Individuals entered into dating and maintained a dating relationship only with partners whom they perceived as supporting their own self-concept of physical attractiveness." Bailey and Kelly did not offer an adequate explanation of why their self/partner attractiveness correlations were not found in the earlier R. Bailey and Price study (1978).

Even though several studies have found significant correlations in attractiveness between members of couples, Kalick and Hamilton (1986) have argued that this may be the result merely of attractive members of both sexes forming couples more readily and thus being removed from the pool of possible dates (as found in their computer simulation study). They suggested that, in the end, within-couple attractiveness across couples at all levels of attractiveness becomes correlated because an individual's attractiveness is negatively correlated with the number of dates required before he or she successfully becomes a boyfriend or girlfriend. Thus they argued that the attractiveness correlations noted in the above studies may well be not so much the result of people choosing at the outset to approach as dates people of a similar attractiveness level to themselves, but more the result of the most attractive individuals being removed quickest from the pool of available partners. Futher research (e.g., of first-year students on a residential university campus) could address this suggestion.

The weight of evidence seems to support the notion that marriage partners may often be similar to each other in facial attractiveness. If this is indeed the case, where does this leave the other suggestion, made above, that facially attractive women frequently marry prestigious, wealthy, high-status men? Similarity in terms of attractiveness would still be found if such men are themselves facially attractive (Chapters 3 and 4 examine this notion). However, let us examine the evidence concerning whether it is facially attractive women who usually marry prestigious men.

Attractive Women and Prestigious Men

Feingold (1981) stated that, "According to the 'equity theory' of interpersonal attraction, persons having romantic partners higher in physical attractiveness than themselves should have more desirable nonphysical attributes than those having less attractive partners." Bar-Tal and Saxe (1976) found evidence that their subjects applied such an equity model when shown a slide of a married couple. When the husband was facially unattractive and believed to be married to a facially attractive woman, he was evaluated as having a higher income, occupational status, and professional success than when he was facially attractive and married to an attractive woman. Such an effect was not found when the stimulus persons were shown individually and subjects were told that they were not married. Bar-Tal and Saxe concluded that whereas for the attractive married couple no further explanation that similarity in facial attractiveness was needed by the subjects, those who saw the unattractive male–attractive female married couple might have inferred that the male must have possessed other highly valued characteristics in order to attract the attractive woman.

So far we have mentioned mere expectation concerning whether attractive women marry prestigious men. Elder (1969) found this indeed to be the case, noting that "girls who became upwardly mobile through marriage were characterized by physical attractiveness." In his (possibly sexist) paper Elder stated that, "The social advantages of hypergamy for the low-status girl—in which she achieves higher status through marriage—appear as status costs for the man, though what he loses in social rank may be surpassed by gains in other forms of status. Equity in this type of exchange would require the woman to be exceptional in other qualities which are defined as desirable in the culture." He further suggested that physical attractiveness would have its strongest influence on the marriage mobility of women "from the working class."

Elder asked married women, who were born in the 1920s and whose physical attractiveness had been rated in their teens, for information about their husbands' occupational status (in 1958) and that of their fathers (in 1929). These occupational standings were classified into one of seven status levels.

The women were then put into an upwardly mobile or nonmobile group. Elder found that, "Mobile women from the middle and working class were rated significantly higher in adolescence on attractiveness . . . than nonmobile women of similar class origin." The correlation between physical attractiveness and husband's occupational status was +.46 and +.35 for working-class and middle-class women, respectively. No significant correlation was found, however, between these women's IQ and their upward mobility. Only for the physically attractive women was their IQ somewhat related to the husband's occupational status. Overall, Elder found for working-class women that their physical attractiveness was more predictive of marriage to a high-status man than was their level of educational attainment. For middle-class women the relative effects of these two factor were reversed, but attractiveness still had a significant effect.

P. Taylor and Glenn (1976) also examined the relationship between females' physical attractiveness, their educational attainment, and their husbands' occupational status. They found the physical attractiveness of daughters of "low-manual workers" to be related significantly to their husband's occupational prestige. However, no such relationship was found for daughters of upper-middle-class fathers or of farmers. The women's educational attainment (i.e., number of years in school) was found to be more strongly related to husbands' occupational status than was their physical attractiveness. However, since the physical attractiveness ratings were made after marriage, and only the women's husbands' occupational status rather than the difference between this and their fathers' was noted, Taylor and Glenn's study is not a full replication of Elder's. Nevertheless, they did concur with Elder in concluding that "attractiveness is more important to the status attainment through marriage of females of low origins than to those of high origins and that education is more important to females of high origin than to females of low origin."

J. Udry (1977) partially replicated both Elder's and P. Taylor and Glenn's studies. Females' attractiveness ratings were obtained at the same time as was information on husbands' and fathers' occupation. Udry found that, "Within origin categories, upwardly mobile women are more attractive than those who are not upwardly mobile, but differences reach statistical significance for only some origin categories," these being white women in the highest of Udry's four status origins and black women from the middle two origins. Udry found that white females' years of education was more strongly related to husband's occupational status than was attractiveness. For black women these two factors were equally predictive of his occupational standing. When the effect of attractiveness was examined for women of different levels of educational attainment it was found that for women of low attainment their attractiveness was significantly related to husband's occupational status. This was also found to be the case for more educated black women. Although such significant relationships were found, Udry wisely decided to examine the amount of variance in husband's occupational status that was explained by wives' attractiveness, and he found, "In no cell in any table does attractiveness explain as much as 10% of the variance in mobility status. In most cells, it does not explain 5%." Thus the impact of attractiveness may be consistent yet rather weak.

J. Udry and Eckland (1984) did not examine the amount of variance that could be attributed to attractiveness when they examined its relationship to marriage. They found ratings of women's facial attractiveness based on high school photographs to be related to husband's income and to his educational attainment. However, since female attractiveness was also found to relate to father's income and occupational status it might not have been the case that the attractive women were more upwardly mobile in marriage. Udry and Eckland examined this question by controlling for father's income; when this was done an effect of attractiveness was still found. An effect of attractiveness was also found for females (although not for males) in terms of a greater proportion of the attractive women being married.

P. Taylor and Glenn noted in 1976 that recently in several societies the opportunities for women to occupy high-status occupations may be increasing. Given this, future research concerning whether people occupying high-status positions do have facially attractive spouses may not be quite so sexist as it has been to date. Udry and Eckland found that husbands' physical attractiveness was negatively rather than positively related to wives' educational attainment.

We began this section on female marriage mobility by mentioning Feingold's equity model. He found in 1981 that physically attractive men were more likely to have physically attractive women as "romantic partners," and in 1982(a) that the more physically attractive were female college students than their boyfriends, the taller were their boyfriends. Women in the 1981 study whose partners were more attractive than they had lower neuroticism scores than did women whose partners were less attractive than they. The former's IQs were higher but not significantly so. No such effects were found for Feingold's male subjects.

From the research on whether attractive women do marry prestigious men it does seem that some evidence exists to support this contention. That being so, one might ask why prestigious men would want to marry attractive women. One explanation might be the men's expectation that individuals will evaluate them more positively if these individuals see that the men have facially attractive wives.

Effects of Having a Facially Attractive Partner

In 1973 Sigall and Landy asked undergraduate subjects to rate another (male) subject whom they had just seen for intelligence, self-confidence, friendliness, likeability, talent, excitement, and physical attractiveness. Half of the subjects were led to believe that the male was the boyfriend of a woman they saw sitting next to him, others were not informed that the male and female were associated. For some subjects the female was made up and dressed to appear physically attractive and for others she looked unattractive. In the unassociated condition the female's physical appearance had no effect on subjects' ratings of the male. However, in the associated condition it had a significant effect on ratings of likeability, friendliness, and self-confidence. Thus when the male (who was of average physical attractiveness) was thought to be the boyfriend of an attractive female he was rated more positively than when his girlfriend appeared to be unattractive. Sigall and Landy concluded that "our results strongly supported the notion that the physical attractiveness of one's girlfriend affects the impressions others form of him. While there was a tendency towards reduced favorability as a function of being associated with an unattractive woman, the most compelling finding was that being linked to a beautiful woman led to enhanced impressions."

The same year also saw the publication by Hartnett and Elder (1973) of a study similar to that of Sigall and Landy. In this study the subjects did not sit in the same room with the stimulus "couple" as they had in Sigall and Landy's study, but instead saw photographs of a supposed married couple. When the wife was physically attractive the physically unattractive male was rated more positively than when his wife was unattractive. Hartnett and Elder suggested that, "The increase in attitude towards the male could be that S's believed he must possess a number of positive traits to attract such a good-looking girl." Ratings of the wife were also affected by partner attractiveness, but in the opposite way. When she was physically attractive she was rated more positively when her husband was physically unattractive than when he was attractive. Hartnett and Elder suggested here that, "by choosing an unattractive mate she demonstrated that . . . her choice was governed by more noble choices than physical appearance." They also suggested that the reversed effect of partner attractiveness for evaluations of the female may have been affected by the fact that all their raters were female. Sigall and Landy used both female and male subjects, but they found no interactions between subject sex and their independent variables.

In a study by Meiners and Sheposh (1977) the male and female subjects saw on video a man with his girlfriend. Her physical attractiveness and "intelligence" (i.e., medical student or coffee-shop waitress) were varied. Using Sigall and Landy's rating scales Meiners and Sheposh found very significant effects of girlfriend attractiveness on all scales of evaluation of the male, whereas the nature of her employment only affected ratings on three of the scales. Similarly, Strane and Watts (1977) found that ratings of a female were affected by the physical attractiveness of her male partner. They concluded that, "Evidence suggests that it is advantageous to be beautiful; however, even if one is lacking in beauty, one may still enjoy the advantages by association with a beautiful partner."

Chapter 7 deals at length with the topic of facial disfigurement, but we should mention here one of our own studies on this topic. Bull and Brooking (1985) found that subjects rated a person with a facial "port-wine stain" (a "strawberry mark") as less attractive than did those who saw this male or female without the disfigurement. However, if the stimulus person was thought to be married (to a partner of average attractiveness) the disfigurement had no effect on the attractiveness ratings.

The studies cited so far on the effects of having a physically attractive partner have employed heterosexual partnerships, and the explanations of the effects found have tended to focus upon mate selection. However, would the effects of being associated with an attractive person be found when the person being judged and the partner are friends of the same sex rather than lovers? Kernis and Wheeler (1981) found this to be the case both for males and females using Sigall and Landy's methodology. Additionally, they found that their targets were rated more positively when seen sitting next to someone they did not know who was *un*attractive. This latter effect they explained via the contrast effect noted by Kenrick and Gutierres (1980). (Such contrast effects are discussed in Chapter 9.)

Geiselman, Haight, and Kimata (1984) found that attractiveness of same-sex friends enhanced the ratings of target (female) attractiveness. They also found in most of their experiments an enhancement effect for the unassociated condition, thus not replicating Kernis and Wheeler's contrast effect. However, whereas in the study by Kernis and Wheeler the target persons had been seen face-to-face by their subjects, in the study by Geiselman et al. photographs were used. Only in their fourth experiment, which alone involved successive presentation of target and context faces, did Geiselman et al. find a contrast effect. However, whether Kernis and Wheeler's "live" presentation of target plus context individuals should be deemed to have involved successive rather than simultaneous presentation of stimuli is open to debate.

From the studies described above on the effects of having a facially attractive partner it would seem that this may be one reason why Nida and Williams (1977) found facial attractiveness to influence judgments concerning a possible marriage partner. Indeed, in their second experiment Sigall and Landy (1973) found that their (male) subjects expected people to evaluate them in a more positive way if they were believed to be with a physically attractive girlfriend.

So much for the possible benefit of having a physically attractive partner. What does research say about possible drawbacks?

Facial Appearance and Marital Adjustment

We described previously a study by Bar-Tal and Saxe (1976) that found that when a wife was physically attractive she was frequently perceived as having more desirable characteristics than when she was unattractive. However, Bar-Tal and Saxe noted that on the dependent measure of marital happiness "the attractive wife received a less favorable evaluation. That is she was rated as being less happily married." Although Bar-Tal and Saxe did not discuss this finding, Hatfield and Sprecher's (1986) suggestion that "if one partner is much more desirable than the other, the more desirable partner is more likely to have extramarital affairs" could be a possible explanation of it. Dermer and Thiel (1975) found that physically attractive women were rated as more likely to have an extramarital affair than were unattractive women. Brigham (1980) found that a facially attractive wife was rated by students as having far greater temptation for extramarital affairs than was an unattractive wife, particularly when the husband was facially unattractive. The male subjects also rated her as more likely to be affected by this temptation, and therefore to be adulterous when she was attractive. No such effect was found for the effects of his attractiveness on ratings of the husband.

From these studies one might conclude that there are indeed possible drawbacks in having an attractive wife, but none, research seems to suggest, from having a facially attractive husband. However, these studies have been concerned merely with students' expectations about hypothetical stimulus persons. What about real-life relationships?

Kirkpatrick and Cotton (1951) found, as Murstein and others have found that members of married couples were rated as similar to each other in physical attractiveness. Those wives who were judged by students who knew them to be in a "well-adjusted couple" were also rated by these students as being more physically attractive than wives in a "poorly adjusted couple." However, here the mean attractiveness ratings for the two groups were very similar (3.69 versus 3.47, respectively) and the sample size very large (n = 678). Nevertheless, this finding was repeated by another, smaller sample (the figures being 3.72, 3.54, and 305). Therefore, at least in 1951, there seemed no support for Bar-Tal and Saxe's subjects' expectation that an attractive wife would be less happily married. Those couples in which Kirkpatrick and Cotton's subjects rated the wife as being the more attractive partner were not judged as being poorly adjusted couples. If anything, it was when the husband was the better looking that couples were more likely to be judged as being poorly adjusted. Kirkpatrick and Cotton's study does, however, contain a serious design fault in the sense that the same subjects who nominated the couples whom they judged to be poorly or well adjusted also rated each member for attractiveness. Nevertheless, they took their findings to suggest that small within-couple differences in physical attractiveness tended to go with good marital adjustment.

J. Peterson and Miller (1980) also found that members of married couples were rated as similar to each other in physical attractiveness. In their study, unlike that of Kirkpatrick and Cotton, the raters were unaware of who was married to whom. In addition Peterson and Miller found that husbands' good marital adjustment (which was self-rated) was positively related to their attractiveness and to that of their wife (as independently rated), but that wives' marital adjustment seemed related neither to independent nor to self-nor to spouse ratings of their attractiveness. Thus, as we concluded above from studies of merely what people expect, Peterson and Miller's data could suggest that being an attractive wife may not relate positively to marital adjustment, but being an attractive husband may do so. That is, attractive husbands may bring largely positive qualities, but attractive wives may bring a balance of positive and negative factors. However, the findings of Kirkpatrick and Cotton point to the opposite of this conclusion.

Murstein and Christy (1976) found no relationship between independently rated similarity of attractiveness and self-rated marital adjustment. However, they did find members of married couples to be similar to each other in physical attractiveness. Self-rated marital adjustment (particularly the husbands') was found to be related only to spouses' ratings of their partners' attractiveness, and clearly these two ratings may not have been made independently. Nevertheless, the relationship is worthy of note.

From the above studies it does seem that Stroebe et al. (1971) may have been wrong when they argued that physical attractiveness is of much less importance regarding marriage than dating. Although the relationship between attractiveness and marital adjustment seems unclear, there seems little doubt that research concurs in finding that members of married couples are often similar to each other in independently rated attractiveness.

R. Bailey and Price (1978), however, concluded that "perceived attractiveness similarity between self and spouse was relatively unimportant as far as the maintenance of a marriage relationship was concerned." They arrived at this conclusion because they found no significant correlation between the self-rating of physical attractiveness of members of married couples and their rating of their spouses. R. Bailey and Kelly (1984) did, in fact, find such a relationship for their engaged and "going-steady" couples. Bailey and Price's conclusion may not be that contradictory to previous research because it was based on self-ratings rather than on independent ratings. Surprisingly, even though Bailey and Price had available independent ratings of attractiveness they seem not to have reported the within-couple correlation for these. Murstein and Christy (1976) and J. Peterson and Miller (1980) also found no correlation between self-ratings of members of married couples. However, as stated above, they did find such correlations for independent ratings. Bailey and Price did find (a) for wives' self-rating a significant correlation with the wives' estimates of their husbands' ratings of their wives, and (b) that most of their subjects' self-ratings for attractiveness differed from those of independent raters. Bailey and Price suggested that perhaps only at the beginning of a marriage are partners' attractiveness evaluations similar to those of independent raters. As time goes by they may change. Indeed, Peterson and Miller found their subjects (who had been married for 40 years) to rate their spouses as more physically attractive than did the independent raters. Again, Gross and Crofton's (1977) notion that "What is good is beautiful" may be relevant here.

Conclusion

Studies conducted in the 1960s and early 1970s suggested that facial appearance (i.e., attractiveness) played a major role in liking and dating. However, most of these studies were conducted in settings so artificial as to make their findings of very limited utility. Subsequent studies, although not usually any more ecologically valid, manipulated other independent variables (e.g., attitude similarity) in addition to facial appearance. In such studies facial appearance was often found still to exert a significant effect, although the power or strength of this effect was rarely mentioned. A few studies took the trouble to find that certain types of individuals seem more affected by facial appearance than do others.

Studies of marriage do imply that facial appearance does play a role. The weight of evidence suggests that individuals do often marry people of similar physical attractiveness to themselves (as independently rated; spouse ratings seem biased by the experience of living together), or those who instead can offer other things (such as wealth, status, and prestige). No consistent relationship between facial appearance and marital adjustment has been found, although there is the suggestion the facial appearance may play a contributory role.

Chapter 3

The Effects of Facial Appearance in Persuasion, Politics, Employment, and Advertising

In 1964 Singer pointed out that, "only recently have psychologists turned specifically to ascertain whether conniving, manipulating strategies do in fact exist as personality syndromes, and, if they do, whether they can be validly measured." In this chapter we shall examine research that has focused on the role of facial appearance in the delivery of persuasive communications, in politics, in persuading someone to offer an employment candidate a job (or a promotion), and in advertising. (The relationships between facial appearance and aspects of social skill other than persuasion are dealt with in Chapter 8.)

Facial Appearance and Persuasion

One of the very first studies designed to see if the facial appearance of a communicator has any effect upon the persuasive power of a communication was published in 1965. In this study Mills and Aronson noted that previous research (not concerned with facial appearance) had suggested that when a communicator is judged to demonstrate a definite intention to persuade others, such a communicator is perceived as less trustworthy and is therefore less persuasive. They argued, however, that if such a communicator happened to be a physically attractive person

> . . . a person whom the members of an audience would very much like to please . . . such a person would be *more* effective if he expressed a desire to influence. If people think that someone whom they like very much wants them to do something, they may be motivated to do it. . . . Thus, a very attractive source may be *more* effective in changing opinions if he openly and honestly informs the audience that he *wants* to change their opinions. [On the other hand,] What if the communicator is unattractive? If the audience does not like the communicator they will not be prone to please him by allowing

their opinions to be changed according to his desire. Thus, a stated desire to
influence will not increase the effectiveness of such a communicator. In fact,
if anything, an unattractive communicator may lead the audience toward
active disaffiliation; hence a stated desire to influence, in this case, might
actually *decrease* the effectiveness of the communication.

In Mills and Aronson's study the opinions of male subjects were gathered
before and after they received a communication on "general versus special-
ized education" from a female who was made up to look physically attractive
or unattractive. In addition, "In the persuade conditions the communicator . . . stated beforehand that she would very much like to influence the
views of others. In the nonpersuade conditions she . . . stated that she was
not at all interested in influencing the views of others." Comparison of the
data for the attractive/persuade and attractive/nonpersuade conditions from
their first experiment resulted in a difference that approached significance, as
did the data from their second, very similar, experiment. When Mills and
Aronson combined the *p* values from both experiments, the resulting (two-
tailed) probability value was "just barely short of the conventional .05 level."
No effect whatsoever was found when comparing the unattractive/persuade
with the unattractive/nonpersuade data. Mills and Aronson concluded that
"an overt, frankly stated desire to influence does *not* influence the effectiveness of the communicator, unless he is attractive. If he is attractive it increases
his effectiveness."

Mills and Aronson not only made the unjustified assumption that what is
found for a female communicator may automatically apply to a male communicator, they also rather overstated the observed effect of attractiveness. Several publications since 1965 have included such overstatement. For example,
Horai, Naccari, and Fatoullah stated in 1974 that, "Mills and Aronson (1965)
have directly demonstrated that physical attractiveness is a usable resource in
social influence. A female confederate made to look attractive was more
effective in influencing a male audience when she told them she wanted to
persuade them than when no mention of intent was made." Such overstatement notwithstanding, Mills and Aronson suggested that persuasive effects of
a communicator's physical attractiveness may relate to perceived trustworthiness and to liking for the communicator. (Chapter 2 contains information on
the perceived relationship between facial appearance and liking.)

Sigall and Aronson (1969) suggested that, "it is more rewarding to please a
physically attractive person than one who is not attractive. If this is true, we
can infer that when one is confronted with a physically attractive person a
greater drive is aroused to be well received." They hypothesized that the
effects, in terms of liking, of an evaluator's positive or negative evaluation
would be greater if she was made up to look physically attractive rather than
unattractive. They found that, "it does not make too much difference whether
one receives a positive or a negative evaluation when the evaluator is unattractive, but there is a world of difference between receiving negative and
positive feedback from a pretty girl." Sigall and Aronson wisely checked to

see whether the apparent effect of attractiveness was mediated by evaluator credibility and they found no evidence for this.

Attractiveness and Credibility

Snyder and Rothbart (1971) also checked that their observed effect of communicator physical attractiveness on opinion was independent of judgments of expertise and trustworthiness since, "an impressive array of evidence has been presented which indicates that expertness, trustworthiness, intelligence, honesty, manipulative intent, and other objective indices of credibility all modify the impact of a communicator's message." They noted that the "most interesting and least studied" communicator characteristic is that of physical attractiveness, and that Mills and Aronson (1965; see above) did not check whether their "less attractive communicator was also perceived as less credible." In Snyder and Rothbart's study male and female high school students listened to "a tape-recorded speech accompanied by a slide projection of either a relatively attractive or relatively unattractive male face identified as the speaker." The speech was a 5-minute talk advocating lower speed limits and after hearing this the subjects filled in a questionnaire. It was found that those subjects who had been presented with one of the (four) attractive faces advocated significantly lower speed limits that did those exposed to one of the unattractive faces. (The speed limit data from those subjects not supplied with a photograph was in between that of the attractive and unattractive groups.) No group differences, however, were found in the recall of factual information contained in the speech. An almost significant effect of attractiveness on liking for the communicator led Snyder and Rothbart to conclude that liking might mediate the persuasive effect of attractiveness in that (a) attractive communicators produce more liking, and (b) people have a "tendency to model the attitude and opinion statements of those whom we like."

Synder and Rothbart found no effect of attractiveness on ratings of expertise and trustworthiness and consequently they ruled out these factors as mediators of the attractiveness effect. In a similar vein Mills and Harvey (1972) suggested that the processes that lead to agreement with a physically attractive communicator are different from those that produce agreement with an expert communicator. They found that the amount of agreement with a communicator's stance was influenced by whether information about his expertise and attractiveness was presented either before or after the communication. However, Horai et al. (1974) pointed out that, "A major weakness in the Mills and Harvey (1972) study is that expertise and attractiveness were not completely manipulated. The attractive source was nonexpert, while the expert source was unattractive." From the point of view of research on facial appearance a similar weakness (i.e., nonindependent variation of the level of attractiveness) exists in a study by Norman (1976), who also suggested that the processes that may lead to agreement with an attractive communicator are different from those applying to communicator expertise.

Attractiveness and Expertise

In their own study Horai et al. independently varied both attractiveness and expertise. Female junior high school students read a "Letter to the Editor" of a newspaper on the value of generalist education in high school. This was accompanied by a photograph of the author and information that he was either a professor or a "teacher's aide" (i.e., high versus low expertise). It was found that attractiveness did not affect the subjects' perception of the author's expertise or vice versa, nor did these variables affect the amount of factual recall. They did, however, affect subjects' amount of agreement with the author's point of view, and their effects were independent of one another. (The no-photograph or no-expertise conditions did not differ from the low-attractiveness or low-expertise conditions.) With an eye on the Mills and Harvey (1972) study, Horai et al. made the valuable suggestion that future research should examine the effects of independently varied attractiveness and expertise being presented at the end of the communication, rather than only at the beginning as in their study. Also of interest was their finding that low attractiveness decreased liking for the author, although Horai et al. concluded that, "Liking, however, may not be the sufficient condition for opinion agreement."

The effects of communicator attractiveness and expertise were also examined by Howard, Cohen, and Cavior (1974). Students saw and heard via video a male who, using makeup, appeared to be of high, medium, or low physical attractiveness and who presented an argument against the televising of courtroom proceedings. No main effects of communicator attractiveness, expertise, self-interest, or subject sex were found on the degree of attitude change (even though attractiveness was successfully manipulated). The only significant effect on attitude change that involved facial appearance was a complex and difficult to interpret interaction between all four independent variables.

No main effect of physical attractiveness. (i.e., varying makeup, hairstyle, and clothing) was similarly found by Altemeyer and Jones (1974) on male and female students' decisions whether or not to accept a female communicator's solution to a problem. Their study's procedure was perhaps more realistic than that used by other researchers. Small groups of students engaged in a variety of problem-solving tasks and, unknown to them, one of their number was the confederate whose appearance was varied from group to group.

A Field Study

Chaiken (1979), however, did find a significant effect of facial attractiveness on persuasion. Chaiken pointed out that previous studies on this topic had been conducted in laboratory settings, and consequently there existed the possibility that "the highly controlled settings of previous experiments made the attractiveness cue more salient than it would typically be in more naturalistic settings, and the context of these experiments may therefore have inflated the importance of the variable as a determinant of persuasion." Chaiken noted that previous studies that had found an attractiveness effect had used photographs, whereas studies finding no effect had used live or videotaped communicators. On the other hand, Chaiken suggested that previous research might have underestimated the effect of attractiveness since "The implicit demands of the laboratory may encourage subjects to adopt a highly logical mode of cognitive functioning. At the same time such demands may discourage subjects from utilizing information such as physical attractiveness."

Chaiken was interested in the possibility that if attractiveness does affect persuasion, then attractiveness may, in reality, be "correlated with other attributes that affect communicator persuasiveness." Previous studies of this topic, because of their design, had kept constant such factors rather than allowed them to vary. To explore this possibility Chaiken trained a large number of male and female communicators drawn from the top and bottom attractiveness thirds of an undergraduate population to orally present a brief argument concerning the provision of meat in the university dining halls. At the end of training the communicators were videotaped in the laboratory presenting the argument. These communicators also completed a number of self-ratings, and produced information on their educational attainments. Each communicator then approached a number of lone subjects on the university campus until two male and two female subjects had been presented with the argument and had then provided a variety of data. Throughout such interactions Chaiken (a) "stood nearby and monitored" the interactions in order to check that the communicators did not deviate greatly from the procedures, and (b) recorded the number of subjects needing to be approached until the target figure of four was achieved.

The data indicated that the subjects did rate the attractive communicators as, indeed, significantly more attractive. They also rated them as somewhat friendlier ($p<.07$), but no more "knowledgeable" (which Chaiken equated with credibility). There was no effect of attractiveness on the number of subjects needed to be approached until four were found who agreed to participate. Communicator attractiveness was found significantly to increase subjects' agreement with the communicators' position. It also had an almost significant effect ($p<.06$) on the number of subjects who agreed at the end of the interaction to sign a petition in line with the communicators' argument. Analysis of the videotapes (recorded prior to the interactions with the subjects) revealed that the facially attractive communicators were significantly more fluent speakers and had a marginally faster speech rate ($p<.07$), but did not smile or gaze more. Although attractiveness did not relate to communicators' locus of control scores, the attractive ones reported higher scores on the Scholastic Aptitude Test. They also rated themselves "as more persuasive" than did the less attractive communicators, although no effect of attractiveness was found for most of the other self-ratings. With regard to these comparisons of the communicator's skills and personal data Chaiken noted that, "These results suggest that while the observed individual differences do not provide a full explanation for the observed effect of attractiveness on persuasion, they may have contributed at least partially to this effect."

This study by Chaiken is clearly one of the better ones concerning facial appearance and persuasion. Not only was a field setting used where "the salience of information about physical attractiveness should approximate its salience in genuine interpersonal situations," but also used was a large number of communicators who were not drawn solely from the extremes of attractiveness.

Chaiken concluded that "while physical attractiveness may be a significant determinant of persuasion, it may not be a particularly important determinant," and that, "credibility enhancement does not typically mediate the attractiveness-persuasion relationship. However, mechanisms such as social reinforcement, cognitive balance, classical conditioning, and perhaps others remain possible and require further evaluation." Perhaps the most important conclusion to be drawn from Chaiken's study is that in genuine interpersonal situations, attractive individuals may be somewhat more persuasive either because they possess characteristics or skills that dispose them to be particularly effective communicators, or because, as Snyder et al. (1977) found, stereotype-based expectations of others tend to elicit and maintain such behaviors.

Chapter 8 reviews research on the possible relationship between facial appearance and social skill, but we should mention here a study on physical attractiveness and selling that was reported by Reingen, Gresham, and Kernan (1980). Students played the role of either the seller or buyer of a house smoke-detector kit. The sellers were provided with a short script about their role as local sales representative of the product. The buyers' script stated that they had recently moved into a new locality and among their "welcome to the neighborhood" package from local merchants was a letter from the seller plus his photograph. The role of the seller was to telephone the buyer to try to arrange an in-house demonstration. Unknown to the buyers and to the sellers the attractiveness of the photographed male was varied.

Before engaging in the telephone conversation the buyers rated the seller on scales "which were selected from the personal selling literature to represent a broad spectrum of characteristics of successful sales-people." Once this had been done, a 4-minute conversation between buyer and seller took place that was recorded. After the sales call each participant rated his partner on a number of scales. Students unaware of the hypotheses heard from the recordings only the voices of the sellers and they rated the sellers on a variety of scales. Similarly, other students heard and rated only the buyers.

Attractiveness was found to affect significantly the buyers' preconversation ratings of the sellers in that they attributed "more favorable images for social skills, personal industry, enthusiasm, tact, but not persuasiveness." After the sales call attractiveness also had an effect in that buyers who believed they had interacted with an attractive seller indicated that they were more likely to grant the demonstration and to buy the product. Additionally, the sellers in the attractive condition (of which they knew nothing) indicated after the conversation that they were more likely to be granted an appointment, and that the buyers had been more friendly/warm toward them. Reingen et al. also noted that, "the sellers' evaluations of the sales call show that the buyers' reactions toward the unattractive sellers was perceived as less typical and more unusual and different from the way people normally react to them." (For further discussion of this notion see Chapter 8.)

The students who listened (blind) only to the buyers' speech indicated that those who believed that they were interacting with an attractive seller seemed more likely to grant an appointment and buy the product. "Similar but only marginally significant results were found for the corresponding evaluations of the seller tapes." Buyers who interacted with a supposedly attractive seller were rated by the listeners as more comfortable, intimate, personal, enthusiastic, and warm/friendly. However, no effect upon ratings concerned with social skills were found. With regard to ratings of the sellers' speech, no effects at all were found, which therefore does not replicate the findings of Snyder et al. (1977). Nevertheless, sellers' supposed attractiveness did influence buyers' stated intentions and therefore it could be deemed to have had a persuasive effect upon them.

Number of Arguments

No support for the notion that attractiveness affects persuasion was found, however, by Maddux and Rogers (1980), who, as in earlier studies, also varied communicator expertise. They tested the hypothesis that varying the number of arguments presented to support an advocated opinion should influence the effectiveness of an expert source more than an attractive source, having pointed out, in terms of theories, that "both functional and reinforcement approaches agree that an attractive source's persuasive impact is not dependent on the provision of supporting arguments." Female students received folders containing a "statement of opinion," a photograph of its source, and information regarding the source's expertise on the topic. Level of expertise and the number of arguments presented had significant effects on agreement, whereas successfully manipulated attractiveness did not, even though attractiveness influenced some of the 13 ratings made of the communicator (which, unfortunately, did not include scales directly relating to liking or to credibility).

Maddux and Rogers suggested that attractiveness may not have had a significant effect in their study because, unlike Chaiken (1979), they used only very extreme levels of attractiveness that, in the laboratory, may have led their subjects to make a "deliberate attempt to prevent the source's beauty or ugliness from influencing their agreement with his position." However, they added that, "Rather than attempt to explain away the nonsignificant effect on persuasion, perhaps we should accept these null findings and conclude that a source's physical attractiveness may not be a robust variable in the field of persuasive communications." They also made the suggestion, "That being unattractive was not sufficient cause to disagree with the source should be comforting to some of us, 'unattractive, middle-aged professors.' " (Of comfort to students may be the finding of Lee, Adams, and Dobson [1984] to the effect that the facial appearance of those on the receiving end of a live attempt at persuasion seems not to influence persuaders' interactional style.)

Maddux and Rogers also made the point that, "We are not suggesting that physical attractiveness is never an important source characteristic. Undoubtedly there are conditions in which the physical attractiveness of a communicator would influence persuasion consistently." They suggested that such conditions might be those in which people can choose whether or not to attend to the communicator's message, and those in which aspects of the communication may not be so concerned with logical or factual information. Commercial advertising is one aspect of life in which people usually can choose whether or not to attend to the message, and therefore here a communicator's facial appearance may have an effect on such decisions. (We shall, later in this chapter, review studies that have examined the effects of facial appearance in this setting.) In political campaigning (also reviewed later in this chapter), which, contrary to some views, may be based as much on emotion as it is on logic, facial appearance may also have an effect on subjects' agreement with the points of view stated.

In attempting to explain why the effects upon persuasion of attractiveness and expertise may be psychologically different Norman (1976) suggested that agreement with a position advocated by an expert source is based primarily upon the acceptance of supportive arguments provided, whereas the influence of an attractive source is relatively independent of reaction to the specific arguments presented in the message. He found that, "The expert source's endorsement of a particular opinion was ineffective in influencing audience agreement unless he provided justifying arguments for the position he advocated. The attractive source, in contrast, was able to bring about significant agreement *regardless* of whether he provided supporting arguments."

Objectivity

Blass, Alperstein, and Block (1974) suggested that in the study of the effects of communicator attractiveness upon persuasion people's tendency to take into account irrelevant attributes of a person could be important. They employed the Blass Objectivity-Subjectivity Scale to perform such a study ("subjective" subjects being those who would be more susceptible to irrelevant effects). In their study a significant effect of attractiveness (i.e., variation in hairstyle, dress, and posture) was found for the subjective subjects, but, as hypothesized, not for the objective subjects. When the communicator was white and attractive this was accompanied by greater attitude change than when she was unattractive. However, attractiveness had the (unexpected) reverse effect when the communicator was black, perhaps because all the subjects were white, although the black female's attractiveness manipulation had a significant effect on their attractiveness ratings of her. In line with previous research, attractiveness had no effect on perceived credibility nor on the recall of factual information contained in the communication.

Pallak (1983) did not cite Maddux and Rogers' (1980) paper, but she also differentiated between persuasion being mediated on the one hand by "information and arguments relevant to the attitude issue," and on the other hand by "factors other than the attitude issue itself." She suggested (a) that the former of these "two routes to persuasion" could be "analogous to the distinction made by Craik and Lockhart (1972) between deep and shallow processing, or to that made by Schneider and Shiffrin (1977) between controlled and automatic processing," and (b) that "Chaiken's (1980) description of systematic and heuristic processing in persuasion" could also be relevant.

Information Processing

In connection with Chaiken's (1980) suggestion, Pallak (1983) pointed out that "when a persuasive communication is processed systematically, the recipient attempts to comprehend and evaluate the arguments and to assess their validity in relation to the conclusion. . . . Alternatively, the decision to accept or reject the conclusion of a persuasive communication could be made on the basis of a relatively simple rule (i.e. a heuristic). When a heuristic information-processing strategy is employed, recipients rely on information that is readily available, such as the characteristics of the communicator." Chaiken (1980) had suggested that one heuristic often employed could be "I generally agree with people I like." If physical attractiveness affects liking (see Chapter 2), then Pallak argued that "the more salient a communicator's physical attractiveness, the more convenient it may be to use" such a heuristic. Thus, "Making a communicator's physical attractiveness particularly salient may induce heuristic processing of a persuasive communication that would be processed systematically if the communicator's physical attractiveness were less salient." Therefore, Pallak hypothesized that strong and weak versions of a persuasive communication were expected to elicit equal agreement in the high-salience conditions. In contrast, reducing the salience of the communicator's attractiveness should enhance the importance of the message characteristics.

In Pallak's study female students read a statement that strongly or weakly argued that people have a responsibility to donate money to support the Arts. This was supposedly written by an art expert, and in the folder containing the statement was a photograph of an attractive male in his 30s. The photograph was either in color (high salience) or was "a low-quality Xerox copy of the photograph" (low salience). Immediately after reading the statement the subjects indicated the extent of their agreement with the communicator and listed "the thoughts they had while reading the communication."

Pallak reported that the salience manipulation was successful in that the distinctiveness of the communicator's physical attractiveness was rated higher in the color photograph condition. As planned, however, the salience manipulation had no effect on how attractive the communicator was judged to be. The data significantly supported the main hypothesis, which was that subjects' degree of agreement with the communicator would only be affected by the strength of his argument in the low salience (or attractiveness) condition. The low salience weak argument condition occasioned significantly less agreement than did the other three conditions, which did not differ. Thus Pallak found facial appearance only to affect persuasion when the communication itself was weak. This is yet another example (as noted throughout this book) of a person's facial appearance assuming importance only when other information about that person is not positive (or is absent).

Examination of Pallak's subjects' written thoughts revealed that they listed significantly more thoughts referring to the communicator when his attractiveness was salient than when it was not, and listed fewer negative message-oriented thoughts when the communicator's attractiveness was salient. In addition, "The salience of the communicator's attractiveness affected the strength of the relationship between the number of negative message-oriented thoughts generated and the degree of agreement. These two measures were negatively correlated when the communicator's attractiveness was not salient, but uncorrelated when the communicator's attractiveness was salient." Thus Pallak concluded that, "the salience of a communicator's attractiveness can influence the strategy used to process a persuasive communication."

This conclusion has a number of implications, one of which relates to political parties' and politicians' attempts to persuade people to vote for them.

The Role of Facial Appearance in Politics

In 1968 Sears stated that, "It is certainly easier to base one's decision on how a person looks rather than on the arguments he is putting forward. One gets the impression that voters prefer to think about politics in terms of individual personalities rather than abstractions. The principal contents of candidate images seem to have to do with personal qualities rather than with policy decisions." Sears suggested that even when political issues are discussed, "all but the simplest implications are quickly lost from the content of the image, even if the affective change is stable." Thus, "the primary purpose of raising issues at all may be simply to provide something for the politicians to talk about."

In *The Selling of the President*, McGinnis (1976) illustrated how the democratic process that elected Richard Nixon to the White House was influenced by the use of the media and the images portrayed. He cited one of Nixon's advisers as saying that "the response of the viewer is to the image. It's not the man we have to change but rather the received impression of him. And this impression depends more on the medium and its use than it does on the candidate himself." Another Nixon aide wrote that, "Most national issues today are so complicated, so difficult to understand that they bore the average man. Few politicians recognize this fact." McGinnis reported another adviser as saying that, "Voters are basically lazy. Reasoning requires a high degree of concentration; impression is easier. Reason pushes the viewer back, it assaults him whereas impression can envelop him without making an intellectual demand. Thus the emotions are more easily aroused, more malleable. Let's not be afraid of gimmicks. Get the voters to like the guy and the battle's two thirds won."

Attractiveness and Number of Votes

Although his paper was not concerned with facial appearance but with character attractiveness, it is worth noting Mishler's (1978) point that "constituency organizations are also attracted to and tend to nominate individuals whom party officials *believe* will be attractive to the voters and thus enhance the party's support at the polls." Support for this view comes from a study by Efran and Patterson (1974) that, rather surprisingly, was not cited by Mishler. In the 1972 Canadian federal election Efran and Patterson asked high school students to rate from photographs the attractiveness of 79 parliamentary candidates who were competing for seats in 21 ridings in the Metropolitan Toronto area. The ratings were carried out about 6 months after the election. The persons shown in the pictures were not identified as political candidates and comments made by the judges at debriefing gave no indication that the slides had been recognized as photographs of politicians. Candidates who obtained attractiveness scores equivalent to or greater than 1 standard deviation above the overall group mean were assigned to the attractive group ($n = 16$), and those with scores equivalent to or lower than 1 standard deviation below the mean were assigned to the unattractive group ($n = 15$).

Efran and Patterson found that the attractive group obtained an average of 32% of the votes cast in their ridings, whereas the unattractive candidates received an average of only 11% ($p < .001$), and that there were seven winning candidates within the attractive group but only one winner within the unattractive group ($p < .05$). Overall the correlation for the 79 candidates between physical attractiveness and the proportion of the vote obtained within the candidate's riding was $+0.4$ ($p < .001$). These rather strong effects could be taken to suggest that facial appearance may have a powerful effect on political voting. However, Efran and Patterson wisely decided to see whether there was a relationship between a candidate's physical attractiveness and whether the candidate was from a major or minor party. They found that, "Only one of those 17 candidates who were not affiliated with the three major parties was above the median in attractiveness for all candidates ($p = .0001$)," and that many of the candidates in the unattractive group were members of minor parties. Efran and Patterson concluded that their results "unquestionably show that physical appearance is an important individual attribute which interacts with the political system. Several issues warrant further study. One of these is the extent to which physical appearance influences the choice voters make between major candidates." (They noted that "one member of Parliament has recently proposed legislation that would make it mandatory election procedure to publish a photograph of each candidate beside the candidates' name on the election ballot.")

Efran and Patterson stated that it was not possible to determine whether the unattractive candidates received fewer votes because of their party affiliation rather than their physical appearance. They also stated that, "it was not possible to analyze meaningfully the effect of appearance with respect to the major party candidates."

However, the major party candidates' facial appearance and the number of votes they received was examined by Bull, Jenkins, and Stevens (1983). This study by Bull et al. replicated some of the findings of Bull and Hawkes (1982), which in turn was partly inspired by a study published by Jahoda in 1954.

Judging Political Inclination from Faces

In his study Jahoda asked members of the general public to sort anonymous portrait photographs of men into two piles depending on whether they thought the pictured person would be likely to vote Labour or Conservative. (In fact the photos were of Labour and Conservative backbench, nonlocal members of Parliament, but fewer than 10% of the observers guessed this.) It was found that the general public were significantly more right than wrong in their assignations of the political inclinations of the men shown in the photos. The observers were also asked to say whether they thought the photographed persons had high, medium, or low IQs, and whether they were "good-looking," average, or not "good-looking." Observers who said that they themselves were Conservatives rated the photos of individuals whom they said were Conservatives as more intelligent and "good-looking" than the pictures of Labour members. Male Labour observers demonstrated the reverse whereas female Labour observers evidenced no significant effect for "good-looks." With regard to social class, in 1954 both Conservative and Labour observers indicated that they believed all the photographed individuals to be of high social class. Jahoda reported that statements such as the following were frequent from Conservative observers: "The ones with breeding in their features are Conservatives. Socialists are rough-looking types;" and from Labour supporters, "The fat and stupid ones are Conservatives. Labour people have a frank and open appearance."

Most voters, and especially the undecided ones, never meet the candidates for their own constituency. They do see on television some politicians presenting arguments as to why a certain political party is worth voting for, but in connection with candidates for their own constituency all that most voters see is the leaflet that comes through the door, posters, and perhaps a photograph with some words in their local paper. Thus here we have a situation in which some voters never have the opportunity to determine whether the candidates have the personalities, attributes, and the like that their photographs suggest.

In Bull and Hawkes' (1982) study photographs of seven Labour and seven Conservative male, backbench members of Parliament were selected from *The Times 1984 Guide to the House of Commons*, which contains details and a photograph of every member of Parliament. These facial photographs were selected according to the following general criteria:

1. All must have a plain background and similar lighting conditions,
2. None of them must show shoulders or body lower than the top of the tie knot,
3. None must have abnormally long hair or be bald or have a beard or moustache,
4. All must represent English constituencies.

Since such things as the candidates' age, sex, and facial expression are likely to be important, as may be physiognomic features, aspects of grooming, and the presence or absence of spectacles, some more specific criteria were also adhered to. For each of these criteria, the following photographs of the first Labour and the first Conservative appearing in the alphabetical order of the *Guide* were selected:

1. No smile, wearing glasses, age more than 60, face straight ahead
2. Smile, no glasses, age more than 60, face straight ahead
3. No smile, no glasses, age less than 40, face straight ahead
4. Smile, glasses, age less than 40, face straight ahead
5. No smile, no glasses, age 40 to 60, face straight ahead
6. No smile, no glasses, age 40 to 60, face turned to left
7. No smile, no glasses, age 40 to 60, face turned to right.

These criteria were important since if all the Conservative members were smiling and wore glasses and none of the Labour members did so, then differences in the judgments of the Conservative and Labour members may have nothing to do with political stereotypes. The 14 selected photographs were shown in random order to a large number of adults who had been residents in Britain for 5 years, the vast majority being born in Britain. The observers were given booklets in which to indicate their judgments of each of the 14 faces. They were not told that the faces were of members of Parliament and when questioned afterward only one observer suggested that this was in fact the case. For each photograph every observer was asked to evaluate the face for intelligence, sincerity, social class, political inclination, and attractiveness. On the final page of the booklet the observers were asked to indicate their age, sex, and political inclination.

The first hypothesis we wanted to examine was whether the political allegiances of Labour and Conservative members of Parliament could reliably be judged by a large number of people from mere facial photographs alone. If such were the case this would then permit examination of a second question, whether judgments of intelligence, sincerity, social class, and physical attractiveness are related to judgments of political inclination. A third hypothesis was whether the political inclination and sex of the evaluators would play a role.

Analysis of the data revealed that there was significant interjudge agreement with regard to the political allegiance allocated to each of the photographed persons. Thus the first hypothesis was supported. Of the 14 faces, 6 had an average political inclination rating under 3.5 and these were deemed to be the "judged as Conservative" group; 5 had an average political inclination rating over 4.5 and these formed the "judged as Labour" group. Of the "judged as Conservative" group, 2 were actually Labour members, and of the "judged as Labour" group, 2 were actually Conservatives.

Having found that observers agreed in their judgments of people's (members') political inclinations solely on the basis of a facial photograph, we next wanted to see if there were any relationships between "judged as Conservative" or "judged as Labour" and evaluations of intelligence, sincerity, social class, and physical attractiveness. With regard to intelligence, those members of Parliament judged to be Conservative (i.e., 4 really Conservative and 2 really Labour) were accorded significantly more intelligence ($p < .001$) than those judged to be Labour. Surprisingly, this was equally the case for both Conservative and Labour subjects. The political inclinations of the persons making the judgments of intelligence had no effect; even Labour supporters rated the photos "judged as Conservative" to be more intelligent than the photos "judged as Labour." We also found that members of Parliament "judged as Conservatives" were accorded a significantly higher social class than those "judged as Labour." This effect occurred irrespective of whether the subjects were Labour, Conservative, or neither. The observers' judgments of how "sincere" the photographed members of Parliament were was not at all affected by whether the members looked Conservative or looked Labour, nor was the political inclination or sex of the observers an important factor. All the members appeared of equal (and in fact average) sincerity. The members "judged as Conservative" were seen as significantly more physically attractive than those "judged as Labour." Here again the political inclinations of the observers had no effect.

Observers' Political Views

Our finding that the political allegiance of the observers had no effect on their ratings came as rather a surprise, especially since Kassarjian (1963) had found a significant relationship between U.S. voters' political beliefs (i.e., Republican or Democrat) and whether they though Jack Kennedy was taller than Richard Nixon. Similarly, R. Johnson (1981) had found that subjects selected the more facially attractive photographs as being supporters of the political party they themselves supported. Just prior to the Canadian federal elections Johnson found in both this experiments that supporters of either the Progressive Conservative Party or the Liberal Party, when asked to select from a booklet of male and female photographs supporters for each of the three major parties, chose as supporters of their own party the more attractive faces. Only supporters of the New Democratic party failed to show such an in-group effect. Johnson concluded that his results were "consistent with the hypothesis that there is a physical attractiveness stereotype whereby members of an in-group see themselves as more attractive than out-group members." He suggested that there could be meaningful individual differences in "cognitive structure" in that people to the "right" of the political spectrum may be more inclined to employ such stereotyping. He also suggested that such a hypothesis could explain the findings of studies concerning women's facial attractiveness and their presumed support for the women's movement (see below).

A Replication

Because Bull and Hawkes (1982) had found no effect of subjects' political affiliation Bull et al. (1983) conducted a replication in which the politicians' faces to be evaluated were obtained from marginal constituencies. Just prior to the 1979 General Election a list was drawn up of the 30 most marginal constituencies in Great Britain in the 1974 General Election. Within each of these 30 constituencies the 1979 candidates from the two political parties that polled the most votes in 1974 were selected for contact. A letter was sent to each of these 60 candidates, this letter suggesting that the sender wished to cast a postal vote in the constituency and desired information about the candidate. The vast majority of candidates replied and most of their replies contained an election address leaflet with a facial photograph printed on it. (It is interesting to note how frequently these leaflets do contain a photograph of the candidate.) In this way facial photographs of the two main contenders in each constituency were obtained for 18 of the 30 constituencies (all faces were male and were of Labour or Conservative candidates). These 18 constituencies were randomly divided into two groups of 9 (group A and group B) and within each group the 18 faces (9 Conservative and 9 Labour) were put in an arbitrary order. The 18 group A faces were shown to 22 adults and the 18 group B faces to a further 23 adults who evaluated each face for intelligence, honesty, social class, political inclination, and attractiveness.

Follow-up questioning revealed that although the raters were asked at the end of the investigation for details of their own political inclinations, they were unaware of the aims of the study and none realized that the photographs were of politicians. Thus, the aims of the present study were first to see whether the results of Bull and Hawkes (1982) were replicable and second to examine whether the ratings of the faces in any way related to the 1979 General Election outcome in each of the constituencies. This latter aim, although perhaps expecting rather a lot, was formulated in the light of the "expert" opinion, current at the time, that the result of the 1979 General Election would be very marginal, the likely outcome being a very small over-all majority in the House of Commons. Those faces that received on the dimension of political inclination a mean rating of greater than 5.5 were deemed "judged as Conservative" and those a mean rating less than 4.5 were deemed "judged as Labour." Within group A, 4 faces were "judged as Labour" (these all, in fact, being Labour candidates) and 5 faces were "judged as Conservative" (3 of these being Conservative candidates and 2 being Labour). Within group B, 7 faces were "judged as Labour" (3 being Labour and 4 Conservative) and 7 were "judged as Conservative" (4 being Conservative and 3 being Labour). The groups of faces "judged as Conservative" and "judged as Labour" were then compared for their ratings of in-telligence, social class, attractiveness, and honesty, with the raters' sex and political inclination being taken into account. For group A the "judged as Conservative" faces were rated as significantly more intelligent, more attractive, and of higher social class. For group B the "judged as Conserva-tive" faces were rated as significantly more intelligent, more honest, and of higher social class. The raters' sex and political inclination had no effects upon these judgments.

In connection with the second aim of the study, to examine whether the ratings of the faces related to the General Election outcome in each consti-tuency, a variety of comparisons and analyses were conducted. In the light of the actual outcome of the 1979 General Election (an uncontrolled variable in this study), which resulted in the largest "percentage swing" in votes cast for the Conservative party in recent decades, little, if any, effect of the variables being examined in this study was expected. (The face evaluations were obtained just prior to the election.) Indeed, this was found to be the case, with none of the facial evaluations examined in this study relating to the voting outcome in the 18 constituencies or to the actual percentage or total number of votes cast. The only noticeable trend was that the more intelligent-looking candidate in each constituency was somewhat more likely to have been elected ($p < .09$).

Thus both of Bull's studies found that although observers agreed, they were not always correct in their allocating of politicians' faces to political parties. Their judgments of which political party a person supported were related to how attractive and intelligent they judged that person's face to be and from which social class they believed that person to come. These judgments were affected neither by the rathers' political inclinations, nor by their sex.

Sex has, however, had an effect in studies that have examined the role of facial appearance in a different part of the political arena, that of support for the "women's movement."

Facial Appearance and Support for the Women's Movement

One of the earliest studies concerning facial appearance and the women's movement found that when asked to decide from a series of women's facial photographs which were and which were not supporters of the women's liberation movement, both male and female subjects significantly assigned unattractive faces to the supporter category (Goldberg, Gottesdiener, & Abramson, 1975). In this study 30 female undergraduates completed a questionnaire concerning their attitudes toward the women's liberation movement. The subjects were also photographed. These facial photographs were rated by students from another campus for attractiveness. No difference in actual attractiveness was found between the females who did or did not support the women's movement. However, when other male and female students were asked to say whether each photographed woman would support or not support women's liberation it was found that both males and females significantly alloted unattractive faces to the support category.

Goldberg, Gottesdiener, and Abramson suggested that since "the feminist movement has aroused strong feelings" the bias they observed (in terms of attractiveness) against supporters of the movement might be explained by the notion that, "Imputing unfavorable characteristics to people whose attitudes we do not like very much is simply one well-evidenced halo effect." However, they found that subjects' own attitudes toward the women's liberation movement were not correlated with the categorization data. The concluded that their results "may provide one more example of the pervasive put-down to which women are subject."

M. Jacobson and Koch (1978) also found data that suggested a stereotypical bias against unattractive women. They investigated whether subjects would attribute different reasons for being in favor of women's liberation to facially attractive women compared to unattractive women. In noting the finding of Goldberg, Gottesdiener, and Abramson they suggested that any observed relationship between unattractiveness and feminism may work both ways in the sense that "many nonsupporters of the feminist movement have the attitude that unattractive women *need* feminism." However, since "it is clear that some attractive women are feminists" how do people "explain the presence of attractive women in the movement?" Jacobson and Koch suggested that, "Under these circumstances, we believe people would feel that the attractive woman is a feminist not because she needs to be, but because she wants to be." They showed facially attractive and unattractive women's photographs to male and female students who were asked to indicate why they thought the woman in the photograph was a feminist by choosing one of eight listed reasons, four of which were positive reasons (e.g., "She's interested in promoting human values") and four of which were negative (e.g., "She hates men"). It was found that significantly more of the attractive photographs occasioned a positive reason than did the unattractive faces. Jacobson and Koch concluded that this "effect of attractiveness is disheartening because it is a severe put-down of unattractive women," because it implies that feminism is seen as "an ideology that is more appealing to and more needed by people who are undervalued in society (i.e. the unattractive)." However, they also pointed out that a halo effect explanation is possible in the sense that "attractive people have good things attributed to them and unattractive people have bad things attributed to them and in this study the 'things' just happened to be reasons for being a feminist."

Reasons for Supporting Feminism

In 1982 Clingman and Lushene replicated Jacobson and Koch's (1978) study. They showed male and female undergraduates the faces of women who were supposedly supporters of the feminist movement and for each face they were asked to rate the extent to which each of the eight reasons used by Jacobson and Koch applied to that woman. The resulting data were factor analyzed and this produced "two separate factors consistent with those reasons Jacobson and Koch referred to as either 'positive' or 'negative'." A significant effect of attractiveness was found in that the attractive women received higher scores on the positive reasons and lower scores on the negative reasons. Clingman and Lushene concluded that "without possessing certain highly valued characteristics, a woman is likely to have her motivations for becoming a feminist impugned . . . it seems reasonable to assume that most women are perceived as having turned to feminism out of want, to make up for some deficit." However, they pointed out that additional study is necessary to determine the accuracy or inaccuracy of these perceptions.

There is, in fact, no evidence that females who support the women's movement are actually less facially attractive than those who do not. Neither Goldberg, Gottesdiener, and Abramson (1975) nor R. Johnson, Doiron, Brookes, and Dickinson (1978) nor Unger, Hilderbrand, and Madar (1982) found support for such a notion. Johnson et al. did find, as did Goldberg, Gottesdiener, and Abramson, that male undergraduates chose as supporters of the women's movement female photographs deemed by other students to be unattractive. However, nonstudent subjects did not assign unattractive faces to the support category. Even more contrary to the outcome of Goldberg, Gottesdiener, and Abramson's study was the finding that the female students significantly assigned the more attractive women to the support category. Additionally Johnson et al. unlike Goldberg, Gottesdiener, and Abramson, found there to be some evidence that subjects' (both male and female) own views about women's liberation bore a relationship to the extent to which they "put down" liberated women by selecting the less attractive photographs as being those of supporters.

Changes in Society

In attempting to explain why most of their study's findings differed from those of Goldberg, Gottesdiener, and Abramson, Johnson et al. put forward a number of suggestions. One of these was concerned with the possibility that "the more recent collection of the present data may account for the discrepancy in the two reports." Even though in some areas of psychology it may be correct to assume that the date of a study is not a relevant characteristic, in social psychology we believe that it would be naive to assume this, particularly for an issue such as women's liberation. In fact, instead of seeing discrepant findings over the years as a problem for psychological science one could possibly use these to chart changes within society, although this, in fact, is rarely done.

Another of Johnson et al.'s points suggested that for nonstudents (for whom there were no significant effects in their study) the issues of women's liberation may not be as "real and immediate" as they are for undergraduates. They also suggested that people's reactions concerning the women's movement may have been different in Atlantic Canada (where their study was carried out) than in the Eastern United States. Thus, again, discrepant findings may not necessarily suggest that studies have been poorly conducted; they may be used as indications of meaningful differences between samples of subjects.

R. Johnson, Holborn, and Turcotte (1979) also found that subject factors were important in this aspect of the social psychology of facial appearance. They used the stimulus photographs from Johnson et al.'s (1978) study, and male and female undergraduates were asked to sort these into "categories for and critics of the Feminist Movement." It was found that both females and males significantly selected photographs of more attractive women as being supporters of the feminist movement. Also, subjects' own "attitudes towards women" correlated positively with the extent to which they assigned attractive faces to the support category.

In a rarely cited paper Agarwal and Prakash (1977) reported that they found in India that both male and female students significantly chose as supporters of women's liberation the more attractive faces. The major, but not the only, cause for this main effect was that the female subjects who expressed support for the women's movement reliably chose as nonsupporters the unattractive faces. Agarwal and Prakash also found, as did Goldberg, Gottesdiener, and Abramson, no relationship between the stimulus person's attractiveness and their actual support for the movement.

A study by Banziger and Hooker (1979) is yet another that failed to replicate Goldberg, Gottesdiener, and Abramson's "put down" of feminists. They showed to male undergraduates photographs of women that had been pre-rated for attractiveness, and these males also completed a questionnaire concerning their attitudes toward feminism. Each photograph was accompanied by statements that suggested whether or not the woman was a supporter of feminism. The subjects were required to rate each face for attractiveness. No main effect of the women's support for feminism was found on the attractiveness ratings; however, a significant interaction revealed that the men who were profeminism rated the feminists as more attractive and the antifeminist men did the reverse. Banziger and Hooker took this finding to suggest "the effect of perceived feminism seems to work through the dimension of attitude similarity, since males rated attitude-similar stimulus persons as more attractive than attitude-dissimilar stimulus persons."

In-Group Bias

R. Johnson, Dannenbring, Anderson, and Villa (1983), however, consistently failed to find any evidence in their four geographically diverse subject samples that subjects' "attitudes towards women" scores related to their choice
of photographs as supporters of feminism. They hypothesized that, "The
perception of supporters of Feminism as being more or less attractive than
nonsupporters may simply be a case of attributing a positive characteristic
(attractiveness) to those like oneself." To test this in-group bias interpretation, as opposed to the notion that a simple stereotype about feminists exists,
Johnson et al. used not only female stimulus persons but males as well. They
argued that, "If some persons stereotype feminists as being less attractive on
the basis of an opinion that unattractive women need feminism, then this
stereotype should apply only to females. If, on the other hand, subjects show
an in-group bias, which includes attractiveness attribution, this bias should
apply to all who share values and attitudes irrespective of sex." Thus it was
predicted that differences in attractiveness between those categorized as supporters and nonsupporters should similarly hold for both female and male
faces.

R. Johnson et al. (1983) asked subjects to pick from a selection of male and
female facial photographs those that they thought would be (a) an outspoken
advocate of feminism, or (b) an outspoken critic of feminism, or (c) a person
believing strongly in feminism but who does not actively campaign for the
movement, or (d) a person who strongly agrees with the critics of feminism
but who does not actively campaign against feminism. The subjects also completed an attitude toward women scale, and they were either students or
nonstudents from Nova Scotia, or students from either Louisana or Florida.
As was found in most studies subsequent to that of Goldberg, Gottesdiener,
and Abramson (1975), no main effect of attractiveness was found regarding
support or nonsupport for feminism. Only the nonstudent sample evidenced
a significant bias against female supporters of feminism by categorizing unattractive female (but not male) faces as supporters. Although Johnson et al.
concluded from these findings that "the present study finds no support for the
first hypothesis, which predicts attributed advocates to be seen as more attractive," the outcome of the analysis of the Canadian nonstudent sample's data
regarding the female faces perhaps should not be so readily dispensed with.

Johnson et al. found a consistent, unpredicted main effect for the variable
of outspoken versus inactive involvement. The faces categorized as outspoken advocates or critics were less attractive than the inactive advocates or
critics and significant interactions revealed that this main effect was largely
due to the faces categorized as outspoken advocates being less attractive than
inactive advocates. No relationships were found between subjects' attitudes
toward women scores and their allocation of faces to categories. Johnson et
al. concluded that their results (a) "seem fairly consistent with an in-group
bias view of the photo-sorting," and (b) "suggest quite strongly that while

advocates of Feminism are no longer viewed as different, and, therefore, stereotyped in terms of attractiveness, outspoken advocates are perceived as less attractive.''

Meta-Analysis

In the light of a series of somewhat contradictory findings concerning the assumed relationship between facial appearance and support for the women's movement, Beaman and Klentz (1983) undertook a meta-analysis of the results of previous studies. They concluded from their analysis that there was overall no evidence for a general attractiveness bias against those believed to be supporters of the women's movement, and they therefore stated that, "We hope that the assumption that an attractiveness bias against feminists exists will no longer be uncritically accepted." They suggested that previous studies' results might best be accounted for by the notion that people rate others with similar attitudes as more physically attractive than those with dissimilar attitudes.

This hypothesis was tested by Beaman, Klentz, and Conrad (1984), who asked male and female undergraduates to rate on a number of dimensions the photographs of males and females who were described either as supporters or nonsupporters of the women's movement, or for whom no such information was given. Nine rating scales, including one for attractiveness, were used, "eight of which were filler items." Each photograph was also rated "on how similar the subjects thought the person's attitudes were to their own." The subjects also completed a "one-item questionnaire . . . to measure their attitudes toward the women's movement." One of the main findings was that the faces believed not to be of supporters of the women's movement were rated as significantly less attractive than those believed to be supporters (the ratings of which did not differ from the "no-information" faces). A significant positive relationship was also found between subjects' own attitude toward the women's movement and their physical attractiveness ratings of the supporters (but not the nonsupporters).

Beaman et al. reasoned that, "If attitude similiarity mediates one's rating of attractiveness, a relationship should also be found between the subjects' attitudes and the supposed attitudes of the persons photographed." This was, in fact, found to be the case, with a positive relationship existing for the photographs of supporters and a negative one for the photographs of nonsupporters. Beaman et al. therefore concluded that people tend erroneously to perceive others who have similar attitudes as more physically attractive. They argued that such an explanation of various studies' findings concerning facial appearance and presumed feminism "offers the heuristic benefit of incorporating these findings . . . into the general body of attitude research." They stated, however, "that the conclusion that a *general* bias against supporters does not exist does not alleviate concerns about stereotyping of dissimilar others. To say that the reduced judgements of attractiveness are mediated by

assumed dissimilarity does not remove the potential injustic of such deduc-
tions."

Thus, if it is true today that most people see value in the women's movement, then they will not assume that women who are feminists are necessarily
facially unattractive. However, active bias against unattractive women may
be taking place in another aspect of life, that of the employment setting.

The Role of Facial Appearance in the Employment Setting

Recently Heilman and Stopeck (1985a) found, with regard to the evaluation
of employees' performance, that being unattractive was a disadvantage for
women believed to be clerical trainees, but it had no effect on the evaluation
of males. Before we examine the (rather sparse) literature concerning employee evaluation, let us examine studies of the effects of facial appearance on
job applicant selection.

Application Selection

As far back as 1934 Husband noted that many employment application forms
require the applicant to provide a facial photograph. In recent times some
societies have frowned upon such a procedure, but in many countries it is a
widespread practice. Even if information about an applicant's facial appearance is not available to decision makers before an interview, it certainly will
be when they come face to face with the job applicants. Husband (1934)
asked students to rate photographs of men and women whom he knew along
a number of dimensions, including "executive ability." He found no relationship between his ratings of the stimulus individuals based on his
knowledge of them and the students's ratings. He ascribed this invalidity
to "two major sources of fallacy which undoubtedly figure to a great extent in
practical personnel work. Two men who were rather handsome . . . were
uniformly given very high ratings."

Springbett pointed out in 1958 that, "there are psychological processes
which underlie decision-making in the interview. If these can be identified,
and prove to be lawful, they may provide the means for understanding, and
perhaps improving, the selective functions of the interviewer." In what can
now be seen as a pioneering attempt at ecological validity, rather than have
inexperience students attempt to evaluate others who pretend to be applying
for a job, Springbett studied real-life employment interviews conducted by six
pairs of staff from four companies who were recruiting staff. Each member of
an interviewing pair was instructed to independently evaluate the applicant at
the beginning of the interview in terms of his appearance and his application
form, to then interview him and to arrive at a final decision. The rating based
on the application form predicted the final employment decision in 81% of
cases, and that of appearance predicted in only 62%. However, when the

interviewers were instructed to rate appearance before rating the application form, appearance had a stronger effect. Springbett noted that "the superiority of application form over appearance ratings holds only when the application form is rated first." In his second experiment, in which three students were interviewed by 18 experienced personnel officers, the effect of appearance was found to be stronger. Springbett concluded that in the job application interview setting those "who are borderline in appearance," or of "dubious appearance," are the ones for whom physical appearance seems to have the greatest effect on interviewers' decisions.

What Has the Greater Effect, Ugliness or Attractiveness?

Carlson and Mayfield (1967), however, came to the opposite conclusion. Their study examined several hundred life insurance agency managers' reactions to either completed job application forms or merely photographs of applicants. Not suprisingly, those managers given the application forms showed greater interater agreement and greater intrarater reliability over time for ratings and rankings of the applicants and decisions whether to employ them than did those who only received applicants' photographs. Carlson and Mayfield found that "favorably rated photographs have a greater effect on employment decisions than an unfavorable photograph, while for the written information just the opposite effect was noted." However, the photographic part of their study was so lacking in ecological validity that it could be ignored. Nevertheless, the managers' reactions to the photographs did show fairly high interrater agreement and intrarater reliability across 4 weeks. Carlson and Mayfield stated that their study found that managers "will make a selection or rejection decision on the basis of appearance alone. Whether they do so in actual practice is deferred to future studies."

A rather more appropriate test of the effect of applicants' facial appearance was conducted by Dipboye, Fromkin, and Wiback (1975). Male interviewers who represented a wide range of companies took part in the study while they were on campus to interview actual job applicants. In addition male undergraduate industrial management students also took part in the "experimental task which was designed to be compatible with the employment interviewing practice of screening applicants' résumés prior to the job interviews." The subjects, who were told that they were taking part in a study, each saw 12 applications for the post of head of a furniture department in a large department store. The applications varied in terms of the applicants' scholastic record (three levels), sex, and physical attactiveness (two levels), and the subjects were required to give an overall rating to each résumé and to rank-order the applicants. Physical attractiveness was found to have a significant effect on the ratings and the rankings, with the more attractive applicant being more positively evaluated. However, whereas appearance accounted for only 6% of the variance in the ratings and 9% in the rankings, scholastic record accounted for 33% and 38%, respectively. Sex of applicant did not interact with the attractiveness effects, nor did type of subject. Dipboye et al. concluded that, "The training and experience of professional interviewers did not give them immunity from the tendency to discriminate on the basis of physical attractiveness." However, perhaps wisely, they noted that since the job description read by subjects stated that, "the position is a very visible one requiring a high degree of interpersonal skill. . . . It is not clear whether the suitability ratings reflect the stereotype of physical unattractiveness as inferior and/or whether the ratings reflect the perception that physically unattractive persons do not meet the requirements set forth in the job description." (Chapter 8 of this book discusses the relationship between social skill and facial appearance.)

In 1977 Dipboye, Arvey, and Terpstra attempted to replicate the 1975 study by Dipboye et al. Unfortunately only introductory psychology students, and not "professional interviewers" (as in the 1975 study) acted as subjects. However, in the 1977 study both males and females participated. The job description was that for a trainee in sales management, and in this study three levels of applicant facial attractiveness were used. The subjects were required to rate their willingness to hire each of the 12 applicants, to state the salary they would provide, to rate each on a series of bipolar adjectives, and to choose the one applicant they would hire. Analysis of the willingness-to-hire ratings and of the salary data revealed a main effect of applicant attractiveness, with increasing attractiveness occasioning greater willingness and higher salaries. Also, there were interactions between applicant qualifications and applicant facial appearance in that the effect of attractiveness was more pronounced if the applicant had low qualifications (a recurring theme throughout this book). Facial appearance also had an effect on the choice of the one applicant subjects would hire. In addition, applicant attractiveness had a significant effect on the bipolar ratings. Sex of applicant and sex of subject made very little difference to these attractiveness effects. No effects whatsoever of subjects' physical attractiveness were found.

Dipboye et al. did not report in 1977 the actual amount of variance occasioned by variations in attractiveness, as was done in 1975; however, they did note that the eta-square values were small. They stated that, since they wanted to vary sex of subject and "given the scarcity of professional interviewers and recruits," they had used students, but they noted that caution must be used in generalizing from the 1977 study to professional interviewers. Dipboye et al. again pointed out that it was not clear "whether bias against physically unattractive persons occurs across a variety of positions or whether it is specific to certain types of positions, such as those that are visible and require social interaction." They also suggested that attractiveness may account for even less rating variance in a realistic interview setting where the interviewer may observe a variety of interviewee characteristics in addition to the limited information contained on a résumé. Nevertheless, they concluded that, "Despite these limitations it seems reasonable to conclude that physical attractiveness biases exist."

Other Information about the Applicant

A study by M. Greenwald (1981) did use a different type of job description from those used by Dipboye et al. In addition, experienced male and female personnel interviewers were used as subjects who were ordinarily responsible for evaluating entry-level clerk typists. These subjects were seen at their usual place of work and each was asked to evaluate eight job applicants for their overall suitability for employment as a clerk-typist and to make recommendations concerning hiring them first on a 7-point scale and then on a 3-point "disposition" scale of "would definitely consider," "undecided," "would definitely not consider." The applicants' facial attractiveness and amount of relevant employment experience were varied on the application form, and their "social performance" was varied by the use of audiocassette tapes. These tapes were recordings of a woman who was seeking a clerical job responding to such questions as "Tell me about yourself." and "Why do you want to work here?" The recordings were evaluated as either good or poor in terms of "level of social performance" and "global social skill."

No effects whatsoever of facial appearance were found. Whereas "social performance" and experience had significant effects, "the proportion of the variance accounted for by the physical attractiveness of the candidates is minimal." Greenwald stated that this lack of a facial appearance effect may possibly have been due to previous studies using more extreme levels of attractiveness than he used. Indeed, he criticized studies of physical attractiveness for manipulating "experimental stimuli vigorously," and for not using stimuli "likely to be seen in an applicant population." Greenwald did check that his photographs (four for each of two levels) did in fact differ in attractiveness, and therefore more likely explanations of his finding may be either that facial appearance has no effect regarding applications to be clerk-typists, whereas it may for other positions; or than when other applicant information is available appearance has little effect.

Type of Job

The nature of the post being applied for was varied by Cash, Gillen, and Burns (1977) in their study of the effects of applicants' facial attractiveness. Male and female professional personnel consultants rated the suitability of applicants for "masculine," "feminine," or "neuter" jobs. Each résumé was identical and the applicant's sex and facial attractiveness were varied. Cash, Gillen, and Burns noted Gillen's (1981) finding that attractive persons are perceived as haivng two types of "goodness," one type being sex irrelevant and the other sex linked. His subjects were asked to fill in the Bem Sex Role Inventory for a number of photographed persons. He found that the assumed femininity scores increased with attractiveness for female stimuli but not for male stimuli, and that the masculinity scores increased with attractiveness for male stimuli but not for female. Both male and female assumed social desirability scores were lower for the unattractive than for the moderately or highly attractive photographs. Thus, attractive persons were presumed to have sex-linked "goodness" as well as general "goodness."

Cash, Gillen, and Burns hypothesized that, "(a) Males are preferred over females for masculine jobs; (b) females are preferred over males for feminine jobs; (c) for neuter jobs, attractive applicants are more favorably evaluated than unattractive applicants (sex-irrelevant goodness); (d) for in-role jobs (i.e. masculine jobs for males and feminine jobs for females), attractive applicants are more favorably perceived than unattractive applicants (sex-relevant goodness); and (e) attractive applicants are attributed greater overall employment potential than unattractive applicants." Each of the personnel consultants evaluated one male and one female applicant for each of six jobs, two of which in a pretest were found to be viewed as masculine (e.g., car salesperson), two feminine (e.g., telephone operator), and two neuter (e.g., motel desk clerk). The evaluation consisted of 9-point ratings on a number of dimensions, including the consultants' confidence in their other ratings (which was high). Hypotheses (a) and (b) were supported by the data from all three rating scales (i.e., degree of qualification for the job, expectancy of success in the job, and strength of hiring recommendation), and sex of consultant had no effects. Hypotheses (c), (d), and (e) were supported only by the "degree of qualification" data, with no effects for the other rating scales (except for a $p < .10$ effect on hiring recommendation regarding the third hypothesis). Cash, Gillen, and Burns also asked the consultants "to assume the applicant's success and failure on each job and to rate the causes of these projected outcomes" on "ability, effort, task difficulty, and luck." They found that

> Attractiveness affected the attribution of job failures to lack of effort. Consistent with sex-irrelevant *and* sex-relevant stereotypes, unattractive employees were seen as less responsible than attractive personnel for negative outcomes on neuter and in-role occupations, respectively. Because consultants thought the attractive applicants to be more qualified for these jobs, any explanation of their negative outcomes would be apt to reflect failure to apply effort sufficient to demonstrate their inherent abilities.

Cash, Gillen, and Burns pointed out that such a conclusion is congruent with research showing that attractive persons are attributed greater control over their outcomes than unattractive individuals (see Bordieri, Sotolongo, & Wilson, 1983; Cash & Begley, 1976; M. Hill & Lando, 1976; A. Miller, 1970b; Pavlos & Newcomb, 1974; Seligman, Paschall, & Takata, 1974; and Chapter 8 of the present book).

A study by Heilman and Saruwatari (1979) also varied, in addition to job applicants' level of physical attractiveness, the the nature of the post and the sex of the applicant. They suggested that the more attractive a woman is, the less suitable she will be judged for occupying a job that is thought to require "male" characteristics, and that "for many jobs falling in the lower ranks of the organizational hierarchy both masculine and feminine skills are believed to provide potential for success. In contrast, however, there seems to be a general consensus that to be successful in the most powerful and prestigious organizational positions (managerial ones) requires almost exclusively male skills." Their hypothesis was that facial attractiveness would prove to be advantageous to males applying either for a nonmanagerial or a managerial job, and for females applying for nonmanagerial jobs, but that it would prove disadvantageous to females applying for a managerial post. Male and female students read either a clerical or managerial job description and they then evaluated a number of applications for these posts in terms of hiring recommendations, starting salary, and the applicants' qualifications for the posts. In addition, a number of bipolar ratings were made of the applicant and they were placed in "ranked preference."

No effects of sex of evaluator were found. The data for the ratings of the candidates' qualifications, for the hiring recommendations, for the starting salary ($p < .10$), and for ranked preference supported Heilman and Saruwatari's hypothesis. They therefore concluded that attractiveness was disadvantageous to women seeking a managerial post, and they noted that their data did not support the notion that subjects would generally evaluate male applicants more favorably than female ones.

The data from the bipolar scales supported Gillen's (1981) findings in that attractive male applicants were judged to be more masculine and females to be more feminine. Analysis of covariance concerning applicants for the managerial post revealed that when the bipolar feminine-masculine ratings were used as the covariate, the effects of attractiveness disappeared. Heilman and Saruwatari argued that this finding lends direct support to the thesis that gender characterizations play an important role in mediating the effects of attractiveness on personnel decisions. Thus, "whether attractiveness is a help or a hindrance to job applicants depends upon the sex of the applicant and the nature of the job." Therefore, it can be concluded from this study that the effects of facial appearance may well be mediated by the perceived fit between assumed applicant attributes and presumed job requirements.

Mediating the Effect of Attractiveness

This notion was examined by L. Jackson (1983a) and by Beehr and Gilmore (1982). In Jackson's study she hypothesized, in the light of the findings of Heilman and Saruwatari (1979), that the influence of attractiveness on judgments of occupational suitability may be mediated by its influence on perceptions of masculinity and femininity. If this assumption is correct, Jackson argued, then "explicit information about masculinity and femininity should eliminate the influence of the physical attractiveness stereotype in situations where gender traits are important, i.e. sex-linked occupations." On the other hand, the sex-irrelevant (general goodness) component of the attractiveness stereotype should continue to have an influence for sex-neutral occupations. Personnel consultants read the résumé regarding an applicant for what Heilman and Saruwatari deemed to be a male job (e.g., operations researcher), a female job (e.g., dietitian), and a sex-neutral (e.g., educational counselor) job. The applicant's facial photograph was attached as was a completed "self impressions questionnaire," which was varied to indicate that the applicant had either a masculine or a feminine or an androgynous profile. The consultants were asked to evaluate the applicant in terms of qualifications, expected success, hiring recommendation, starting salary, and overall employment potential.

Jackson found, as hypothesized, that applicant sex-role (i.e., their self impression profile) had a significant effect on several of the dependent variables, and that attractiveness had one effect for the sex-neutral occupations. However, this significant effect of attractiveness on starting salary also applied to the masculine and to the feminine occupations. Jackson attempted to explain this finding by stating that, "It may be that attractive applicants are seen as having more occupational alternatives and a higher starting salary is therefore necessary to attract them to the employment." This effect of attractiveness notwithstanding, Jackson concluded that, "Consistent with research on the psychology of prediction, the presence of individuating target case information (in this case, the sex role information) overshadowed the use of prior probabilities (stereotypic assumptions) in making predictions about an individual (Kahneman and Tversky, 1973; Tversky and Kahneman, 1977)."

Beehr and Gilmore (1982) varied the facial attractiveness of male applicants and the presumed relevance of attractiveness to managerial job performance. Male and female students read one of two types of job description, an application for the job, and a transcript supposedly of the applicant being interviewed for the post. The prerated job description was for a management trainee who would, or would not, be required to work with others in face-to-face situations. The students were required to say how likely they would be to hire the applicant, to select a starting salary, to rate his ability for the job, how well his personality would fit the job, and his expected performance. In addition, they evaluated the applicant on "a 13-item, 7-point semantic-differential type scale." Beehr and Gilmore argued that if a general, halo effect of attractiveness were in operation then the effects of their attractiveness factor should not interact with job type. However, since such interactions were present they concluded that attractiveness only has an effect when the evaluators' assumptions about the abilities possessed by attractive people are job relevant.

Beehr and Gilmore made the further point that attractiveness may not have much of an effect in situations where qualifications and experience regarding the job in question are varied. Even though their own study held these constant, eta-squared analysis revealed that the amount of variance attributable to attractiveness was very small. They argued that future studies should vary not only the nature of the job, but also other aspects of applicants in addition to their facial appearance. In this way it would be much easier to determine whether evaluators' decisions reveal irrational effects of facial appearance, or evaluators are making assumptions based on applicant appearance that may be rational to some extent. (Many parts of this book are concerned with just how valid such assumptions might be.)

Job Status

Waters (1985) varied the nature of the job applied for in her study of the effects of facial appearance. In this study photographs were taken of eight women before and after they received makeovers (changes in hair color and style and facial cosmetics), and experienced personnel interviewers evaluated some of these job applicants on the basis of their résumés (plus photograph). Waters hypothesized that the higher the level of skill a job requires the less would be the effect of increased attractiveness. The applications (and therefore the résumés) were for the posts of either secretary (deemed the lowest skill level), editor (mid-level skill), or financial analyst (higher level of skill). Waters found that "the variable of physical appearance did play an important role in the hiring process on all skill levels. Furthermore, as expected, the greatest differences were on the lowest skill level."

Boor, Wartman, and Reuben (1983) examined the effect of the attractiveness of applicants for what could be viewed as a high-skill job, that of "medical residency," and found it to have no effect. In a praiseworthy attempt to conduct a study that had ecological validity they noted the ratings that two faculty members gave during "the standard selection interview" to applicants to a "general internal medical residency training program," and they related these data to those independently gained from ratings of the applicants' photographs and from observations of their behavior made by "receptionists." It was found that ratings of attractiveness did not significantly correlate overall with any of the interviewer ratings, but there was for the female candidates "a nonsignificant trend toward a relationship with final candidate rankings ($rho = .32$, p $< .10$)." However, the ratings of neatness and grooming did significantly correlate, for the females, with the final rankings of the candidates. More strongly related to the outcome of the selection process, both for female and for male applicants, were the receptionists' ratings of professional demeanor, and the interviewers' ratings of social skills and of overall commitment to becoming professional providers.

Boor et al. (1983) concluded from these findings that "physical appearance may have less effect on interview evaluations and subsequent selection decisions than previous research suggests, and professional demeanour may have greater influence on these evaluations than is generally recognized."

Nonfacial Information

Cann, Siegfried, and Pearce (1981) also examined whether other applicant characteristics might have a greater effect than facial appearance. They suggested that since "It has been well documented that interviewers are greatly influenced by first impressions and tend to make their decisions very quickly

. . . when superficial characteristics such as sex or attractiveness are negatively perceived initially it seems likely that the final decision will reflect these biases." The aim of their study "was to determine whether the discriminatory effects of physical attractiveness and applicant sex could be reduced by forcing evaluators to attend to specific items of information before making a summary judgment to hire or not to hire. Specifically, raters indicated a hiring decision either before evaluating individual items or after." They hypothesized that "sex and attractiveness would affect summary judgments only when these ratings were not preceded by careful consideration of specific individual items." Undergraduates received a folder that contained a job description ("department manager"); the applicant's two-page résumé, which included a photograph; and three references regarding the applicant. The main independent variable was the order in which subjects made their evaluations. Some completed the page concerning their ratings of the applicant's "overall qualifications" and "how much they favored hiring the applicant" before the evaluation page dealing with "individual ratings" (i.e., "educational background, work experience, personal interests, and reference letters"), whereas other subjects completed the two-page evaluation in the reverse order. A third page, which was always given last, contained a question concerning the subject's perception of the extent to which the applicant's physical attractiveness affected his or her evaluation of the applicant's qualifications.

The design of this study seems not to be as commensurate with Cann et al.'s stated aim as one would wish. It may well have been much more worthwhile to vary, during the time that subjects were making their various evaluations, the moment at which they saw the applicant's photograph. Cann et al. found that subjects' impressions of how much their various judgments had been influenced by the applicant's physical attractiveness revealed a main effect of attractiveness. The more attractive the applicant the more did subjects indicate that attractiveness had influenced their evaluations. The order in which the evaluations were made did not meaningfully interact with this effect. However, attractiveness (high, medium, and low) had an effect on neither the "individual ratings" nor the evaluations of applicant qualifications. It did have an effect on how much subjects favored hiring the applicant in that the high-attractiveness applicants were favored over the low-attractiveness applicants. Only for applicants of medium attractiveness was the order of the evaluation pages important. Applicants of medium attractiveness were as favored for being hired as were those of high attractiveness if the hiring judgment was made prior to the individual ratings. If the order of evaluations was reversed then the applicants of average attractiveness were treated no differently from those of low attractiveness.

Cann et al. concluded that extreme levels of attractiveness had a more powerful effect than did the order in which the evaluations were required to be made. However, as stated above, a far better designed study seems warranted concerning the moment when information about applicant facial appearance is made available during the employment decision process.

Nevertheless, Cann et al. (who did question the ecological validity of their study) made the possibly worthwhile suggestion that applicants should "moderate the impact of unattractive appearance by demonstrating strong social skills and directing the interviewer's attention to other strengths." (Readers interested in the topic of social skills should see Chapter 8.)

This overview of studies of the effects of job applicants' facial appearance suggests that its effect may be strongest when other employment-relevant applicant characteristics are kept constant. When these are varied the effects of facial appearance per se may often be weak or nonexistent. Let us now see if the same conclusion is arrived at by studies involving evaluations not of those applying for employment but of those already employed.

In-Post Evaluation

A study in which all ecologically valid factors were free to vary was conducted by J. Ross and Ferris (1981). They studied several hundred male employees of two accountancy organizations and they found in one organization that independently rated employee physical attractiveness had a significant relationship with supervisors' recorded evaluations of "personal effectiveness" but not with salary or recorded technical and professional effectiveness, or supervisors' estimated likelihood of the employees being offered a partnership. In the second firm of accountants attractiveness had an almost significant relationship ($p < .10$) with estimated likelihood of being offered a partnership, but did not relate to any other of the measures. The employee factors found to be most strongly related to the above measures were whether they had a postgraduate degree and the length of their employment. In the light of previous research on the effects of facial appearance Ross and Ferris stated that they were "surprised to find that photo attractiveness did not have a very strong impact on evaluations." However, they did point out that, "Very few field tests of the impact of physical attraction in organizational settings have taken place." They concluded that further study of the effects of physical attractiveness in the employment setting is needed.

Although Ross and Ferris did not cite the work of Sparacino (1980), his findings are of some relevance here. Sparacino related the attractiveness ratings of males based on their university graduation photographs, and on their photographs taken 25 years later, to their "occupational prestige scores," to their final level of educational attainment, and to the class of their bachelor's degree. He found "no indication whatsoever that more attractive men excelled over the less attractive ones." In fact, the correlations between attractiveness at graduation and the above three measures were negative ($-.11$, $-.12$, and $-.08$, respectively; although small, these correlations were significant because of the very large sample size; the correlations with 25-years-on attractiveness ratings did not even reach significance, the largest being $-.04$). Sparacino suggested that "attractiveness is a variable whose period of primary effect is extremely limited. While it it may exert immediate effects on raters, particularly when they do not deal with a real person, but a photograph, additional interaction may yield considerably more information which in effect obfuscates the effect of attractiveness."

Although Sparacino did not find a positive relationship between facial attractiveness and occupational prestige, Hatfield and Sprecher (1986) reported an unpublished study by Quinn that found males' and females' physical attractiveness to be related positively to both occupational prestige and earnings. However, since the interviewers who asked the questions about occupation and income also rated attractiveness, bias could have crept in.

Female Employees

Most of the (few) studies that have sought to examine the possible effects of facial appearance on employee evaluation have, contrary to Sparacino's suggestion, merely required raters to react to photographs of supposed employees whom they have never met and about whom little of the information varies from evaluator to evaluator. One such study was conducted by L. Jackson (1983b), who examined not only the effect of males' facial appearance (as had Sparacino [1980] and Ross and Ferris [1981]) but also the effect of females' facial appearance. Jackson suggested that discrimination may have a greater effect regarding female stimuli, and many studies reviewed in the present book do suggest, as least prior to the 1980s, that female facial appearance may have greater effects than that of males. Jackson also suggested, in the light of research by Beehr and Gilmore (1982), Cash, Gillen, and Burns (1977), Heilman and Saruwatari (1979) and Jackson (1983a) (see above), that any "advantage of attractiveness for women may be limited to gender-congruent occupations," and that "explicit information about masculine and feminine traits should eliminate the influence of gender and attractiveness in situations where gender traits are important, that is, sex-linked occupations." However, for sex-neutral occupations Jackson hypothesized a positive effect of facial attractiveness. In her study personnel consultants were asked to assume the role of employer and were provided with a photograph of a supposed employee together with this employee's masculinity/femininity self-impression questionnaire profile, résumé, and academic record. Subjects evaluated their stimulus person with regard to each of four vignettes that were concerned with either promotion, being sent on a special training program, being assigned to a challenging or routine job, or taking prolonged leave of absence for child care. For each vignette a masculine, a feminine, and a sex-neutral occupation was specified.

The data supported Jackson's hypothesis that facial appearance would have no effect regarding sex-linked occupations. However, contrary to her hypothesis it also had no effect for the sex-neutral occupations. In criticizing her own study Jackson quite rightly pointed out that the "consultants were asked to evaluate one employee for three quite different occupations, an unlikely, and potentially confusing set of tasks." If she had varied more the employee's details this problem might have been avoided. As it was the employee's résumé and academic record were both good, and this could explain why Jackson noted that even though her preratings of facial attractiveness had clearly suggested that the unattractive faces she used were indeed so, these were rated as being of average attractiveness by the consultants. Previously we pointed out that the provision of positive/negative information about a person could well modify subjects' evaluations of their facial attractiveness (Gross & Crofton, 1977). This interesting possibility could have accounted for Jackson's lack of effect of attractiveness. However, this possibility would seem to have to apply to her sex-neutral as well as sex-linked occupations. Another possible explanation of the lack of effects of facial appearance may be that "the attractiveness stereotype does not influence the treatment of employees once entry into the organization has been secured." This is, of course, what both Sparacino (1980) and Ross and Ferris (1981) found, and since Jackson argued that a necessary next step to establish the external validity of her results was to test these hypotheses in field settings, it is surprising that in her paper she cited neither of these two field studies.

Type of Job

Heilman and Stopeck (1985a) also failed to cite these two field studies of male attractiveness even though they hypothesized that physical attractiveness might influence "how rewards are allocated in work settings." Like Jackson (1983b) they hypothesized that attractiveness could be an asset for both men and women in sex-neutral occupations such as many nonmanagerial posts, but in managerial posts for which "masculine qualities are considered to be requisite for success" it may only be advantageous to men and may be disadvantageous to women. Male and female graduate business students read employee summary performance reviews supposedly from a large manufacturing organization. Each subject read four fairly similar summaries, two male and two female, with one of each sex having an attractive photograph, the other an unattractive photograph. For half the subjects the person was described as holding a management trainee position, for the other half a clerical trainee position. The subjects were asked to evaluate the employee's performance and potential for advancement, to suggest a pay raise, and to characterize the employee on a series of bipolar adjective scales. No effects of males' attractiveness were found for performance evaluation. For the females being attractive led to more positive performance evaluations but only for the clerical position, the reverse being the case for the managerial position. The same outcomes applied to evaluations of employee potential for advancement, and to suggested pay raises. Analyses of the adjective scale data revealed that attractiveness increased the femininity ratings of the female stimuli but had no effect on the masculinity ratings of the male stimuli.

In the light of their finding that attractiveness enhanced the femininity ratings of the female stimuli Heilman and Stopeck (1985a) conducted a partial analysis of covariance that found that when stimulus femininity-masculinity was covaried out no effects of facial appearance were evident. Thus they concluded that "it is the gender characteristics which arise from appearance which mediate its effects." Heilman and Stopeck suggested that their "results underscore the limitations of the 'what is beautiful is good' arguments, and point dramatically to the instances when attractiveness is not at all good for women in work settings." However, they wisely pointed out that real-life employee evaluations are not usually conducted in the way undertaken in their study, and therefore studies of real life seem warranted. However, we should point that there are some organizations in which final decisions concerning employee evaluations are made by staff who do not know and may not meet those they are evaluating.

Speed of Success

In 1985 Heilman and Stopeck also published another study of employee evaluation. In this study (1985b) the type of post occupied by the stimulus person was not varied. However, whether his or her rise to the position of assistant vice president had been rapid or not was varied, as was the sex and facial attractiveness of this person. Heilman and Stopeck pointed out that causal attribution theory would suggest that "when success is consistent with expectation it is attributed to stable internal causes, that is, on individual's ability. But when success is unanticipated it is deemed unstable or temporary and assumed to derive from sources other than the individual's ability." They also suggested that when succeeding at a masculinely sex-typed job attractive women should be disadvantaged by their appearance, and their success will not be attributed to internal causes, particularly if their rise to a senior post has been uncommonly rapid. In their study working men and women read a short description of an employee's career. The employee was female or male, and of high or low facial attractiveness; his or her rise to a senior managerial position was described as normative or rapid. The subjects were asked to rate how responsible they believed each of a number of factors was for the career progress, and to characterize the individual on a number of bipolar adjective scales. It was found for attractive women that their success was attributed less to ability and more to reasons other than their job-related skill or talent. (No effects of subject sex were found.) For male stimuli there was no such prejudice; the attractive males' success was attributed to their ability and they were rated as more capable than were the unattractive males. However, the attractive stimuli (both male and female) were also seen as having "exercised less diligence but more interpersonal savvy in advancing their careers."

Heilman and Stopeck (1985b) concluded that "specter of beautyism can be expected to follow the successful woman right up the career ladder." However, whether there is in reality a relationship between female facial appearance and in-post empolyment factors waits to be assessed since Sparacino (1980) and Ross and Ferris (1981) only examined this relationship for males.

There is in fact some evidence that a female's attracti᾿
evaluations of her work. Murphy and Hellkamp (1976᾿
who were led to believe that the work they were evalua
tive woman rated a painting more positively than those
of an unattractive woman. They suggested that "an
have a more favorable influence on other people t᾿᾿
attractiveness," and although the more recent research on the eᴜᴄᴄ᾿
appearance on general persuasion, in politics and in employment suggests
that this statement may be considered rather naive, in a particular area of
persuasion (that of advertising), do marketers believe in this simple statement?
Murphy and Hellkamp stated that their study's "result related to what the
field of advertising has in mind when an attractive female is paired with a
certain brand of cigarette, hair spray, etc., believing sales would be higher
than if a company tried to sell its product on its own merit or through a more
'average' looking person." It is to the role of facial appearance in advertising
that we now turn.

Facial Appearance and Advertising

In 1982 Joseph pointed out that the use of physically attractive models in
advertising had increased considerably in the preceding years. He stated that,
"Evidently, advertisers believe that the beautiful are also credible, and that
physically attractive sources can contribute to a communication's effectiveness. However, the empirical evidence, to date, on the persuasive advantage
of using highly attractive communicators is both modest and far from conclusive." Our above review of the relevant literature would support Joseph's
latter sentence. The evidence is rather contradictory, although when one takes
into account first Gillen's (1981) notion of attractiveness being a determinant
of two types of goodness, and second subject factors, the picture becomes
somewhat clearer in that attractiveness per se seems to have little effect.
Joseph suggested that the available empirical evidence was not only modest in
amount, it was also rather ecologically invalid, being more concerned with the
reactions of students who may have been adopting in the psychological
laboratory a form of logical cognitive functioning not so readily found in the
real world of advertising.

Just this type of cognitive functioning may have taken place in a study by
M. Baker and Churchill (1977), who conducted what they considered to be a
"unique" study in that they manipulated the physical attractiveness rather
than bodily sexiness of a person seen in an advertisement. From the perspective of attribution theory they suggested that a physically attractive person
may be viewed as having more freedom of choice over his or her actions than
an unattractive person. Thus, if an attractive person endorses or is paired with
a product this may be seen as resulting more from his or her own volition that
it would for an unattractive person. From a naive reinforcement theory

ach, again pairing a physically attractive person with a product could d to greater sales. Furthermore, if attractive persons are stereotypically elieved to be more trustworthy then again advertisements employing them might be more effective. On the other hand, some of the studies of the effects of sexual photographs on advertising had found these to lessen advertisement effectiveness.

Baker and Churchill varied the physical attractiveness and sex of a person who held the product in a photographed advertisement that was accompanied by a brief written statement endorsing the product. Also varied was the nature of the product (coffee or cologne) and the sex of the subject. Undergraduates evaluated a male and a female advertisement along a number of "affective, cognitive and conative" scales. Physical attractiveness was found to have a significant main effect on the effective scores (i.e., "appealing, impressive, eye-catching") but no effect on the cognitive evaluations (i.e., "believable, informative, clear"). For the conative scales (i.e., "seek out, buy, try the product") only the physical attractiveness of the female stimulus had an effect and this was upon males' intentions. Whether attractiveness had a positive or negative effect on stated intention was influenced by whether the product was cologne or coffee, respectively. Baker and Churchill concluded regarding evaluations of the attention-getting, liking/aesthetic value of advertisements that there is reason to believe that attractiveness will have a positive effect. However, with regard to behavioral intentions they suggested that attractiveness may by no means always have a positive effect.

Type of Processing

The nature of any advertising attractiveness effect is likely, as Joseph (1982) pointed out, to be a function of the type of cognitive processing subjects employ. We made a similar point in this chapter's earlier section on the role of facial appearance in politics. This notion was examined in a study by Pallak, Murroni, and Koch (1983), who varied in a magazine advertisement the facial attractiveness and expertise of a male endorser. The endorser's written statement supporting the use of a headache relief product was either rational or emotionally toned. Pallak et al. noted Maddux and Rogers' (1980) point (see this chapter's earlier section on persuasion) that the persuasive effect of communicator attractiveness might be enhanced by using an emotionally toned message rather than an information-based rational message. They suggested that "the tone of the message may determine whether an audience focuses on the message content or on the communicator, and as a result, whether the message is processed systematically or heuristically." Chaiken (1980) had argued that when a message is processed systematically it is the reactions to its contents that determine receivers' reactions, whereas when a message is processed heuristically simple decision rules (or heuristics) are used. Pallak et al. noted that typically heuristics are based on characteristics of a communicator (e.g., attractiveness), particularly if the message is emotionally rather than rationally toned. They further argued that "opinions based on systematic processing may tend to be more highly correlated with behavioral intentions than would opinions based on heuristic processing," and that "opinions of students reading a rationally toned message would be influenced by the communicator's expertise and that the opinions of students reading an emotionally toned message would be influenced only by the communicator's attractiveness."

After having read either the rationally or emotionally toned message and seeing either an attractive or unattractive face of a doctor or lawyer, the female students were required to evaluate the product, to "list all thoughts that went through your mind while reading/looking at all the material presented," and to respond to questions concerning their behavioral intentions regarding the product. The data concerning evaluation of the product and behavioral intentions revealed more favorable judgments of the product when it was associated with a facially attractive communicator, but only for the emotionally toned message. Attractiveness had no effect for the rational message, and thus Pallak et al. arged that the emotional message is likely to have been processed heuristically whereas the rational message occasioned systematic processing. Their analysis of the thoughts listed by the subjects supported this contention. (No effects of communicator expertise were found.) Therefore, we can conclude from the study by Pallak et al. that studies and theories concerning the social effects of facial appearance should not ignore factors relating to subjects' cognitive processes, even though there is debate regarding the extent to which people can validly describe their own though processes (Nisbett & Bellows, 1977; Nisbett & Wilson, 1977).

Kahle and Homer's (1985) study of the effects of facial appearance in advertising also attempted to address the issue of systematic versus heuristic processing. However, their suggestion that subjects who have "high involvement" would process an advertisement systematically through a "central route," and those who have "low involvement" would process heuristically through a "peripheral route," was not adequately tested in their study. Nevertheless, they did find endorsers' (celebrities') physical attractiveness enhanced attitudes and behavioral intentions regarding the product (a disposable razor). Contrary to their argument concerning "peripheral" versus "central" route processing, subjects' recall of the persuasive message's arguments (and the brand product) were significantly affected by attractiveness in both the high and low involvement conditions. Kahle and Homer suggested that, "many consumers may only glance at an advertisement for a second or two before moving to the next source of information. . . . If this hypothesis is true, the information obtained in that second or two will be the only information to have an impact. Name of the product and the visual impression of the celebrity may be all the information conveyed: the arguments in the copy, whether strong or weak, cannot influence the consumer." Thus for some advertisements endorser facial appearance may not so much affect the processing of the message as it could influence whether or not people bother to process the message at all.

Ecological Validity

Whatever the effects of facial appearance may be, few studies have attempted to assess its effects on real-world buying behavior rather than on the answers to questionnaires concerning product evaluation and mere behavioral intentions. The only published study that we have found concerning the effects of physical attractiveness on actual purchasing behavior was conducted by Caballero and Pride (1984). In this study a random sample of 30,000 subscribers to the magazine *Christianity Today* received through the post a three-part direct mail advertisement for a book on religion. "Prominently displayed on the left side of the detachable order blank was a photograph of the stimulus person (or a blank space for the control groups)." The male or female stimulus person was of high, medium, or low facial attractiveness. No other aspects of the three-part mailing (e.g., the sales message) were varied. Although less than 1% of the sample returned an order form to purchase the book there was a significant effect of attractiveness that was caused by the highly attractive female condition. The medium and low levels of attractiveness did not differ in sales, and the no-photograph condition sales figure was in between the high and medium/low figures. Female purchasers in particular were affected by female endorser high facial attractiveness.

No effects of sex of subject were, however, found by Patzer (1983), who stated that

> The results of existing physical attractiveness research can be summarized into four generalizations. (1) Physically attractive people have greater social power than their unattractive counterparts. (2) Physically attractive people are perceived to possess more favorable personal and nonpersonal characteristics, including intelligence, personality traits, and success in life. (3) Physically attractive people have more positive effects on other people and receive more positive responses from others, including work requests, and requests for help, than do the physically unattractive. (4) Physically attractive people are more persuasive than physically unattractive people.

The present book shows that these claims, particularly the final one, may not be in line with all the evidence. Patzer made an attempt to investigate whether in advertising any influence of facial attractiveness may be mediated by its effect on endorser liking or trustworthiness or expertise. Subjects saw a printed advertisement (for a pain reliever) on which the message remained the same but on which the sex and facial attractiveness of the endorser were varied. They were required to rate the endorser for the above three characteristics, and it was found that attractiveness had a significant enhancing effect on all three scales. However, other studies (see this chapter's section on persuasion) have claimed that any effects of facial attractiveness occur independently of expertise. As in Caballero and Pride's (1984) investigation, the no-photograph condition in Patzer's study (which is more fully reported in Patzer [1985]) occasioned more positive responding than did the low facial attractiveness condition. Patzer (1985) also examined, as had M. Baker and

Churchill (1977; see above), the effects of facial apperance on subjects' affective ("interest, appeal, eye-catching"), cognitive ("believable, impressive, informative"), and conative ("try, buy, seek the product") responses. Attractiveness was found to have a significant positive effect on all three of these components, as it did on what Patzer termed subjects' belief component responses (i.e., the product provides relief from headache and minor pains, is fast and strong). However, attractiveness had no effect on subjects' recall of advertisement facts or details and no effect on subjects' views about the quality, price, and uniqueness of the product.

Summary

From the above research on advertising we can again conclude that the evidence concerning the social psychological effects of facial appearance suggests that although aspects of appearance (e.g., attractiveness) may enhance ratings or expectations, there is little evidence that actual behavior is affected. (For further discussion of the role of the media in the perpetration of stereotyping based on facial appearance see Chapter 8.)

General Conclusion

From this chapter's review of the published research on the effects of facial appearance in persuasion, politics, employment, and advertising we have to conclude that the evidence by no means consistently agrees with Patzer's recent proposition (1985) that, "The physical attractiveness of a communicator determines the effectiveness of persuasive communication, and ultimately, physical attractiveness of the communicator influences overall marketing outcomes."

Chapter 4

Facial Appearance and the Criminal Justice System

The Extent to Which People Expect a Relationship Between Facial Appearance and Criminality

Although Mueller, Thompson, and Vogel (1988) concluded that at present we do not have sufficient findings with which to answer the question of whether criminal stereotyping might affect witness identifications, there is some evidence that people do at least possess such stereotypes.

Many decades ago, back in the early days of criminology and of psychology, many people held the belief that criminality and people's physical appearance were related. It was then believed that one could often pick out from a group of people "the criminal type" and that, in fact, this judgment was veridical. However, more recently it has been argued, for example, by Liggett (1974) that, "Modern criminologists do not believe that criminals belong to a single physical type." Nevertheless, the first author of the present book has argued (Bull & Clifford, 1979) that the general public may still believe in the stereotype and that such beliefs may influence their behavior. Similarly, B. Clifford and Bull (1978) have argued that witnesses of a criminal incident may unwittingly permit their expectations to play a role in their identification of a suspect. That is, for example, when witnesses attempt to pick out a person from an identification parade they may merely pick out the person who best resembles their expectation of what a certain criminal should look like. If the general public do not have such expectations then this argument is of little value. On the other hand, if such expectations do exist then a number of important effects may result from them.

Shoemaker, South, and Lowe (1973) stated that "stereotypic conceptions of what a particular suspect 'should' look like, or does not look like, could influence the selection of 'the one who did it' by an eyewitness to a crime, particularly when that eyewitness did not have a good, clear look at the offender." They asked a group of students to pick out from an array of male photographs the faces most and least likely to be a murderer, or a robber, or a homosexual, or someone who had committed treason. Strong interstudent agreement was found for the choice of faces, with different faces being chosen for the different categories. A second group of students was asked to evaluate the guilt or innocence of photographed men who were described as having been involved in certain activities. Those students who saw a photograph chosen by the first group as being likely to have committed a certain crime produced more "guilty" responses when the photograph was paired with the crime chosen by the group 1 subjects, except for homosexuality (no effects for "least likely" and judged innocence were found). Shoemaker et al. concluded that their findings indicated that "facial stereotypes of criminals would have some influence on the determination of guilt or innocence by a trial jury, especially when the evidence for or against the defendant is ambiguous or fragmented."

Shoemaker and South (1978) went further than this by suggesting that, "The literature on impression formation (person perception), stigma and labeling theory, along with that of stereotyping, all contain elements which, if taken collectively, would predict differential treatment of persons by the criminal justice system." They noted that, "Since 1922, when Walter Lippman described stereotypes as 'pictures in our heads', a large body of literature has developed on stereotypes, their social and psychological consequences, and the stereotyping process. . . . For our purposes, an important question is whether there is significant consensus among the general population as to what 'bad' people in general or specific kinds of deviants look like and whether these ready-made images might influence criminal justice procedures."

Photographs of Criminals

Research on the true relationship between criminality and physical appearance is sparse, one major reason for this being the understandable difficulty of obtaining suitable photographs of criminals. In Germany in 1962, Kozeny obtained photographs of 730 convicted criminals that he then divided into 16 categories depending upon the type of crime that had been committed. From each of these 16 groups of photographs a composite portraiture was made and the resultant physiognomic character was demonstrated to be significantly dependent on the respective category of crime from which the criminals' pictures had been taken. Thus there may be some relationship between physical appearance and criminality.

G. Thornton (1939) selected from the files of the Nebraska State Penitentiary the case records of 20 criminals, deliberately avoiding seeing the photographs of the criminals until the selection had been made. Since he was going to ask people to indicate which crime the particular individual had committed by looking at a facial photograph of the criminal, Thornton wisely wanted to avoid selecting criminals whose photographs matched his own expectancies of what a certain type of criminal should look like. (In this way he avoided the possibility of a biased selection of photographs about which observers might agree solely because the investigator had specially selected the photographs in the first place.) These photographs were shown one at a time to a large audience of adults who were required to note down which of four crimes each photographed individual had committed. The observers' judgments were found to be correct more often than was accountable by chance alone, but not overwhelmingly so. Thus the observers could fairly often, but by no means always, correctly assign a face to the crime.

Bull and Green (1980) attempted a replication of Thornton's study but we were (perhaps understandably) not given permission to use official photographs of convicted individuals. Therefore we used photographs of non-criminals. This may have been a blessing in disguise since the use of criminals' photographs would have provided us only with the faces of persons convicted of crime and not with a random sample of the faces of those who commit crime. Because people were going to be asked to match the photographs to certain types of crime (in order to see whether the general public do share common beliefs about criminal appearances) it was important that the photographed persons were all of a similar age so that age alone could not be used to pair a face to a crime. Each of the 10 photographs used was of a male between 27 and 33 years of age, each of the photographs having the same background. The amount of the photograph occupied by each face was similar and all the faces were (by design) bland and expressionless. The subjects were asked to say which of 11 listed crimes each of the 10 persons had committed. These observers were allowed to allot more than one face to a particular crime. Statistical analysis of the data revealed that for the crimes or arson, theft, rape, and burglary no face was chosen significantly more frequently than any other. However, for the crimes of mugging, robbery with violence, company fraud, soliticing, taking and driving away, illegal possession of drugs, and gross indencency, one of the faces was chosen much more frequently (and statistically significantly) than the others. Furthermore, different faces were chosen for different crimes: that is, it is not the case that for every crime the observers merely chose repeatedly the same face.

A similar study was conducted by Goldstein, Chance, and Gilbert (1984), who also found that people consensually selected different faces as being of a mass murderer, an armed robber, a rapist, a medical doctor, or a clergyman. Other subjects then rated the faces most often chosen by the first group as being of criminals or of "good guys," and significant differences were found for dirty-clean, insane-sane, brash-cautious, excited-calm, cruel-kind, vulgar-refined, bad-good, and unfriendly-friendly, with the faces chosen by other subjects as being of criminals being associated with the former of each pair of words. Goldstein et al. concluded that "the degree to which a particular individual's face invites facial stereotyping may influence the outcomes of any legal process in which they become involved." This stereotyping may not only affect the general public, it may also influence criminal justice professionals.

Police Reactions

In the study by Bull and Green (1980) the subjects were either members of the public or police officers and both groups produced similar evidence of stereotyping, suggesting that police officers are not immune from these effects. Indeed, research by Piliavin and Briar (1964) found that youths "whose appearance matched the delinquency stereotype were more frequently stopped and interrogated by patrolmen," and Hartjen (1972) made the point that "In making . . . decisions, in determining how and when to intervene, the police engaged in a characteristic mode of behavior, that of stereotyping." A book by a senior London police officer (Robinson, 1978) informs new policemen that in response to the frequently asked question, "How can you possibly say that a person looks like a criminal?" he would answer, "Several policemen talk about the ability to 'feel' or 'smell' a criminal, or to have a 'sixth sense' about a person. What they are really talking about is the ability to see a criminal when they come across one. It is basically a question of being able to categorize or stereotype a person." Robinson was further of the opinion that "the most skilful policeman will therefore not only be able to recognize a criminal when he sees one, but will often be able to state what type of previous conviction the particular criminal has." Another senior London policeman advised police officers to observe in court persons in custody for the theft of cars to "see to which category they belong. This will help you slant your mind to the general type of person you must watch for when patrolling" (D. Powis, *Thieves on Wheels*, cited in B. Clifford & Bull, 1978).

Yarmey (1982) pointed out that such acts of stereotyping are examples of a person-centered approach to the understanding of cognitive processes.

> This approach assumes that the way that observers process, store and retrieve information can contribute to stereotypic beliefs, and ultimately, in judgements and behaviour toward social groups. . . . [A] distinguishing characteristic of stereotypes is the illusory relationship between the observer's beliefs regarding group membership and psychological attributes. Thus, for example, the statement that 'criminal suspects look tough' does not only mean that only villians . . . are frightening. . . . Enough evidence is now available to show that people attend to and encode such co-occurances of variables. As a consequence these encodings are possible sources of distortion when memory is searched at a later time for recall.

Evidence supporting Yarmey's line of reasoning, although not cited by him, comes from a study by Shepherd, Ellis, McMurran, and Davies (1978), who asked 40 women to construct a "photo-fit" resemblance of a man's face that they had just previously seen in a photograph. Half of these subjects were led to believe that the man was a murderer, the other half that he was a lifeboatman, whereas, in fact, all subjects saw the same photograph. The resultant 40 "photo-fits" were shown to 20 female students who received no information regarding murderer/lifeboatman. These subjects were asked to rate the 40 "photo-fits" on nine scales. A significant murderer/lifeboatman effect was found, with the murderer reconstructions being rated as less intelligent and less good-looking than were the facial reconstructions made by the women who were told that the face was of a lifeboatman. (We should note that Bull [1979] found rated unattractiveness, rated dishonesty, and amount of facial scarring to covary together.) Shepherd et al. concluded that "differences in the constructors' impressions of the two characters were translated into physical differences in the constructions they made from memory."

Yarmey (1982) stated that although many people assume (e.g., Shoemaker) that "a stereotypical relationship exists between recognition accuracy and negative criminal features, no research to my knowledge has been published which actually tests this hypothesis." In this chapter's following section we will discuss studies that have examined the effects of certain aspects of facial appearance (e.g., attractiveness) on recognizability (some of which were in fact published before 1982). Here we will note the findings of two of Yarmey's 1982 studies. In the first Yarmey's subjects saw a series of slides portraying a violent assault and theft of a wallet. The assailant was a male in his early twenties who, by prior determination using other subjects, had a guilty- or innocent-looking appearance. No effect of this factor was found on subjects' recognition performance. In Yarmey's second study the appearance of the one, three, or five assailants and of a young adult male bystander were varied. No effects of assailant appearance were reported, but bystander appearance had a significant effect on the elderly subjects', but not the young adult subjects', frequency of falsely identifying the bystander as an assailant, with the guilty-looking bystander being identified more frequently by the elderly subjects.

The Effects of Facial Appearance on Recognizability

Another aspect of the social psychology of facial appearance that began to be researched empirically only fairly recently is concerned with whether certain sorts of faces are more memorable than others. Since facial attractiveness is one of the major appearance factors examined in this book we shall focus on its effects upon recognition. Readers interested in how other aspects of faces (e.g., eyes versus nose) affect recognition should consult Davies, Ellis, and Shepherd (1981) and Ellis, Jeeves, Newcombe, and Young (1986).

In 1971 Cross, Cross, and Daly asked subjects to indicate from an array of 12 female and male faces which ones they considered to be attractive. The subjects then did this for several other arrays of faces. Without having been warned that their memory for the initial array of faces would be tested, the subjects were presented with the 12 faces from the original array and 12 faces that they had not seen before. It was found that the faces that subjects had indicated as being attractive were better recognized than those deemed unattractive. Cross et al. described their study so briefly that it is not possible to tell exactly how they arrived at this conclusion. However, they did point out, regarding the effect of attractiveness, that a simple explanation in terms of differences in exposure time could be ruled out because "Our S's often spent more time scrutinizing the faces of doubtful beauty." They did, however, note that, "Instructional set probably played a part in the results." As we shall see, the debate concerning whether some faces are more memorable than others revolves around whether some faces are, in fact, of themselves easier to remember or whether certain faces occasion more effective cognitive processing than other faces.

In 1973 Shepherd and Ellis pointed out that some studies in verbal learning had found that words evaluated as "good" were recalled better than words rated as "bad," which in turn were more memorable than neutral words. This suggested to them that not only might faces deemed "good" (i.e., attractive) be better recalled than "neutral" faces, but also that faces deemed "bad" (i.e., unattractive) might also be better recalled than "neutral" ones. They further suggested that one of the factors that could account for such a finding would involve arousal, and that arousal effects may be more marked with delayed than with immediate recognition. Subjects were shown 27 female faces (which had been rated by other people as being of high, medium, or low attractiveness) and were then asked to indicate for 27 pairs of faces which face was the one they had seen previously. Nine of these recognition pairs were used for an immediate memory test, another 9 were used at a delay of 6 days, and the remaining 9 after 35 days. Although the subjects were warned before the initial presentation of the target faces that their immediate memory would be tested, they were not aware that delayed testing would also take place.

The mean number of faces correctly recognized (out of 9) at immediate testing was 8.1, at 6 days 7.3, and at 35 days 6.4. This delay effect was found to interact with attractiveness in that after 35 days the faces of medium attractiveness were recognized at only chance level, whereas those of high and low attractiveness were recognized at significantly above chance level (with no difference between high and low); the same level of performance was found for all three types of face after a delay of 6 days, and for immediate testing. That is, only the faces of medium attractiveness showed a significant delay effect for 6 versus 35 days. For this finding Shepherd and Ellis offered an arousal interpretation and/or one suggesting that attractive and unattractive faces have more distinctive features than neutral ones.

Going and Read (1974) examined the effect of uniqueness of faces on recognition. A large selection of faces was rated on a 7-point scale of uniqueness (no further details of this independent variable were given; in particular no mention was made of attractiveness). Subjects were shown 28 male and female faces (14 high and 14 low in uniqueness) and told that they would be required to recognize them after a minimal delay. Fifty-six of the distractor faces were of intermediate uniqueness, 14 were of high uniqueness, and 14 of low uniqueness. It was found, using a recognition test that presented one face at a time, that subjects were significantly better at recognizing faces high in uniqueness than low, and that distractor faces low in uniqueness led to more false positives than did high-uniqueness distractors. In attempting to account for their findings Going and Read suggested that uniqueness may occasion a greater number of eye fixations and that these may lead to better recognition.

A study by Fleishman, Buckley, Klosinsky, Smith, and Tuck (1976) also found attractive and unattractive female faces to be better recognized than "neutral" faces. In their study the subjects were shown a number of faces and were asked to rate them for attractiveness. They were also told that their recognition of the faces would be tested subsequently. Two hours after having rated the faces the subjects were shown 12 of the initial faces (4 each of high, medium, and low attractiveness) together with 10 distractors. Faces high and low in attractiveness were recognized equally well and at a level significantly above that for faces of medium attractiveness (which were recognized at chance level). Like Shepherd and Ellis, Fleishman et al. offered as explanations of their finding an arousal and/or a distinctiveness explanation.

Yarmey (1977) attempted to compare the effects upon face recognition of attractiveness and of feature saliency (likeability was also studied). Yarmey stated that "faces differing in their level of physical attractiveness, feature saliency, and likeability" were studied by subjects for 2 seconds each. Sufficient details are not given of how these stimuli were chosen, and although one can assume it was the rating of these faces by others that led to their being chosen for this study, no comment is made concerning whether the three factors of attractiveness, feature saliency, and likeability are in fact independent of one another (i.e., were faces high in attractiveness also rated high for feature saliency?). During the 2-second presentation of each face "S's were required to judge each face's level of attractiveness or distinctiveness or likeability and to encode it for a later memory test." (Presumably one group of subjects judged attractiveness, another group distinctiveness, and another group likeability.) Recognition testing occurred immediately or after 7 or 30 days. Yarmey found that "the recognition of targets was best for faces judged for their likeability, followed by those judged for physical attractiveness, and poorest for those considered for feature analysis," but in fact the differences were not great either for hits (0.82, 0.81, and 0.76, respectively) or for false alarms (0.7, 0.6, and 0.6, respectively). Delay had a significant effect, with hits decreasing (0.89, 0.83, and 0.68, respectively) and false alarms increasing (0.04, 0.06, and 0.09, respectively) over time. Yarmey noted that "when males and females judge faces for their attractiveness high attractive females and low attractive males are most easily identified. When faces are inspected for feature saliency, female faces low in distinctiveness and male faces high in distinctiveness are best remembered." Thus here we have a suggestion that the effect on face recognition of attractiveness may not be synonymous with that of feature saliency/distinctiveness. Yarmey concluded that, "The present study shows that what is remembered in facial recognition are faces that are beautiful and likeable, if female, but not male." It is interesting to note that in the studies mentioned above that have reported effects of attractiveness on recognition, those by Fleishman et al. (1976) and by Shepherd and Ellis (1973) used only female faces. However, those by Going and Read (1974) and by Cross et al. (1971) used both female and male faces (and they did not report any interactions between attractiveness and sex of face).

Male faces were used by Light, Hollander, and Kayra-Stuart (1981), who took Galton's (1907) comments on his composite faces to suggest that attractive faces are more similar to each other than are unattractive faces. (This assumption is, of course, unwarranted since Galton's composite photograph procedure could have led to the resultant faces appearing beautiful simply because the procedure merely removed facial abnormalities.) They then hypothesized, assuming similarity may impair performance, that "more attractive faces should be harder to remember." How they could form this hypothesis in the face of the findings of previous research is rather surprising, since they do not cite the work of Yarmey (1977), whose study had been the only one that had found an inverse relationship (and then only for males) between attractiveness and recognizability. In their first experiment Light et al. asked subjects to rate faces for "typicality," and then a day later they were given an unexpected recognition test. In their second experiment the subjects were asked to remember a set of faces for a recognition test 3 hours later. In the third experiment subjects were required to say whether each face's gaze was to the left or right, or to rate each face for likeability, with an unexpected recognition test being given 3 hours later. The fourth experiment replicated the third, save with a 5-hour delay and some subjects being warned that a recognition test would occur. Attractiveness ratings for all the faces used in these experiments had been gathered from 31 other male subjects. Light et al. found that the relationship between attractiveness and recognizability was negative, in most of their experiments significantly so. In no case did they find a curvilinear relationship between attractiveness and recognizability, as had Shepherd and Ellis (1973) for their long-delay condition.

Going and Read (1974) had concluded that uniqueness aids recognition, and a similar conclusion was arrived at by Light et al. (1981), who found in their regression analyses that similarity was commonly the first variable to enter the regression equation. They found a negative correlation between similarity and recognizability (i.e., faces judged as similar to other faces used in the experiments were not recognized so well), and the correlation between similarity and attractiveness ratings was found to be +0.57. They therefore stated that, "Typicality (or ordinariness) is highly correlated with judged attractiveness." However, a mutual variance of 34% is not that high, and some readers may find Light et al.'s statment rather counterintuitive in the light of their own life experience concerning facial attractiveness and typicality. Light et al. were aware of this, and they ran a successful check to ensure that the faces that they had used had not merely varied in attractiveness from only low to medium (which could explain a positive correlation between attractiveness and similarity). They were, however, at rather a loss to explain why their results differed from those of Shepherd and Ellis (1973), but they failed to note one possibly important difference between the two sets of studies. Whereas Shepherd and Ellis had employed female faces, Light et al. had used male faces. It was stated previously that Yarmey (1977) had found a positive relationship between attractiveness and recognizability for female faces, yet the reverse for male faces. Yarmey offered no explanation of this sex difference, but we should note that he found distinctiveness to correlate positively with recognizability for males faces, and negatively for female faces. Light et al. also found for their (male) faces that there was a negative correlation between similarity and recognizability. Thus perhaps the nature of the relationship between attractiveness and recognizability depends upon how typical/similar/nondistinctive/nonunique the particular subjects in a study find the attractive faces. Some studies may use subjects who are used to seeing attractive faces and therefore deem them to be typical/similar/common, whereas other studies may use subjects who more rarely experience attractive faces.

Courtois and Mueller (1981) found distinctiveness to aid recognition. Their male and female subjects (college students) saw 10 faces previously rated at the two extremes of being "typical of college seniors." The recognition test trials presented each target along with three distractors (which were also high or low in distinctiveness). Target and distractor distinctiveness both had significant effects (across the three delays used) and did not interact with each other. Typical faces (i.e., nondistinct) led to poorer recognition performance than atypical (distinct) faces, and to more false alarms. Sex of face had few effects, except that whereas for male faces target typicality interacted with distractor typicality, it did not for female faces. That is, typical male targets presented at testing with typical male distractors led to the worst performance. Courtois and Mueller's finding that "the best recognition occurred when a distinctive target was paired with other distinctive faces as distractors" corroborates Light et al.'s (1981) finding for similarity, but since Courtois and Mueller make no mention of facial attractiveness, no support is offered for Light et al.'s view that similarity is positively correlated with attractiveness.

Mueller, Heesacker, and Ross (1984) found rated likeability to reduce face recognition both for male and female faces. Since they found a strong positive correlation between likeability and attractiveness one could take the results of their study as suggesting that facial attractiveness would be correlated negatively with recognizability.

Thus the literature contains some studies that suggest a negative correlation between attractiveness and recognizability (e.g., Light et al. [1981], Yarmey [1977, for males], and Mueller et al. [1984]), some that suggest a positive correlation (e.g., Cross et al. [1971] and Yarmey [1977, for females]), and some that suggest a curvilinear relationship (Shepherd & Ellis [1973] and Fleishman et al. [1976]). A correct explanation of why attractiveness may affect recognizability (via arousal, and/or distinctiveness, or some other factors) obviously awaits reconciliation of the disparate findings presented above. One possible explanation for the disparity may be concerned with the actual range of attractiveness used in the various studies. Even if from each study's population of faces the extremes or entire range were used, there is no guarantee that the faces employed in one study occupy the same span of "real-world," "true" attractiveness as used in other studies. Again we find that for empirical, well-conducted studies on an aspect of the social psychology of facial appearance that produce contradictory results we have no way of checking whether a face deemed in one study to be of high attractiveness would have been similarly labeled in another researcher's study.

In addition to finding that their attractive/likeable faces were harder to remember, Mueller et al. (1984) noted that "the present data suggests that likeable looking suspects *may* be more apt to escape detection than their unlikeable counterparts. This outcome is in accord with the notion that a witness may seek someone who looks like a criminal (i.e. unpleasant) and thus possibly overlook a more pleasant suspect." (Mueller et al. also noted that the data for their target-absent cases did not support this notion.)

Although the study by Klatzky, Martin, and Kane (1982) was not cited by Mueller et al, their findings could be taken as supporting Mueller et al.'s notion. Klatzky et al. found male faces that observers could consensually assign to one of 13 occupations. Some of these faces were presented to subjects simultaneously with a congruent or incongruent occupational category. These subjects were then presented with a series of faces and were required to indicate which had previously been presented to them. The results indicated that faces that were rated as more stereotypical were more recognizable, and there was some limited evidence that congruent occupational labeling led to better recognition. Klatzky et al. remarked that, "Just what makes stereotyped faces more memorable remains unclear." They suggested that the features of stereotyped faces may be more distinctive, and that their effects of stereotypy may be judged to contrast with those of Light et al. (1981), who found among a collection of faces from a single category (male high school seniors) that atypical rather than stereotypical faces were better remembered. However, they pointed out that, "Typicality effects may have been masked by competing effects that arose because of the use of such a homogeneous stimulus pool in Light et al.'s experiment. In this case, atypical faces could gain an advantage because of discriminability, which would outweigh the advantage of stereotypicality." Klatzky et al. concluded that

> The finding of categorically induced errors in face recognition is of obvious interest from the applied point of view. . . . facial stereotypes that are encoded along with the physical features of a particular face could be the basis for false recognitions on later tests. On the more positive side, the present studies indicate that there are physiognomic factors that make certain faces more memorable than others. Further research might determine the nature of these factors.

Mueller, Thompson, and Vogel (1988) examined whether faces they considered to fit a stereotypical "criminal type" would be easier or more difficult to recognize. They used as targets and distractors male and female college yearbook facial photographs that were rated high or low for honest/trustworthy. Subjects initially saw 16 target faces (8 high, 8 low) and after 25 minutes they saw 32 four-face arrays during a recognition test. On each recognition trial all the nontargets were either "honest" or "dishonest." No effects were found for sex of photo or sex of subject. Rated honesty did not have a pronounced effect on the number of hits, but the "honest target–dishonest distractor" arrays did yield significantly fewer hits, largely because the subjects incorrectly indicated that in such arrays none of the faces was the target. For the subjects' confidence ratings regarding their responses significantly greater confidence accompanied (a) hits when distractors were honest rather than dishonest, (b) correct "not present" responses for dishonest rather than honest arrays, and (c) incorrect identification of an honest, as opposed to a dishonest, distractor from a target-absent array. Mueller, Thompson, and Vogel considered two possible explanations of why rated honesty might affect facial recognition. "One concerned the relationship between honest appearance and other dimensions of the face (specifically distinctiveness), whereas the other concerned the influence of observer expectancies or stereotypes about honest people." They took their data as supporting the former of these two explanations, and added that since rated honesty correlated positively with likeability ($+0.8$) and with attractiveness ($+0.6$) and negatively with typicality (-0.6), distinctiveness would be the more likely explanation of their findings. They suggested that the face label "common" could be synonymous with "honest." However, one reason why they found very limited support for the effect of observer expectancies/stereotypes could have to do with the ecological validity of their study. They correctly pointed out that undergraduates looking at facial photos in a standard "laboratory-based" recognition task may not occasion factors that operate in real-life criminal indentification situations. In addition, one should note that the mean ratings for their extreme honest and dishonest faces did not differ very much (4.8 versus 3.4, on a 7-point scale). Mueller and Thompson concluded that "the safest conclusion would seem to be that the jury is still out on the influence of the criminal stereotype on face memory."

Is There, in Fact, a Relationship Between Facial Appearance and Criminality?

In the previous section we reported on studies that support the notion that people expect there to be a relationship between facial appearance and criminality. However, does such a relationship actually exist? In 1974 H. Cavior, Hayes, and Cavior suggested that "low physical attractiveness contributes to careers of deviancy." Similarly, N. Cavior and Howard (1973) stated that, "This and other evidence suggest that facial attractiveness may be causal in delinquency," and they suggested that since physical attractiveness may well play an important role in various dyadic and group processes, unattractive people may be rejected by others, this rejection leading to delinquency.

Cavior and Howard formed two hypotheses. The first was that juvenile delinquents would be less facially attractive than nondelinquents, and the second was that there would be differences in unattractiveness across Quay's (1972) four behavior dimensions of juvenile offenders (these dimensions being [a] socialized-subcultural, [b] neurotic-disturbed, [c] inadequate-immature, and [d] unsocialized-psychopathic). In their first study photographs of 103 white, male delinquents and 78 white, nondelinquent students were rated by white students on 5-point scales for attractiveness. It was found (a) that the faces of nondelinquents were rated as significantly more attractive than three of the four groups of delinquents (the difference between the non-delinquents and the socialized-subcultural delinquents reached the $p < .10$ level of significance); and (b) that the four groups of delinquents significantly differed among themselves (the order shown above of the four groups show-ing decreasing attractiveness). Cavior and Howard wisely ensured that the photograph raters knew nothing about the study; however, the photographs of the nondelinquents "were printed on different paper" from those of the delinquents. This methodological weakness was somewhat offset by the fact that one group of students rated the photographs of delinquents and another group of (similar) students rated the nondelinquents. The possibility that the use of different photographic paper caused the difference in ratings be-tween delinquents and nondelinquents is difficult to deny, but this weakness could not account for the predicted difference between the subgroups of delinquents.

In their second study Cavior and Howard used photographs of 56 black, male delinquents and 56 black, nondelinquent students. These were rated by black and white students who each saw both groups of photographs (which again appear to have differed in terms of the paper on which they were printed). The black raters evaluated the nondelinquents as more facially attractive than the delinquents, but no differences were found between the four delinquency subgroups. For white raters no significant differences were found (not even the suggestion of a trend). Cavior and Howard con-cluded that "delinquents are significantly lower in facial attractiveness than non-delinquents," that, "this finding. . . is congruent with the findings of Kurtzberg, [Safar, & Cavior] (1968) on the effectiveness of plastic surgery in reducing recidivism," and that "a lack of facial attractiveness may . . . reduce the probability that the offender will receive a suspended sen-tence."

H. Cavior, Hayes, and Cavior (1974) noted that no studies had been re-ported examining the effects of the degree of attractiveness of female offend-ers. They asked white males to rate the facial attractiveness of 44 black and 31 white, female offenders (mean age 19 years) who had served an average of 10 months at a minimum security prison. It was found that attractiveness was significantly related (a) positively to frequency of permitted trips into town (much more so for whites than for blacks), and (b) negatively to frequency of receiving reports of undesirable prison behavior regarding the use of violent aggression (with frequency of reports regarding threatening to use violence producing a nonsignificant relationship). No relationship was found between attractiveness and (a) type of offense for which the females had been committed (although four of the total of five committed for aggressive offenses were rated as unattractive), (b) frequency of reports of good prison behavior, and (c) the reason for the inmate leaving the prison. Cavior et al. concluded

> . . . it is clear that physical attractiveness affected a number of measures which may have an important impact on the incarcerated female. . . As of yet, the exact mechanism of the effects of physical attractiveness has not been determined. It seems likely that the differing environmental consequences for attractive versus unattractive individuals may shape divergent behavioral repertoires. The relationship between aggression-based behavior and physical attractiveness is perhaps one such example. If attractive individuals are reacted to more positively they may find less reason for recourse to violent means to achieve their goals. Conversely, unattractive individuals may experience more frustration due to their relative lack of access to important reinforcing events, thus increasing the likelihood of aggression.

Although not cited by Cavior et al., a study by A. Miller, Gillen, Schenker and Radlove (1974) provided some support for their idea that female unattractiveness may relate to predictions of aggressivity. Miller et al.'s subjects experienced a vivid verbal and visual description of Milgram's (1963) original obedience experiment and were then asked to indicate what maximum level of shock they thought each of 24 photographed people would have administered in Milgram's experiment. It was found that unattractive females (rated in a prior study) were assigned significantly higher shock levels than attractive females (but there was no difference for male stimuli). Miller et al. therefore suggested that unattractive people are associated not only with undesirable personalities (as many previous studies have shown), but also with undesirable deeds.

Unger et al. (1982) hypothesized that unattractive females and males would be judged as more likely to be involved in minor forms of social deviancy than would attractive individuals. They found females rated as facially unattractive by one group of students to be judged by other students as "deviants (feminists, political radicals, homosexuals and those aspiring to stereotypically masculine careers)," and unattractive males to be rated as more likely to be politically radical, as aspiring to stereotypically feminine careers, and to be homosexual (only by female, not male, raters). Whether or not one agrees with Unger et al. that these judgments do, in fact, denote social deviancy in any derogatory sense, their findings seem worthy of note.

A more direct test of the hypothesis that facial appearance and social deviancy are related was undertaken by Agnew (1984), who suggested that delinquency would be higher "among physically unattractive, poorly groomed, and poorly dressed individuals." He argued that "if appearance is related to delinquency, . . . efforts might be made to reduce the discrimination against unattractive people by sensitizing individuals such as teachers and police to the stereotypes they hold."

The data Agnew collected were from a longitudinal survey of adolescent boys conducted by the University of Michigan. Each of the boys had been interviewed on two occasions and among the data collected by the interviewers were their ratings of each boys' "general appearance" (i.e., "pay attention to physical appearance, dress, and grooming"). Even though factors other than facial appearance were noted to have contributed to these ratings (e.g., being overweight, being "not as physically mature as the attractive boys"), facial complexion and facial attractiveness seemed to have contributed to the general appearance ratings. Having been interviewed, the boys then provided three self-report measures of delinquency, these being one on "seriousness of delinquency," one on "trouble with parents," and one on "delinquent behavior at school." Agnew hypothesized that, "Given the argument that attractiveness is most important in first impression situations, we would expect bias against the unattractive to be greater at school than at home. For this reason, we predict that attractiveness will have a greater effect on school-related delinquency than on family-related delinquency." Agnew examined these delinquency data for the boys rated as having the best ($n = 186$) or worst ($n = 105$) appearance out of the total sample (of around 2,000). Significant relationships between the appearance ratings and all three delinquency measures were found and, "As predicted, appearance had a greater effect on school-related delinquency than on family-related delinquency." Appearance was found not to be related to the boys' race, although it was to socioeconomic status (SES).

Although the relationships between appearance and delinquency were significant, this conclusion may have been driven more by the sample size used than the strength of the relationships. Agnew reported that, "After race and SES are controlled, appearance explains 4% of the variation in seriousness of delinquency, 4% of the variation in trouble with parents, and 9% of the variation in delinquent behavior in school." Thus the significant relationships found between appearance and self-reported delinquency are not strong. Another reason why Agnew's study may not be taken as necessarily supporting the hypothesis that delinquency and facial appearance are meaningfully related is the way in which appearance data were gathered. Although the appearance raters were, quite rightly, blind to the actual delinquency data, they did perform these ratings at the end of 2-hour-long interviews with the boys. Thus, following the findings of Gross and Crofton (1977) that the good may be seen as beautiful, the appearance ratings may have unwittingly been influenced by information that the boys divulged in the interview. Agnew was aware of this possibility and he did take the trouble to calculate an interviewer appearance rating correlation. However, this was not very high (.38) and he therefore suggested that future research should be concerned to have unbiased appearance evaluations.

Agnew suggested that his finding of a relationship between delinquency and physical appearance lent support to the notion of "programs designed to improve the appearance of delinquents." It is to a review of research on such programs that we now turn.

Facial Surgery and Deviancy

In 1973 Longacre stated that, "The high value placed upon personal appearance in our culture today has intensified the impact of facial deformity upon the individual so afflicted, oftentimes leading to deviant behavior. . . . With juvenile delinquents there is a great opportunity for the plastic surgeon to modify the physical handicap which may have played a major role." Several studies have been conducted in North America in an attempt to determine whether the notions of the Caviors and of Longacre concerning a relationship between unattractive facial appearance and undesirable behavior can be supported by examination of the recidivism rates of prison inmates who have received facial surgery.

In 1966 Spira, Chizen, Gerow, and Hardy attempted to evaluate some aspects of the use of plastic surgery in the Texas prison system. Their work was supported by the Director of the Department of Corrections, O.B. Ellis, who held the opinion that "there can be no question of the fact that physical deformities, especially facial defects, develop inferiority complexes which make employment difficult and, in the final analysis, may contribute to criminal behavior. Correction of these defects enhances the chance of an inmate making a satisfactory adjustment to society after release." At the main prison at Huntsville, Texas, 17 beds were allocated to plastic surgery. Spira et al. reported that, "The programme has become increasingly popular within the prison system. Inmates voluntarily make requests for a number of cosmetic and reconstructive procedures which, by word of mouth and personal contact, are familiar to them. Often a prison official will make the convict cognisant of his defect and will suggest the service which is available to him." An inmate who requested such treatment was first seen by a prison doctor and if this doctor believed surgery to be warranted, the inmate was then seen by the plastic surgery staff. Spira et al. stated that "infrequently, the prisoner will present with a minimal defect and surgery will be deemed unwarranted. Occasionally, because of an obvious neurotic overlay, surgery is considered ill advised." However, "in the majority of cases surgery is performed and, after a reasonable convalescent period the patient is discharged to his initial place of detention. . . . Most prisoners in need of this surgery realise that this type of work is unusual in penal systems; and they exhibit a most appreciative attitude, making excellent patients."

Spira et al. found in the mid-1960s that in 22 of the states in the United States some type of plastic/reconstructive surgery was being carried out on inmates in the state prison systems. Eight federal prisons also had similar programs. Rhinoplasties and septoplasties (i.e., nose operations), scar revisions, hand repairs, and removal of head/neck tumors were the most common operations. No formal assessment of the effects of these operations was undertaken, but Spira et al. did conclude that, "Most surgeons and officials directly involved in these activities are of the opinion that a needed service is being provided which has contributed materially toward prisoner rehabilitation. Although no definite conclusions can be drawn as to the specific effectiveness of the surgery relative to recidivism, a few have expressed at least guarded optimism on this point." Spira et al. also made the point that, "One can argue with regard to the role of physical appearance in antisocial activity, that appearance alone would suffice to propel a normal individual into a life of crime. As a general statement, this appears reasonable; examples of individuals who have overcome varying degrees of physical impairment to achieve success are abundant; yet, who can deny that there might be occasions on which a person with a facial deformity would be denied an opportunity otherwise available to him." Spira et al. reported that of a group of prisoners who received plastic surgery 17% returned to prison with a new sentence within a few years, whereas 32% of the general prison population did so. Of course, valid comparisons of this nature are difficult to achieve because one should take into account types of crime committed, length of sentence, and the like. Nevertheless, Spira et al. concluded that they were encouraged by the results.

One year after the publication of Spira et al.'s paper there appeared a paper by Masters and Greaves (1967) in which they claimed that at that time there was "little objective evidence that surgical correction of a defect of body image will affect an abnormal personality trait, or that there is a significant increase in the incidence of physical deformity among those individuals who are emotionally disturbed." Masters and Greaves wanted to examine the incidence of facial abnormality in the criminal population and to compare this with that found in the general population. They felt that psychologists, sociologists, and criminologists had paid only lip service to the concept that there may be a relationship between facial deformity and crime, and they believed that most people saw the so-called criminal type as a figment of the imagination of detective fiction writers and movie makeup artists. With the cooperation of the police departments of Kansas City, St. Louis, Baltimore, Miami, and Los Angeles a study was carried out by Masters and Greaves to try to determine objectively whether the incidence of facial deformity was greater in the criminal population. Utilizing the police file photographs (front view and profile) of 11,000 criminals, the incidence and type of facial deformity was catalogued and compared with "a cross section of the general public." (No information is given on how this control group of the general public was obtained.) For their criminal group Masters and Greaves chose the following categories of crime: homicide, rape, prostitution, sex deviation, and suicide "since there could be little doubt concerning the personal or social maladjustment of the individual" in these cases. (Some psychologists may not agree with this claim.) Overall, the results showed a significant difference in the incidence of correctable facial deformity in the criminal group compared with the control group. Masters and Greaves noted that, "Critical evaluation [it was not stated how this was achieved or how reliable it was] of over 11,000 photographs reveal that 60 per cent of the criminals have surgically correctable facial defects, as compared with 20 per cent of the general public."

At first glance this difference between the two groups in the incidence of facial deformity seems meaningfully large. However, Masters and Greaves give *no* information concerning the methodology of their research and to what extent the photographs of the general population were similar in backgroup, lighting, and facial expression to those of the criminals. If the persons who examined the photographs could tell whether they were of a criminal or not, this could well have had an influence on whether they judged a deformity to be present or absent. This study needs repeating but with a far higher standard of procedural control. (The finding of a 20% incidence rate of facial deformity in the general public also seems surprising.) Nevertheless, we cannot easily ignore the major finding of this piece of research which was that "60 per cent of the criminals have surgically correctable facial defects, as compared with 20 per cent of the general public." However, Masters and Greaves may have been wise to conclude that, "The high incidence of facial deformity among criminals whose social maladjustment is unequivocal is not conclusive of the fact that defects of body image do play a role in an individual's reaction to himself and society. The 40% differential incidence is significant evidence only that a difference between the general public and the criminal exists. By no means can this be interpreted that a given individual's facial defect led him into a specific crime or that correction of the deformity might have prevented this crime or in any way limited his criminal activity."

In 1974 Lewison reported a study of over 20 years of plastic surgery involving over 900 Canadian prison inmates with facial disfigurements, the vast majority of whom were serving sentences of less than 2 years. He was particularly interested in examining the possibility that abnormalities of facial appearance may be related to, or even cause, antisocial behavior and he was of the opinion that "improving the inmate's appearance as well as his functional ability, and bolstering his self-image, might facilitate his social integration," especially in the habitual offender for whom "Current methods of rehabilitation have so far not been very effective." Commencing in 1953, inmates requesting facial surgery were selected for treatment. Those with minimal facial deformities and those who "may be severely impaired emotionally by plastic surgery" were rejected, although on only two occasions was surgery refused on the latter grounds. Rarely was treatment refused on the grounds that an individual was using facial deformity as a "crutch" on which to rest a life's disappointments, even though Lewison was aware of the common but probably fallacious argument that, "The sudden withdrawal of this crutch may leave the individual without defenses against his inadequacy and may plunge him into deep depression." (Our own research on society's reactions to facial disfigurement [described in Chapter 7] does, in fact, suggest that deformed individuals may not be fantasizing when they say that people act in a nonpositive way toward them because of their deformity.)

Lewison reported that following facial surgery the inmates' within-prison behavior improved significantly, but his main index of the value of the surgery was recidivism rate. He admitted that in his early studies (up to 1965), which found a recidivism rate of 42% in those who had received within-prison facial surgery compared with a rate of 70% in those who had not, no adequate control groups were used. However, in his major study (of 1966) of 200 inmates seeking facial surgery 100 were randomly selected for treatment. For those who received facial surgery the recidivism rate (presumably up to 1974) was 48% and that for the control group was 69%. This considerable reduction in the recidivism rate was not found in all types of minor offender. Narcotics offenders had a higher postsurgery recidivism rate than did other types of offenders.

Kurtzberg, Safar, and Cavior (1968) also investigated the effects of plastic surgery on prison inmates by making operations available to some prison inmates who had various visible "defects that might handicap their social and vocational rehabilitation after discharge from prison." Kurtzberg et al. reported that the majority of inmates' surgery requests were for the "correction of non-functional stigmatizing deformities," and that the inmates felt that their deformities caused people to "stereotype them as boisterous, mean, aggressive." The subjects in a study by Kurtzberg, Lewin, Cavior, and Lipton (1967) were short-term male inmates (mainly chronic petty offenders) in New York. Of the 1,570 inmates who volunteered for surgery several hundred were judged to have reparable defects. Not all of these, however, were offered surgery. It was reported that 12% of those with nasal deformities were refused surgery for "excessive focusing" (i.e., having too strong a belief, judged by the research team, that surgery would "solve my problem" or "change my life"). That surgery was refused to this group was, from the scientific methodology point of view, a pity since the hypothesis that surgery could be harmful by withdrawing the "crutch" Lewison (1974) referred to could not consequently be tested. Of the inmates who were judged suitable for surgery several dozen subsequently received it (the 1968 paper by Kurtzberg, Safar, and Cavior suggests that this surgery may have been performed in a civilian hospital upon the inmates' release from prison), whereas others in this group were randomly allocated to nonsurgery control group. Subjects (both surgery and nonsurgery) completed the Minnesota Multiphasic Personality Inventory (MMPI) and, somewhat surprisingly, it appears from Figure 5 of Kurtzberg et al.'s 1967 paper that the no-surgery inmates differed somewhat on a number of personality dimensions (e.g., paranoia) from those due to receive surgery. Nevertheless, at least Kurtzberg et al. (1967) did attempt randomly to allocate subjects to the control and experimental groups. In their 1968 paper Kurtzberg et al. compared the recidivism rates of the groups of inmates. Of the group receiving no surgery some received "social and vocational services" and others did not. Similarly, in the surgery group some also received these services while others did not.

During the 1-year follow-up period those who had previously been in prison for heroin offenses (and for whom the majority of deformities were needle tracks or tattoos) seemed not to have benefited from the surgery since, although 79% of the no-surgery/no-services group recidivated and 67% of the surgery/no-services group recidivated (i.e., an apparent surgery recidivism reduction of 12%), the no-surgery/services and surgery/services group recidivated at 48% and 50%, respectively. This stronger effect of services than surgery was not found in the recidivism rates of those convicted for other offenses (for whom the majority of deformities were facial). The rate for the services/no-surgery group was 89% (although here the sample was small) whereas that for the no-services/no-surgery group was 56%. The rates for the no-services/surgery group and for the services/surgery group were 30% and 33%, respectively, and so Kurtzberg et al. (1968) were able to conclude that "the findings did indicate that plastic surgery can serve as an important aid in the rehabilitation of disfigured offenders," especially those with facial disfigurements. They further pointed out that the financial "cost of plastic surgery, although relatively high, can be considered negligible if the offender is helped to remain out of prison for even one year."

It would seem from the studies described above that a case has been made for some association between facial appearance and criminality. Indeed, the *British Medical Journal* stated in 1965 in one of its Leading Articles that, "There is no need to justify the correction of cosmetic and other surgical disabilities in offenders." However, not all studies have found plastic surgery to be beneficial. Schuring and Dodge (1967) found no effect of plastic surgery on recidivism rates and they suggested that this may be either due to the fact that many of the treated deformities were of a minor nature or, as Meyer, Hoopes, Jabaley, and Allan (1973) noted, that, "With a more serious deformity, years of maladjustment superimposed on the original problem precluded curing the criminality by surgery." Pick (1948) suggested that disfigured juvenile delinquents would perhaps be the group most likely to benefit from plastic surgery since they had not yet become hardened criminals. Meyer et al. (1973) set out to test Pick's hypothesis in what they admitted was a pilot study. They collected data of a behavioral kind (school or job performance, number of formal charges of delinquency) and a psychological kind (self-esteem, body image, etc.) concerning 21 individuals aged between 12 and 20 years who had been either formally designated as delinquent by the authorities or who "were from a population socially and culturally displaying high risk" (no further description than this is given). Of these individuals 14 were given plastic surgery and 1 year later follow-up data were gathered. For each of the 21 individuals an overall improvement score (on the behavioral and psychological measures) was calculated and no difference in this score was found between the experimental and control groups. Meyer et al. took these few data from this small and poorly controlled study to indicate that "unoperated patients did as well as the operated ones in subsequent improvement of their psychological and behavioral parameters."

Whether there does exist a strong, causative link between facial appearance and criminality awaits the results of future research, as does the question of what to do if such a relationship is found. In 1938 (i.e., prior to almost all of psychology's research on this topic) Straith and De Kleine stated that the facially disfigured child "is most likely to be deprived of many things commonly sought after for their supposed value: for example, money, friends, esteem, beauty, amusements and romance." Research conducted since 1938 may be viewed as largely serving to confirm this expectation and as supporting Straith and De Kleine's view that "such children . . . are apt to do many useless, foolhardy or even dishonest things to attain their desires."

Little research has been conducted on the question of whether children of abnormal facial appearance do, in face, engage in behavior that society would react to in a negative way. However, some evidence relating to this question was gathered by Waldrop and Halverson, who in their 1971 extensive study of minor physical anomalies and children's hyperactive behavior claimed to have found evidence that "hyperactive behavior is related to the presence of certain minor physical anomalies in young children." They noted "when we saw hyperactive play behavior we frequently found that the boys involved also had more minor physical anomalies (such as head circumference out of the normal range, widely spaced eyes, and adherent ear lobes) than boys not displaying hyperactive behavior." The findings for girls were inconsistent in that in some studies relationships were found between abnormal play behavior and physical appearance but in others no such relationships were observed. However, their replication studies did confirm the relationships for boys. Some of the behavioral variables that correlated highly with the presence of physical anomalies were described by Waldrop and Halverson (1971) as "negative interaction," "opposition to peers," and "an inability to delay."

These researchers also performed a follow-up study in which physical anomaly and hyperactive behavior data were obtained for children aged 7½ years who had originally been studied at age 2½ years. The ratings of physical anomaly and of hyperactive behavior were performed independently by judges who had not taken part in the original study. Waldrop and Halverson concluded that

> . . . these data demonstrate that: (a) the weighted anomaly score tended to be stable over the five years, (b) children with high anomaly scores tended to be more frenetic and have less behavioral control than children with few anomalies, (c) children at seven and a half with high anomaly scores tended to be clumsy, (d) children at seven and a half with more than the average number of minor physical anomalies had lower than average IQ scores, (e) frenetic fast-moving behavior showed continuity over the five years, (f) the children at seven and a half with high physical anomaly scores were hyperactive at age two and a half.

In another part of their study Waldrop and Halverson asked 15 teachers to give the names of three children in their classes who were the most hyperactive and three children whose behavior was in the normal range. Of the hyperactive children 75% were male. When all the children had been rated (blind) for physical abnormalities it was found that the hyperactive children had significantly more anomalies than did the nonhyperactive children. Furthermore, the more hyperactive a boy was reported to be, the more physical anomalies he had. Waldrop and Halverson concluded that "these findings make us wonder if children with high physical anomaly scores are insensitive, tough little kids." This may be so. However, hyperactivity could be related to attendant CNS dysfunction which, together with physical anomaly, could have a genetic cause. If this were so, physical anomaly may not play a causative role.

Lowenstein (1978) examined 32 children who had been consistently bullied by other children. Each of these bullied children was matched with the child of the same sex who sat nearest in the class but who was not involved in bullying. It was found that the bullied children were significantly less physically attractive than the controls and that they displayed more physical handicaps and odd mannerisms.

Whether facially abnormal children are more often the instigators of agression than the recipients is not clear, but it does seem from the studies of Waldrop and Halverson and of Lowenstein that facially abnormal children may be more frequently involved in aggressive and possibly transgressive situations than are children of "normal" facial appearance. Such findings as these may serve as support for statements such as that made as long ago as 1938 by Straith and De Kleine (in the absence of any relevant data) that "these are children who may develop distinctly objectionable social behavior, since they often cannot obtain desirable employment, may not succeed in matrimonial measures and will not maintain friendships. As a result they may resort to criminal activities."

We began this section by asking whether, in fact, there is a relationship between facial appearance and criminality. Although the breadth and depth of the literature on this topic is rather inadequate, the suggestiveness of some of its findings is hard to ignore. However, as with most other areas of psychological research, it is impossible to know how many unpublished studies have failed to find such a relationship.

Facial Appearance and Attributions of Responsibility

J. Rich (1975) suggested that unattractive persons may be judged as having a more external locus of control than attractive persons. If this is so one might expect unattractive people to be judged as less responsible for their behavior. Similarly Seligman et al. (1974) suggested that since an attractive person "is evaluated more favorably, more is expected of him, and a more stringent moral code applies to him," and that "attractive persons would be seen generally as more responsible for their fates." In their study male and female students saw a photograph of an attractive or unattractive woman who had taken a job as a secretary knowing that in 6 months the government would make a decision to expand, terminate, or continue its present contract with the company. Half the subjects were told that in fact the government considerably expanded the contract and the woman was promoted to the position of administrative assistant, the other half that the government terminated

the contract and she therefore lost her job. The subjects were asked to estimate the woman's responsibility for the outcome and it was found that those
who saw an unattractive photograph attributed to the woman more responsibility for the bad than for the good outcome. However, for those who saw the
attractive photograph the reverse was found.

Seligman et al. took the absence of a main effect of attractiveness on attributed responsibility to run counter to the suggestion that attractive people
may be judged as having more external control. However, since it was clear to
their subjects that the government was very involved in the outcome, their
study may not be an appropriate test of this notion. Seligman et al. took their
findings to be supportive of a "balance" model in which desirable (i.e., attractive) persons should be associated with desirable things (e.g., promotion),
and vice versa. They concluded that, "Perhaps not only what is beautiful is
good, but what is beautiful is responsible for what is good, and what is not
beautiful is responsible for what is not good."

Data supporting this conclusion were found by Turkat and Dawson (1976),
who used both female and male faces that varied in attractiveness. Male and
female students were asked to imagine that there had been an airplane crash
that had set fire to the apartment building in which the photographed person
lived. Half of the subjects were told that the person's apartment was not
damaged, the other half that it was burned out. The subjects were asked to
indicate how responsible they felt the person had been for what happened as
the result of the fire. It was found that unattractive persons were judged as
more responsible for the burned out apartment than were attractive persons,
but that the reverse applied for the other outcome condition, thus supporting
the conclusion of Seligman et al.

Pavlos and Newcomb (1974) varied the attractiveness of a female student
whom male students were told had attempted suicide by taking an overdose
of pills. Half the subjects were told that the female had been informed by her
physician that she had terminal cancer, the other half, treatable cancer. The
ratings of the justification for the suicide attempt were found to be affected by
attractiveness, but again an interaction was found. When the medical prognosis was "terminal" the attractive woman was rated as more justified than
the unattractive woman, but when the prognosis was "treatable" the unattractive woman was rated as more justified. Whether this finding also fits in
with Seligman et al.'s conclusion is not easy to say since one has to relate
justification to responsibility, and also to decide whether attempted suicide in
the case of terminal cancer is a "good" or "bad" outcome.

An outcome about which there should be less debate concerning what is
"good" or "bad" than for attempted suicide is that of being raped. Seligman,
Brickman, and Koulack (1977) suggested that, on the one hand, "To the
extent that people believe that a beautiful woman, because of her beauty per
se, triggers a rape attempt, then a beautiful woman would be seen as more
causally responsible for being victimized than a physically unattractive
woman," but, on the other hand, on the basis of attribution theory, "If peo-

ple believe it is likely that an attractive woman might be raped, and she is, there is no need to assume she may have behaved provocatively. However, if . . . an unattractive woman is raped then one may conclude that the victim must have acted in some way to encourage the rape." In their study male and female students read a newspaper story of a rape or a mugging or a robbery and saw an attractive or unattractive photograph of the female victim (a nurse). The subjects were asked to indicate "what they thought was the likelihood of the nurse being victimized in the way described in the newspaper story." As predicted, only for the rape was there an effect of attractiveness, with the attractive woman being judged as more likely to be victimized. The victim's responsibility for her plight was assessed in two ways. First, the subjects were asked how much the nurse was to blame for the incident, and no effect of attractiveness was found. Second, the subjects were asked to indicate if the nurse "might have somehow provoked the man into treating her the way he did." Only for the rape was there an effect of attractiveness, with the unattractive victim being thought to somehow have provoked the rape. No effect of victim attractiveness was found for severity of punishment for the criminal. Seligman et al. suggested that individuals have a need to believe in a "just world," and in order to do this blame victims to a certain extent for their misfortunes. Since an attractive woman is believed to be more likely to be raped, then this in itself is a sufficient explanation of why she was raped. However, if she is unattractive, since the world is just, she must have behaved in a provocative way. Feild (1979) suggested that, "For an attractive victim, jurors might conclude that 'the poor guy was so overcome with passion he couldn't help himself' . . . jurors may also reason for an unattractive woman 'she's so homely, who would want to rape her?'"

No support for this argument appears to come from a study by Calhoun, Selby, Cann, and Keller (1978), who found attractive females to be judged ($p < .06$) as more to blame for being raped. Male and female students read an account of a rape and they rated the attractive woman "as playing a greater role in her own rape." However, since the "blame" score in the study by Calhoun et al. involved a composite score ("the extent to which her behavior precipitated the assault, the extent to which she is the kind of person who gets herself into these types of situations, and the extent to which the victim's appearance contributed to the likelihood of her being raped") that combined Seligman's scales of (a) likelihood of being victimized (where attractiveness led to an increased score) and (b) provocation (where attractiveness led to a decreased score), the outcomes of these two studies may not in fact be in opposition. One important point that emerges from a comparison of the studies by Seligman et al. and by Calhoun et al. concerns the rather arbitrary use in studies of the psychological effects of facial appearance of various types and combinations of dependent variables. When various studies employ different operational definitions and measurement of factors such as responsibility/ blame/provocation, it may not be that surprising that the resultant conclusions do not accord one with another.

Similarly, although the explanations offered by Seligman et al. run counter to Rich's idea that what happens to unattractive people is believed to be more outside their control than events that happen to attractive people, they serve again to remind us that the effect of facial appearance may not always be of the same form but may crucially depend upon other aspects of a situation or event.

The Effects of Facial Appearance on "Jurors"

The Facial Appearance of Victims—Rape

B. Thornton (1977) hypothesized, as had Seligman et al. (1977), that a rape victim's physical attractiveness would influence people's notions about her. He also hypothesized that her attractiveness would influence people's decisions concerning the rapist. Thornton noted Dermer and Thiel's (1975) suggestion that a rape victim might experience additional difficulty in securing a conviction of the accused when she is attractive. He pointed out that, unlike the situation in trials for many other crimes, in a rape case aspects of the victim play a very central role. In this study male and female students read a short account regarding the rape of a woman whose photograph (attractive or unattractive) was attached to the account. Contrary to the finding of Seligman et al., no effect of her attractiveness was found on the rated responsibility of the victim. Also, no effect of attractiveness was found for victim credibility or on the accused's guilt/innocence. The sentence length suggested by females was similarly unaffected by victim attractiveness (11 versus 8 years) but that suggested by males was significantly longer (16 versus 10 years) when the victim was attractive than when she was unattractive, respectively. Thornton noted that his study found few effects of attractiveness, but he nevertheless concluded that an offense against an attractive person may elicit a greater desire for retribution, especially from men when a woman is the victim.

Shaw's (1972) suggestion that people believe in a "just world" could be used to explain Thornton's significant finding. Shaw suggested that "people come to believe that the world is a just and predictable place, and that people get what they deserve. Since the victim of a crime receives a negative outcome, this reasoning implies that people will expect that he probably deserved it. A logical extension of this notion is that the perceiver's bias that the world is just will be stronger when confronted with an unattractive rather than attractive victim." Shaw therefore proposed that subjects will ascribe more responsibility for an unpleasant outcome to an unattractive victim and will therefore punish the perpetrator less.

Feild (1979) examined the effect of rape victim physical attractiveness. No main effect was found, and attractiveness entered into only a few significant, but very weak (omega-square $< .06$), three-way interactions with other variables. Thus little evidence was found by Feild to support his conclusion that, "From the view of a rape victim, this study also points to discriminatory treatment by jurors on the basis of several extra evidential factors, namely her . . . physical attractiveness."

Similarly, Villemur and Hyde (1983) found no main effect of rape victim attractiveness, but only significant three-way interactions. However, Villemur and Hyde's interactions may be more interpretable since they found female subjects to give more guilty verdicts when the victim was unattractive, whereas males gave more guilty verdicts only when the unattractive victim was "old." When she was "young" the males gave more guilty verdicts when she was attractive.

Deitz, Littman, and Bentley (1984) also found a subject factor to influence decisions about defendant guilt in a rape case. The subjects in their study completed a rape empathy questionnaire and it was found that only for those subjects low on empathy was their certainty of guilt affected (in fact, lowered) by victim unattractiveness. The low-empathy subjects were also the only ones who rated the unattractive victim as having more likely encouraged the rape.

Findings such as those Deitz et al. point to the need for research on the psychological effects of facial appearance to consider individual difference factors when investigating subjects' reactions. In addition, studies should always vary other variables along with facial appearance. Best and Demmin (1982) did the latter when they contrasted the possible effect of rape victim physical attractiveness with that of victim prerape behavior. They, like Deitz et al. (1984), were interested to see if support could be found for Calhoun et al.'s (1978) notion that a physically attractive victim would be judged as more to blame for the rape. Surprisingly, Best and Demmin did not cite the suggestion of Seligman et al. (1977) and of Feild (1979) that jurors would believe that if an unattractive woman is raped then she must have behaved in a provocative way. Students read a story that described the events prior to a rape. The story victim had been either "drinking alone in a bar" or "studying alone in the library." (Students who did not take part in the main study rated the victim's behavior as significantly more "provocative" in the former condition). Students in the main study read one of these two stories, and the victim was described "as either 'quite attractive' or 'unattractive'." The provocative behavior victim was rated as significantly more blameworthy for her rape, but victim attractiveness had no effect.

A similar outcome (i.e., a null effect of physical attractiveness) was found by Kanekar and Kolsawalla (1980), who found that whether a raped woman was described as "very good-looking" or "not at all good-looking" had no effect on assigned blame or defendant punishment, whereas dressing "in a sexually provocative manner" did so. The findings of Kanekar and Kolsawalla (1980) and Best and Demmin (1982) could be taken as suggesting that when other ecologically relevant independent variables are included in a study then little effect of physical attractiveness may be found. However, neither of these studies, unlike that by Deitz et al. (1984), reported that any check had been performed to determine whether the independent variable of physical attractiveness had, in fact, been successfully manipulated. Nevertheless, our survey of the literature suggests that there is little evidence that the facial attractiveness of a rape victim is of great consequence. However, we should bear in mind that the literature is based on simulations and not real-life decision making.

Victims of Other Crimes

What of other crimes? Does victim facial appearance play a strong role here? It seems not. No effect of female victim facial attractiveness on a male burglar's or swindler's rated guilt, recommended term of imprisonment, and crime seriousness was found by Singleton and Hofacre (1976) who used female and male students as subjects. Similarly Kerr (1978) found no effect of female victim attractiveness on judgments of defendant guilt when the owner of a car that was stolen had left the keys in the ignition ("careless"). He did find victim attractiveness to make conviction significantly more likely if the victim had locked her car doors and steering wheel ("careful"). No effect of victim attractiveness on attributions of responsibility was found. Employing an analysis of the data that differentiated between verdict effects due to differences in the valuation/integration of evidence and those due to differences in conviction criterion, Kerr concluded that when the victim who had been careful was attractive, less evidence of guilt was required by the subjects for conviction than when she was unattractive.

A methodology similar to that used by Kerr (1978) was employed by Kerr, Bull, MacCoun, and Rathborn (1985). In addition to the victim variables of attractiveness and care, a third variable of victim disfigurement was used in which the victim had either (a) a large scar on her face caused by the car's antenna as it was being stolen, or (b) the same scar that was not caused by the car theft and an arm scar that was, or (c) no facial scar, but stated in her testimony that she had a large arm scar caused by the theft. No effects of victim attractiveness on verdicts were found save that when the victim was unattractive and facially scarred prior to the car theft the effect found in the remainder of the study for careful/careless was reversed.

We can conclude from these "simulated juror" studies of the effects of victim facial appearance that there exists at best only weak evidence that this factor has any main effect. In fact, facial appearance seems to be more likely to enter into interactions with other factors such as victim past behavior. Storck and Sigall (1979) found that victim prior victimization modified the effect of harm-doer attractiveness on the punishment given by subjects to the harm-doer. However, in this study the harm-doer's attractiveness was not varied by using facial appearance. It is to studies of the effects of harm-doer's facial appearance that we now turn.

The Facial Appearance of Defendants

In 1969 Landy and Aronson published the first study that employed defendant attractiveness as an independent variable. They found that their simulated "jurors" sentenced the unattractive defendant to a greater number of years of imprisonment. This study employed a paradigm that purported to simulate the decision making of real juries by having students read in the classroom a brief account of a criminal offense, and one that (although Landy and Aronson varied defendant character rather than physical appearance) has been rather slavishly copied by most of the subsequent studies of the effects of defendant facial appearance.

One of the first published studies in which defendant facial appearance was varied was that of Efran (1974), who made the point that, "Numerous reviews suggest the importance of extralegal influences on judicial processes but these are based on anecdotal and case history material rather than controlled research." Efran also suggested that whereas people (but not the law) may believe it appropriate for jurors' decisions to be influenced by a defendant's character, they may be far less likely to agree that defendant facial appearance should be considered by jurors. Indeed, in a survey he found that whereas 79% of students believed that jurors should be influenced by a defendant's character, only 7% believed that physical attractiveness should play a role. In his study male and female students were "given a folder containing a set of instructions, a paragraph representing the judge's instruction to the jury, a fact summary sheet and a verdict sheet. The instructions described a hypothetical college which had initiated a student-faculty court to handle problems such as faculty misconduct and student cheating. The subject was asked to play the role of a student member of the court. The court was said to be hearing the case of a student accused of cheating on an examination." The defendant was facially attractive or unattractive and of the opposite sex to the subject. Attractiveness was found to lead to significantly lower ratings of guilt and punishment from male subjects but not from female subjects. (Efran stated that, "only the differences for male subjects are significant.") In attempting to explain why the effect of facial attractiveness was significant only for male subjects (i.e., female defendants) Efran noted that whereas the male subjects' ratings of defendant physical attractiveness were similar to the prestudy scores obtained from other students, those from the female subjects for the (male) "attractive" condition were not. The male subjects' mean ratings were 5.8 and 3.6 for the attractive and unattractive conditions, respectively, and whereas the female subjects' mean rating for the unattractive condition was the expected 3.5, that for the attractive condition was not significantly higher at 4.1. Efran's explanations of why the female subjects did not rate highly the "attractive" defendant do not include the notion that reading an account of possible cheating may have led the females not to find physically attractive the male faces rated as attractive by other females who received no information about cheating. If there is some validity in the belief that "What is beautiful is good," then it seems entirely reasonable to suppose that "what is bad (i.e., cheating) is not beautiful." This explanation of the lack of an attractiveness effect upon female subjects seems at least as likely as the suggestion put forward by Efran to the effect that for some reason the females did not attend to the attractiveness cues.

In reporting Efran's study authors have not emphasized the contribution to his data of sex of subject. For example, Sigall and Ostrove (1975) reported that Efran "has recently demonstrated that subjects are much more generous when assigning punishment to good looking as opposed to unattractive transgressors," and Sigal, Braden, and Aylward (1978) stated that in Efran's study "attractive defendants of both sexes received more lenient sentences."

Although S. Jacobson and Berger (1974) employed both male and female subjects, they did not report any sex of subject effects. In their study physical attractiveness was manipulated by having just one photograph for each of the levels of attractiveness, whereas Efran tried to make the results of his study more generalizable by using two different faces (i.e., 2 male and 2 female) for each attractiveness level (each subject, of course, seeing only one face). However, a worthy aspect of their attractiveness manipulation was that the same person appeared in both photographs, in one wearing a coat, and glasses and having neatly groomed hair and in the other wearing a t-shirt and jeans with his hair combed in a "loose style" (the former of these two being rated by subjects as significantly more attractive than the latter). In addition to varying physical attractiveness in this way, Jacobson and Berger varied in the case résumé concerning causing death by dangerous driving the amount of repentance shown during the trial by the defendant. Their analysis of data regarding recommended years of imprisonment (the subjects having been told that the defendant had been found guilty) was complicated by their finding that their two independent variables were not, in fact, independent of one another. As well as sentencing the defendant the subjects were asked to rate the amount of repentance shown and the attractiveness of the defendant. Jacobson and Berger noted that within the high-repentance condition the attractive defendant was rated as more repentant than the unattractive defendant, and within the attractive condition the repentant defendant was rated as more attractive than the nonrepentant defendant. Their finding that the effects of subjects' ratings of attractiveness occasioned by their attractiveness variable were affected by other aspects of their study coincides somewhat with our previous explanation of Efran's lack of defendant attractiveness effect on females. Jacobson and Berger found that physical appearance had no effect on sentencing. Schwibbe and Schwibbe (1981) also found defendant facial attractiveness to have no effect on sentencing. In trying to explain why attractiveness had no effect Jacobson and Berger suggested that either their manipulation of attractiveness was not powerful enough (but they did note its significant effect on subjects' ratings of attractiveness) or that their 212 subjects, who were not undergraduates (as is often the case in research on this topic) but members of a parent-teacher association, were unaffected by a successfully manipulated attractiveness variable.

Instructions to Be Impartial

Friend and Vinson (1974) purposely manipulated, along with attractiveness, whether or not the subjects received strong instructions to ignore defendant characteristics when recommending severity of sentence. They noted Landy and Aronson's (1969) finding that the unattractive defendant received longer sentences, but they added that, "Some trial judges, however, are aware of the effects of their biases on the ability to judge fairly and may try to consciously battle their biases in coming to a decision. This attempt to be impartial might cause a judge to lean over backwards to be partial." They hypothesized that the condition in which subjects were instructed to be impartial by agreeing to "completely disregard the personality and characteristics of the defendant," and that, "Your judgment should be based solely on the evidence presented to you," would lead to an attractive defendant being judged more harshly than an unattractive defendant. Subjects who received no such instructions were hypothesized to produce data in line with that found by Landy and Aronson. The subjects read about a criminal case that was "essentially the same as the one constructed by Landy and Aronson" save that the defendant was female rather than male. Attractiveness was manipulated by the defendant being described among other things as having a physically attractive appearance and a friendly personality, or no such details being given ("neutral defendant"), or as being physically unattractive with a criminal record. The subjects' likeability ratings for the attractive defendant were higher than those for the neutral and unattractive defendants, which, rather surprisingly given the nature of the unattractive description, did not differ. An interaction between impartiality and attractiveness was found ($p < .06$) for length of prison sentence. In the "no commitment to impartiality" condition the attractive defendant was sentenced significantly less severely (5 years) than the unattractive defendant (8.6 years), with the neutral defendant receiving 6.6 years. The effect of attractiveness was reversed in the impartiality condition, with the attractive defendant receiving 8.4 years and the unattractive defendant 5.5 years (the neutral defendant receiving 9 years). From these data Friend and Vinson concluded that judges "may be aware of irrelevant dimensions and may compensate by giving unattractive defendants more lenient sentences." They pointed out that jurors, in response to questions from judges and lawyers, often publicly state that they will be impartial and therefore may be unlikely to be harsh on unattractive defendants. From the point of view of real-life criminal justice this may be an important conclusion. It is a pity that Friend and Vinson's manipulation of attractiveness included so many different personal attributes because the attributes that actually caused the reversal of the attractiveness effect cannot easily be identified.

The Nature of the Crime

Sigall and Ostrove (1975) also varied along with defendant attractiveness a factor that may be important in real life, the nature of the crime of which the defendant was accused. They suggested that the findings of some of the early work on the effects of physical attractiveness could be explained with the help of a reinforcement-affect model of attraction that would argue that "beauty, having positive reinforcement value, would lead to relatively more positive affective responses toward a person who has it" and that these would occasion less punishment for attractive defendants. On the other hand, they suggested that a more cognitive explanation could involve people usually assuming that attractive defendants are less likely to transgress again, being more likely to be successful in socially acceptable ways or to be rehabilitated. They contrasted these two suggestions by manipulating the nature of the crime so that although one (burglary) did not encourage the notion that the female defendant's attractiveness might increase the likelihood of similar transgressions in the future, the other (a swindle) possibly did so. They suggested that for a swindle in which the defendant may have been judged to have purposely used her beauty to advantage (she "ingratiated herself with a middle-aged bachelor and induced him to invest money in a non-existent corporation") a cognitive explanation could hypothesize a reversal of the effects of attractiveness, whereas a reinforcement-affect explanation would not.

In their study Sigall and Ostrove varied the physical attractiveness of the defendant's photograph. They were able to gather some data regarding the assumption that the swindle might be assumed to be attractiveness related and the burglary not so by looking at the physical attractiveness ratings given to the defendant by subjects who had not been provided with a photograph of her. These subjects rated the swindler as significantly more physically attractive than the burglar. Those subjects who saw an attractive burglar sentenced her to significantly fewer years (2.8) than those who saw an unattractive burglar (5.2), with the no-photograph burglar receiving 5.1 years. The reverse effect was found for the swindler, who when attractive received 5.5 years but who when unattractive (or no photograph was provided) received 4.4 years, although these differences were not significant. Sigall and Ostrove concluded that "when the crime is attractiveness-related, the advantages otherwise held by good-looking defendants are lost," and they further pointed out that although their manipulation of unattractive appearance was successful, the unattractive defendant was treated no more harshly than the defendant for whom no photograph was provided. Sigall and Ostrove also made the point that their study had little ecological validity.

Even though the studies of the effects of defendant physical appearance published prior to 1976 had very little ecological validity, Solender and Solender (1976) assumed that in real-life court cases attorneys "should be concerned also with the effects their client's physical appearance will have on the trier of fact in a courtroom." Even though it may be true, as Solender and Solender pointed out, that it is extremely difficult to study the effects of defendant physical appearance in real-life court cases, this should not be used as an excuse for blindly assuming that effects found in very artificial situations employing simulated jurors making decisions that real jurors rarely make (e.g., length of prison sentence) would apply in real life.

Solender and Solender (1976) did attempt to make their study more ecologically valid than many studies concerning defendant physical appearance by having their subjects (students) deliberate in groups of 10 concerning their verdict and suggested punishment for a defendant accused of stealing examination question papers. The students saw a photograph of the defendant and read details of the case in which the defendant, when describing the incident in question, made many or few "self-experience references" (i.e., used the first person to describe what happened). No main effects were found for either verdict or punishment, but a significant verdict interaction indicated that in the testimony condition that involved self-experience references the unattractive defendant was rated as more guilty. Thus physical attractiveness only had a significant effect when the defendant made self-experience references. Solender and Solender attempted to explain this complex finding by suggesting that when not making such references the unattractive defendant distanced himself from the situation while suggesting that what happened to him could have happened to the subjects (who were also students). Their conclusions that, "An individual's unattractive appearance can have an adverse effect on the jury," and that, "Having decided that the client is physically unattractive . . . the attorney should, of course, do what he can to change the client's physical appearance to one which will be less offensive" seem to go beyond the evidence available in 1976.

Publication of Null Effects

R. Greenwald (1975), among others (see Bull, 1982) has made the point that it is difficult to get null findings published, but in 1976 Boor reported (although not fully in a referred learned journal) that he had not found any effects of attractiveness in his replication of Sigall and Ostrove's (1975) study (described above). Similarly, Sigal et al. (1978) found, for judgments of guilty versus innocent, no main effects or interactions for physical attractiveness (manipulated in the way that Jacobson and Berger had done, who also found it to have no effect). Their study was accepted for publication in a learned journal perhaps because other factors, such as motivation for the crime, were found to have a significant effect, or because they reported that ratings of the male photographs made by subjects not involved in the first main study had shown them not to differ significantly in terms of attractiveness. However, the male photographs used in Sigal et al.'s second study did differ in rated attractiveness, yet here again no effect of attractiveness on guilt/innocence decisions was found. Sigal et al. noted that studies that have found some effect of physical appearance on simulated jurors have found this more so with female than with male defendants. The also noted that their failure to find an effect of attractiveness may have been due to the fact that their dependent variable employed only two possible levels (guilty/not guilty), whereas other studies have used rated guilt (e.g., on a 7-point scale) and/or severity of sentence. However, they pointed out that their dependent variable has greater ecological validity.

An ecologically valid dependent variable having more than two levels was used by Stephan and Tully (1977), who examined the effects not of a criminal's facial appearance but of that of a plaintiff in a civil suit for damages. Students read a synopsis of court case involving a personal injury suit resulting from an automobile incident. The subjects found in favor of the attractive plaintiff significantly more often, and the (male or female) attractive plaintiff was awarded significantly higher financial damages. (No interaction between attractiveness and plaintiff sex was reported.)

In Piehl's (1977) study students were asked to decide what jurors usually do not decide, that is, the length of prison sentence in a case involving a car driving incident. However, a valuable aspect of this study was that Piehl varied the consequences of the defendant's driving behavior such that some students read that the woman's driving had caused another driver to crash and be killed, some read merely that the other driver's car was "written off," and others read that the incident had no serious consequences for the other driver. Those subjects who "were led to believe that the offender was physically attractive" suggested a prison sentence overall no different from that suggested by those led to believe she was unattractive, or from those given no information about her appearance. There was, however, an interaction between defendant attractiveness and outcome seriousness in that while the attractive offender was treated significantly more leniently in the two less serious outcome conditions; when the outcome involved death the attractive defendant was treated significantly more harshly. (It may be worth noting that in the cases reviewed above where attractiveness led to leniency, the seriousness of the "offenses" was often low.) Piehl made the very worthwhile point that "it seems reasonable that the relative importance and weight of attractiveness may change depending on the conditions and contexts in which judgments are made. Future research may be directed toward specifying these conditions."

In addition to defendant physical attractiveness Leventhal and Krate (1977) also varied crime seriousness (crimes against the person, crimes against property, or victimless crime). Some students were asked to sentence each of 24 male and female defendants (one for each of 24 crimes, with 8 crimes in each crime seriousness category), whereas others merely rated the 24 faces for attractiveness. (The photograph that accompanied each crime was varied across subjects.) A significant negative correlation of 0.42 was found between mean attractiveness rating and mean sentence, demonstrating that the attractive defendant received shorter suggested sentences. Even though less than 18% of the variance in sentencing related to physical appearance, Leventhal and Krate made the important point that, "This simulation clearly demonstrates the necessity for empirical identification and investigation of those extralegal interacting factors found within the sentencing procedure and process."

Unfortunately, far too few studies have explored the effects of defendant facial appearance in actual judicial sentencing. Nevertheless in her 1977 overview of legel aspects concerning defendant appearance Lown suggested that it may not be too speculative to assume that defendant facial characteristics may influence real jurors. She cited a 1965 U.S. court case in which it was argued that the ecologically invalid studies conducted by psychologists should not be ignored merely because ascertaining the effects of certain factors in real-life court cases is very problematical. Lown made the point that, "The possibility that a jury would stereotype a defendant on the basis of his or her physical characteristics raises a constitutional question concerning the accused's right to a fair trial. If stereotyping has a significant effect on guilt determinations, then criminal procedure will have to make adjustments in such cases to ensure that the defendant receives a fair trial." She also pointed out that impressions jurors or judges may form of the defendant based on physical appearance are not likely to be "susceptible to cure by procedural safeguards" since it is not possible to know in real courts if such impressions have been formed. One of her solutions to this problem that Lown admitted would be rather "radical" was for jurors not to be exposed to the defendant's physical appearance. However, we should ask, before any such steps are contemplated, how strong is the evidence for defendant physical appearance being an important factor in court? Up to the date of Lown's paper (i.e., 1977) we believe that the evidence was rather weak.

Poor Studies?

In their 1977 overview of this topic Gerbasi, Zuckerman, and Reis arrived at a similar conclusion, not so much because they cited several studies that had not found a strong effect of facial appearance, but because they were of the view that, "Much of the cited research suffers from methodological and sampling problems, making psychologists and legal professionals justifiably skeptical." They noted that studies had used varying methods of quantifying independent and dependent variables, had used as subjects samples not representative of real juries, and had asked these subjects to do what juries are not usually asked to do. Gerbasi et al. concluded that "unless it is also possible to demonstrate that the data gathered in the laboratory are to some extent generalizable to real juries, these studies will remain without much practical value or external validity."

Kulka and Kessler (1978) attempted to make their study of the effects of physical attractiveness on "jurors" more ecologically valid than preceding studies by having their subjects (again, students) hear, rather than read, an hour-long edited version of a negligent car driving civil trial, and concomitantly see slides of the relevant speakers. Although the present book's review of research up to 1978 would not necessarily lead readers to agree that "there is now ample evidence to suggest that this variable [physical attractiveness] may have a significant effect on the perceptions and decisions of jurors in a courtroom," Kulka and Kessler thought that there was. However, they wisely pointed out that in previous studies "one serious consequence of using written materials which present only a bare-boned account of the situation is to significantly increase the relative importance of an independent variable, since its manipulation then constitutes a much larger share of the total stimulus than in a real trial." Kulka and Kessler compared the data from subjects who had seen an attractive plaintiff plus an unattractive defendant with data from those who had seen an unattractive plaintiff plus an attractive defendant. The former condition led to significantly more decisions in favor of the plaintiff and to larger compensation being awarded. In addition, the defendant was rated as less negligent when attractive. Somewhat to their surprise Kulka and Kessler found that physical attractiveness had no effect on ratings of honesty, goodness, conscientiousness, or trustworthiness, although when attractive the defendant was rated as more likeable. Because of reported problems concerning the missing data from the other two possible conditions in their study (i.e., attractive defendant plus attractive plaintiff, unattractive defendant plus unattractive plaintiff), they were not able to ascertain what separate roles defendant and plaintiff attractiveness played. They did, however, suggest that perhaps the effect of defendant attractiveness on rated negligence was responsible for the significant effects found on compensation, and on jurors finding in favor of the defendant. Kulka and Kessler made the worthwhile point that although controlled studies of the effects of facial appearance on jurors lack ecological validity, this should not lead us to assume that facial appearance has no effect in real-life courtroom. What could lead us to conclude this is our previous review, which demonstrates that by no means all published studies (and what about unpublished ones?) have found a significant effect of physical appearance.

No effect of defendant physical appearance in a swindle case was found by E. Smith and Hed (1979), but they did find defendant attractiveness to reduce recommended sentence length in a burglary case. They suggested, as did Sigall and Ostrove (1975), that the lack of an attractiveness effect for the swindle could be due to their subjects' assuming that the defendant had used her good looks in an unfair way. (The mean difference within the swindle condition was in the same direction as that found by Sigall and Ostrove). Although Smith and Hed did not take the trouble to use subjects who were representative of real jurors but instead used female students, they did at least make an attempt at ecological validity by having subjects deliberate in groups of three and arrive at a collective decision.

Support for an ameliorative effect of defendant physical attractiveness was found by Solomon and Schopler (1978), who observed (using students arriving at individual decisions) in a case of theft that for the attractive defendant shorter sentences were recommended. Solomon and Schopler suggested that even though subjects may judge attractive defendants more leniently, they may also feel pity for an ugly defendant such that a defendant of average attractiveness may be treated the harshest. They found some (limited) evidence to support their hypothesis in that the mean sentence lengths, with increasing attractiveness, were 11.8, 19.4, and 18.5 years, respectively. However, we consider their evidence that the relationship between physical attractiveness and punitiveness is curvilinear to be rather weak. Nevertheless, their hypothesis does suggest that studies of the effects of facial appearance should employ more than two levels of this factor. Rather more noteworthy was Solomon and Schopler's finding that attractiveness did not affect ratings of crime seriousness or defendant responsibility.

Relevant Theory

Izzett and Sales (1979) reviewed the behavioral science literature concerning jurors' reactions to defendants, and they pointed out that no prior reviews had attempted to systematically integrate this literature from a theoretical perspective. They argued that equity theory may be useful in this respect, describing equity theory as being concerned

> with the just distribution of outcomes in a social exchange relationship. Whenever two or more people enter into an exchange they bring with them certain investments or inputs. . . . Individuals also experience various rewards and costs. . . . The net result of rewards minus costs experienced in an exchange are referred to as the outcomes of an exchange. . . . When an individual experiences an inequitable relationship, he/she experiences distress and attempts to restore the relationship to one of equity. . . . Equity restoration may take one of two basic forms. The individual may engage in compensation or justification.

Izzett and Sales suggested that "there is evidence that third party observers to an inequitable exchange react similarly to the participants and attempt to restore the situation to an equitable one," and that, "Since equity theory would predict that our desire to influence the outcomes experienced by others (either favorably or unfavorably) will relate to the nature of the outcomes they cause us to affectively experience, one might expect subject-jurors to be more lenient towards defendants whose social, physical, attitudinal, behavioral or non-verbal inputs result in more favorable or less unpleasant outcomes for the subject juror." They cited findings "that attributing positively evaluated inputs to a defendant as opposed to negatively evaluated inputs will cause subject jurors to treat that defendant more leniently." However, they did not cite the variety of outcomes we have reviewed above regarding the effects of defendant attractiveness. They concluded that, "These results fit nicely into an equity theory framework" because "the physical attractiveness of the defendant can be conceived of as one of many defendant inputs in the equity formulation. The outcome (affective reaction) experienced by the perceiver is likely to be much more pleasant and favorable when viewing a physically attractive target. From an equity perspective the subject jurors will have less of a need to adversely affect the outcomes (sentence) experienced by the physically attractive defendant than the unattractive one."

Izzett and Sales expanded their argument by noting that Izzett and Fishman (1976) had hypothesized and obtained results indicating that a socially attractive defendant with no strong justification for his embezzling behavior would

be sentenced more harshly than a socially unattractive defendant with no justification. Izzett and Fishman reasoned that in the absence of any justification, the attractive defendant would be behaving in the ways that violated the
juror's expectations of him. Upset by such an expectancy violation, the juror
experiencing these intensified feelings of inequity would then dispense more
negative outcomes (sentences) to the socially attractive defendant than usual.
Even though Izzett and Fishman's arguments and reasoning may not be sufficient to constitute a theory as opposed to a notion, theirs was a promising
initial, and rare, attempt to integrate some of the literature, even though in a
footnote they noted that because of the ecological invalidity of the literature
"the external validity of the results of these studies may be limited."

Michelini and Snodgrass (1980) also reviewed some of the existing literature and suggested that at least two explanations were available for why "Research has demonstrated that attractive defendants receive more preferential
treatment than do less attractive defendants." (Like Izzett and Sales, Michelini and Snodgrass tended to ignore studies that had not supported this
finding.) One explanation was the "liking-leniency model" or reinforcement-
affect model of attraction, and the other was the causal inference model,
which argued that "information about a person is used to infer whether his/
her actions are intended and characteristic." These two explanations were
examined in 1975 by Sigall and Ostrove [see above].) In their own study
Michelini and Snodgrass varied defendant character, and whether the character traits were relevant to the likelihood of committing an alleged traffic
felony. They found that only when the character traits were crime relevant
did their manipulation have a significant effect on jurors' guilty or not guilty
decisions. On the other hand, decisions concerning severity of punishment
were affected by character trait manipulation irrespective of their crime relevance. Michelini and Snodgrass took these findings to suggest that "the liking-
leniency and causal inference models may be applicable to the same situation
in complementary ways," with the causal inference model describing how
subjects decided guilt and the liking-leniency model describing how subjects
decided severity of punishment. This is an interesting suggestion that may
account for why some studies have found an effect of defendant facial appearance on one of these outcomes but not on the other. Michelini and Snodgrass
suggested that whereas decisions concerning guilt may be more "objective,"
those concerning sentencing may be more "subjective." Consequently we
would predict that studies of defendant facial appearance would be more likely to find effects on sentencing than on decisions of guilty or not guilty. Our
above review of the literature does suggest that this may well be the case.

Consequences for the Defendant

D. Wilson and Donnerstein (1977) also found it worthwhile to differentiate
between defendant guilt and recommended punishment. In addition they examined whether students acting as "jurors" would be influenced by whether
their decisions would, as in most research, have no real implications for the

defendant or whether their decisions would actually determine what happened to the defendant. Wilson and Donnerstein stated that "we must be concerned with whether or not current methods of studying juror behavior provide us with data that is externally valid," and that, "It should perhaps be noted at this point that the usual 'simulated' jury study is in fact not a simulation at all. . . . Use of the word 'simulation' may imply realism in the experiment that does not truly exist. Perhaps . . . it would be better to call the subjects 'laboratory' jurors." They found defendant character attractiveness to influence judgments about guilt only when subjects believed their decisions to have no real consequences for the defendant. The guilt decisions of those students to whom Wilson and Donnerstein suggested that their decisions would affect whether another student was merely admonished or expelled were not affected by defendant character attractiveness. Unfortunately, Wilson and Donnerstein performed no checks to determine whether the subjects in the "real" implications condition actually believed this to be the case. Regarding severity of punishment, both groups were influenced by defendant character attractiveness. Wilson and Donnerstein concluded that because no effect on guilt verdicts was found for the (assumed) "real"-consequence subjects "current findings from hypothetical jury studies may be misleading." However, they did not fully dichotomize prior studies in terms of whether the dependent variable had been a two-choice guilty/innocent decision or a recommended severity of punishment scale. If they had done this they may not have believed that prior studies had replicated each other.

In their third study Wilson and Donnerstein found no effects of defendant physical attractiveness on guilt or punishment, and that their subjects accurately recalled more of the evidence in the "real" than in the hypothetical condition. In their second study they found no effects of defendant physical attractiveness on guilt or punishment (they suggested that physical attractiveness may have had a greater impact if the defendant was seen in person).

Thus previous research on the effects of defendant facial appearance may be called into question by Wilson and Donnerstein's finding that it only seems to have an effect when those subjects affected by it are aware that their decisions have no real implications for the defendant. The effect of defendant facial appearance may also be qualified by subjects' views concerning the effectiveness of judicial punishment. In McFatter's (1978) study the subjects received instructions to follow one of three sentencing/punishment strategies (retribution, rehabilitation, or deterrence) or no such instructions, and they were informed that the photographed man was guilty. They read an extremely brief (less than 40 words) description of each of 10 crimes and attached to each was a different facial photograph deemed (by prior study and by the subjects' ratings) to be attractive or unattractive. There was an overall significant effect of attractiveness, with the attractive males receiving sentences that were on average 9 months shorter than those given to unattractive males. An interesting significant "attractiveness × crime" interaction for the amount of blame for the crime that could be assigned to "accidental circumstances" revealed that these were blamed much more regarding attractive manslaughterers (causing death while drunk driving) than unattractive manslaughterers. (For the other crimes attractiveness had little effect on the judged contribution of accidental circumstances.) Also of interest is the finding that unattractive offenders were rated as more psychologically abnormal and as more likely to commit crime again in the future. These latter findings relate to similar points made elsewhere in the present book, namely that unattractive people may be blamed more for negative outcomes, and that they are judged as being more likely to consistently transgrees. However, as with many of our reviewed studies, McFatters' was rather lacking in ecological validity.

Real-Life Cases

Stewart (1980) was aware of the criticisms that had been made of previous so-called simulations of juror decision making and he set out to examine whether defendant physical attractiveness would have an effect in real-life criminal court cases. He also wisely decided to examine the effects of physical attractiveness separately both on decisions about guilt and decisions about sentences. Previous studies could be criticized for asking their subjects to do what is not normally done by jurors in criminal cases, that is, decide upon severity of sentence. That previous studies had found physical attractiveness to influence decisions about sentence more so that decisions about guilt could be taken to suggest (a) that only judicially inexperienced people's sentencing decisions would be influenced by physical attractiveness, and (b) that experienced judges' (or magistrates') sentencing decisions may not be influenced by physical attractiveness (although in some instances they may, following proper legal practice, be influenced by defendant character). Stewart had observers attend criminal trials in Pennsylvania and rate defendants on nine 7-point scales including one for physical attractiveness. Interobserver correlations of rated attractiveness were significant ($+0.7$), and rated attractiveness was found to correlate significantly with actual sentence given, with the more attractive defendants receiving more lenient sentences. Although physical attractiveness was not found to be related to guilt decisions, it did significantly correlate with crime seriousness. This relationship is most interesting in itself and relates to points made in this chapter's section on physical appearance and criminality. However, when the effect of crime seriousness was partialled out there was still a significant, although weaker, inverse relationship between physical attractiveness and length of sentence.

From his findings Stewart concluded that "laboratory studies showing similar results must have some degree of ecological validity," and in the light of his findings this is something with which we are led to agree, even though respected lawyers such as Stone (1984) have fairly recently stated of work using mock juries in mock trials that, "Such research may be expected not to establish any fundamental laws of general application to court processes in the future, any more than it has done so far." One worthwhile conclusion that we may arrive at concerning defendant facial appearance is that although the evidence that it affects decisions concerning guilt is weak, the evidence that it affects decisions about sentencing is stronger. If facial appearance does, in fact, really affect this latter type of decision, is this so surprising given that it may be taken (even erroneously) to be a guide to character and that defendant character may affect, and be by society (if not the law) expected to affect, sentencing decisions?

Kerr (1982) pointed out that as the experimental literature on juries has grown, so has concern for its external validity. As had Stewart (1980), Kerr examined the relationship between defendant physical appearance and outcomes in real-life trials. Kerr had access to data concerning the personal characteristics and behavior of principle characters in a number of felony trials that had been gathered by students in the Judicial Administration Program of San Diego State University. Students in groups (or sometimes alone) each recorded for several trials a wealth of information including the hairstyle and attire of defendants and victims. In all, data for 113 criminal jury trials were available, and correlations were computed between trial outcome and the other data collected. (Since a large number of correlations was computed, and since a significance level of $p < .10$ was employed, the possibility of Type I errors was increased.) None of the defendant or victim characteristics or behaviors was found to correlate with trial outcome. Kerr (who did not cite Stewart's [1980] study) concluded that, "It seems likely that defendant and victim characteristics are secondary to evidentiary considerations in most jurors' deliberations."

Evidentiary Factors

Evidentiary factors were varied by Baumeister and Darley (1982). Their two studies showed that the effect of defendant attractiveness (varied not by facial appearance but by written character description) was reduced by increasing the amount of factual material pertinent to the case that was given to the subjects. Only when the facts of the case were "vague" as opposed to "clear-cut" did defendant attractiveness result in more lenient punishment.

Baumeister and Darley suggested that where attractiveness had been found in previous research to have an effect this may have been "the result of a reasonable set of inferences about the details of the incident that are not clearly set forth in the case description." They noted that, "Perceptual research has suggested that bias caused by expectation and prejudice is most potent when the objective stimuli are incomplete and ambiguous."

Worthy though these suggestions are, Baumeister and Darley did not find in the "vague" condition that subjects made "rational attempts to resolve the uncertainty." Rather, they found that when some "facts relevant to the case were left out, subjects simply judged the defendant based on what kind of person he was." For example, in the "vague" condition subjects rated the defendant's transgressive behavior as more "typical" for the unattractive defendant. (For further discussion of this specific point see Chapter 5.)

Evidentiary factors were also mentioned by Dane and Wrightsman (1982) in their review of the effects of defendant characteristics. Although they cited far fewer studies of defendant physical appearance than we have mentioned here, they concluded that, "Our thorough review of the literature completely supports the premise that jurors do react to defendant characteristics." However, they added that, "It is not enough to state that extralegal character- istics have an impact upon jurors' decisions. One must also attempt to asses the extent of that impact. How much do these characteristics effect jurors? Unfortunately, the question is considerably easier to ask than to answer." Dane and Wrightsman made the important point that no single theoretical approach had been successfully used to account for the observed effects of defendant appearance. (We should add that any such theory must attempt to encompass the null effects as well.) They also pointed to some of the ecologi- cally invalid aspects of psychologists' research on this topic, particularly (a) the decisions on which the so-called jurors are asked to focus, (b) the people used as "jurors," (c) the generalizing of findings of effects on recommended sentences to assumed effects on verdicts, and (d) the requirement that "jurors" who may have decided that the defendant was not guilty sentence him anyway.

Bray and Kerr (1982) also focused on methodological considerations of research on the topic of defendant appearance, including the fact that in the majority of studies the proportion of variance accounted for by the indepen- dent variables (e.g., defendant appearance) may be an overestimation of the proportion of variance accounted for in real life, but they pointed out that unrealistic simulations do have certain advantages in terms of experimental control, costs, and ethical factors. They also stated that simulations offer "methodological advantages" that "include the ability to obtain uncon- founded and multiple replications," and although this point is true it serves to highlight the fact that on the topic of defendant facial appearance even the published studies have by no means replicated one another.

Overall Conclusion

The research described in this chapter suggests that many people may well expect there to be a relationship between facial appearance and criminality. However, the evidence supporting the actual existence of such a relationship is not strong. Similarly, as yet no firm conclusion can be offered concern- ing whether facial attractiveness has a consisten effect on recognizability. Also replete with contradictory findings is research on the relationship between facial appearance and attributions of responsibility for crime and other out- comes.

The substantial literature on the effects of defendant facial appearance also is not consensual. At the present time it seems that the simpler the study the more likely it is that an effect of facial appearance will be found. However, in saying this one should not ignore Stewart's (1980) finding that defendant facial appearance seems to have had an effect in real-life court cases.

Chapter 5

The Effects of Facial Appearance in the Educational System

Many studies mentioned in this book have suggested that the social psychology of facial appearance is an important topic. However, Sorrell and Nowak (1981) pointed out that "Developmentalists have virtually ignored appearance variables in their empirical research." This chapter will examine the effects of facial appearance, particularly attractiveness, in the educational setting. We will examine whether teachers (and others) expect attractive students' behavior and academic performance to be different from that of un-attractive students, and whether evaluations of academic work such as essays are influenced by the facial appearance of the supposed authors of this work. Then we will look at those few published studies that have sought to deter-mine whether *in reality* there actually does exist a relationship between facial appearance and academic competence. The effects of teachers' facial appear-ance will also be examined. The focus of the following chapter will move from the educational setting to more widely examine the effects of facial appear-ance on children. In this chapter we have organized the literature so as to be able to differentiate between studies that have merely examined expectations and those that have tested for "real" effects of facial appearance.

In 1968 Rosenthal and Jacobson published a book that created a great deal of discussion. One of their main arguments was that teachers' expectations could have an influence on children's academic performance. This suggestion, in itself, was not that surprising; what caused rather a stir was the power of the effects of teacher expectation that they found in some of their studies. In one study primary-level schoolchildren were given an IQ test and their teachers were told that this test assessed "intellectual blooming" (i.e., that it revealed which children would soon show a marked increase in intellectual functioning). The teachers were then informed of the names of the 20% of their children who had been found to be intellectual bloomers. (The names of these children had, in fact, been chosen at random.) One year later the IQ test was readministered and the results of this revealed that those children labeled as bloomers had shown far greater improvement in scores than had their classmates. This study was subsequently criticized on the grounds of methodology, data analysis and, understandably, ethics. However, it did suggest to M. Clifford and Walster (1973) that perhaps other aspects of schoolchildren might affect teacher expectation.

The Effects of Facial Appearance on Teachers' Expectations

In Clifford and Walster's (1973) study several hundred schoolteachers received a report card concerning a student with whom they were not familiar. The teachers were asked to take part in a project concerned with the usefulness of such cards. The covering letter explained that the informativeness of a variety of types of report card was being examined. The report card used was always, in fact, the same and it provided a fair amount of printed information about a child of somewhat above average ability. The pupil's grades for reading, arithmetic, language, science, art, social studies, music, and "physical attitudes" were reported, as were absences from school. Attached to the report card was a photograph supposedly of the child, and this was the only factor that varied from teacher to teacher. (In the schools at which the teachers in this study worked photographs usually did accompany report cards, and so the presence of a photograph was not unusual.) Photographs of six attractive (three male, three female) and six unattractive children were used. Each teacher was asked to complete an "opinion sheet" regarding the pupil whose report card she or he had received. Four items were included on the sheet and these were concerned with the teacher's estimate of the child's IQ, social relationships with classmates, parental attitudes toward school, and for how long the child would remain in full-time education.

Over 80% of the 500 teachers completed the opinion form they had received. The attractiveness variable was found to have a significant effect upon each of the four items, with attractiveness occasioning more positive ratings (and not interacting with sex of pupil or sex of teacher). However, although the differences in scores between the high and low attractiveness conditions were statistically significant this may have been due to the large sample sizes used rather than any ecologically important effects. The mean IQ scores attributed to the two conditions of attractiveness are not stated explicitly in Clifford and Walster's paper, but from inspection of their Table 1 and examination of their paper's method section, it can be determined that the mean IQ for the high attractiveness condition was 108 and that for the low attractiveness condition was 106! Nevertheless, Clifford and Walster concluded that "Educators as well as parents should be sensitive to the unusual impact a child's attractiveness may have on the way he is treated by others. Unlike such biasing factors as race or socioeconomic status, many of the variables that contribute to physical attractiveness can probably be manipulated with relatively little difficulty. . . . teachers will want to make certain that the child's physical features do not operate as an unwarranted detriment to his intellectual development."

Readers may be wondering what the true IQ scores were of the children whose photographs were used in Clifford and Walster's study. These authors reported that the scores of most of the girls were not available, but for the boys the mean for the (three) attractive ones was 117 and the mean for the (two of the three) unattractive ones was 136.

Expectations and Their Communication

A flurry of studies was published after Clifford and Walster's. Kehle, Bramble and Mason (1974) pointed out that the "Pygmalion in the classroom" effect reported by Rosenthal and Jacobson may consist of at least two aspects, the first being the actual existence of expectations and the second the communication of these expectations and their effects upon pupils. Even though it would seem important to separate out the two parts of the latter aspect, most of the studies published soon after Clifford and Walster's focused only on the first of these. This could be attributed to the obvious necessity of demonstrating whether the effect of physical attractiveness on expectations is a robust phenomenon before embarking upon more complex studies that could examine whether such expectations (a) are meaningfully large and (b) do actually have any effects. However, one has the suspicion that most studies on this topic have investigated merely whether such expectations exist because this sort of study is rather easy to conduct, whereas assessing the effects of such expectations is much more difficult.

Kehle et al. (1974) asked 96 teachers to evaluate a child's temperament in terms of stability/instability and to assess the child's essay. The teachers were provided with a "two-page psychological evaluation" that described the child as being average with respect to temperament. The child's IQ was given as either 110 or 80, and an attractive or unattractive photograph (which was either female or male, black or white) was included. An essay of "average" standard on "What I Think About" was attached. The effects on temperament rating and essay evaluation of physical attractiveness sex, race, and IQ were examined. The factors of race and IQ had no main effects and no effect of physical attractiveness on temperament rating was found. There was, however, a significant attractiveness by sex interaction for essay evaluation. The essay supposedly written by an attractive female was (as could be expected from the studies reported below on essay evaluation) rated higher than when it was believed to have been written by an unattractive female. The effect of attractiveness was actually reversed (and smaller) for the male author but, unfortunately, Kehle et al. did not report whether this atypical effect of attractiveness (for the male) was significant or not. They concluded that "the present study lends support to the position that the formulation of teacher expectations may not be as pervasive as once was feared."

Are Other Factors More Important than Facial Appearance?

A similar conclusion regarding physical attractiveness was arrived at by LaVoie and Adams (1974), who sensibly varied, in addition to physical attractiveness, another pupil factor, conduct, which may in real-life influence teachers' judgments. They noted that in 1972 Dion reported severe behavioral transgressions committed by a physically attractive child to be judged as less likely to reflect an enduring disposition toward antisocial behavior than those of an unattractive child. (Details of this and other studies relating physical appearance to asocial behavior are mentioned in Chapter 6).

In the study by LaVoie and Adams 350 teachers evaluated a student whose progress report card they received. The teachers were told that the study was focusing on how useful and informative such cards could be. The report card was of the above-average student in reading, language, mathematics, art, and music. The information regarding the conduct of the child and the attractiveness of the child's photograph were varied. "Grades in personal and social growth, work habits and attitudes were for the good conduct student mostly A's and B's with some C's, whereas the poor conduct student's grades were C's and D's with a few F's." The attendance record of the two students also differed. "The good student's attendance record showed few absences or times tardy while the poor conduct student was frequently absent or tardy. These manipulations were designed to present a student who was either well adjusted to the school regime or had a conduct problem." The photograph on the report card was of high, medium, or low attractiveness. The teachers were asked to rate the child for IQ, grade point average, percentile rank in class, leadership potential, type of vocation, and the highest level of education expected of the pupil.

No effect of physical attractiveness on any of these ratings was found, whereas conduct affected ratings of IQ, percentile rank, level of education, and leadership potential. LaVoie and Adams pointed out that these effects of conduct could create self-fulfilling prophecies, as could attractiveness if this latter variable were to have an effect. They made the worthwhile statement that, "The failure to replicate the attractiveness effect reported by Clifford and Walster (1973) was probably the result of several factors. Since the teachers in the Clifford and Walster study were not provided with information on the child's conduct the attractiveness variable was not pitted against conduct, a most pervasive factor in teacher evaluation." LaVoie and Adams also suggested that Clifford and Walster may have found an effect of attractiveness because the teachers Clifford and Walster used were accustomed to seeing photographs on pupil's report cards, whereas those employed by LaVoie and Adams were not. However, this does not seem an adequate explanation of why these two studies arrived at different conclusions regarding the effects of attractiveness. One could just as easily argue that teachers accustomed to seeing a photograph on a child's report card would be less likely to be influenced by it. Another factor mentioned by LaVoie and Adams concerned how extreme Clifford and Walster's photographs were regarding attractiveness compared with theirs. They made the valuable point that apparently similar studies concerning physical attractiveness may not arrive at the same conclusions if somewhat different levels of attractiveness are used.

In 1974 these two authors also published some of the other data gathered in their study described previously.. In this paper (Adams & LaVoie, 1974) the teachers' predictions of the child's peer relations, popularity, study work habits, and in-school behavior, plus parental interest in the child's school performance were examined. It was found that whereas the teachers' predictions on all measures were significantly influenced by the child's conduct, facial attractiveness exerted little effect. Only for the teachers' evaluations of study work habits and of in-school behavior were effects of attractiveness found. It was the medium level of attractiveness that led to the highest ratings of study work habits, followed by the low level of attractiveness, with the high level of attractiveness receiving the lowest ratings. For in-school behavior the unattractive children received the highest ratings. In attempting to account for their findings Adams and LaVoie suggested that, "Through past experience teachers may have observed that unattractive students compensated for their deficiency in physical attractiveness by more concerted effort in school." (This may be one explanation of why, in the Bull and Stevens [1979] study, reported below, the unattractive female author who took the trouble to type her essay received high marks.)

Concerning the lack of effects of attractiveness found in their study LaVoie and Adams (1974) concluded that "interpersonal factors such as conduct, warmth and personality are much more influential determinants of teacher assessment than external factors such as physical attractiveness," and that "as teachers interact with students over a period of time, interpersonal factors such as conduct become more influential in teacher evaluation because these factors are given greater weight in the teachers' cognitive system."

In 1975 Adams and LaVoie published a further study that employed the same methodology as that used in their 1974 studies. This time the raters were parents who were asked to make predictions concerning a child whose student progress report they had received for IQ, grade point average, percentile rank in class, likely highest educational attainment, work habits, school attitudes, creativity, peer relations, popularity, election as a class representative, in-school behavior, leadership, teacher involvement with the child, teacher permissiveness toward the child, parental interest in the child, social class of the family, parental discipline practices, parental permissiveness toward the child, and pleasantness of an outing with the child. The parents were told by letter that the purpose of the exercise was to enable researchers to assess the amount of information gained by parents from student progress reports. Adams and LaVoie found, as they had done in their previous studies, that conduct had a much greater effect than physical attractiveness. Conduct had significant effects on many of the ratings, whereas attractiveness had only limited effects. Attractiveness led to higher popularity ratings, to greater likelihood of being elected a class representative, and to higher vocational attainment ratings for good-conduct boys and poor-conduct girls. Poor-conduct children, if attractive, were rated higher on in-school behavior. For boys, but not for girls, attractiveness led to higher ratings of social class and to predictions that parental discipline practices would be based more on the use of reasoning than physical punishment.

Adams and LaVoie concluded that

> Among parents, the physical attractiveness stereotype does not seem to influence greatly their expectancies. . . . These findings do not conflict necessarily with the physical attractiveness stereotype, rather it appears that this stereotype is more apparent in certain situations . . . [and it] may bias parents to the extent that they provide more encouragement for their attractive children to participate in social activities. This differential reinforcement resulting from physical attractiveness undoubtedly may influence self concept formation.

However, Adams and LaVoie pointed out, when offering an explanation of why conduct seems a more pervasive factor, that physical attractiveness may initially influence expectancy, but when certain additional information is available this information may well reduce or obliterate the attractiveness effect.

Adams and Cohen (1976a) found that certain sorts of information did not obliterate a physical attractiveness effect. They had 490 teachers read a cumulative report card of a child who was "working at slightly above average level." Details of the child's "home climate" were also provided, the climate being either "deprived" or not deprived. Attached to each card was a photograph of an attractive or unattractive boy or girl, who was described as being either high or low in verbal ability. The teachers were asked to predict the child's "(a) probability of becoming a classroom representative, (b) being seen as an enjoyable person in an interpersonal experience, (c) family size, and (d) social status." Adams and Cohen found that, "Physical attractiveness emerged as a relatively strong variable. Physically attractive, in comparison to unattractive, children were expected to be more likely to become class representatives, to come from smaller families, and to hold higher social status." In their analysis they wisely took the trouble to determine the values of omega-square since

> The reality of analysis of variance is that this statistical tool is quite powerful when factorial designs are used, but the sensitivity to pick up significant differences (particularly when the sample size is large) does not imply large differences. This sensitivity is created somewhat artificially by the large sample size and multiple factors which pull variance from the error term, resulting in large, but potentially meaningless F values.

The percentage values for omega-square for the three significant effects of attractiveness were 2, 24, and 11, respectively, thus demonstrating that whereas facial appearance had a very weak effect on likelihood to become a class representative, its effect on social status and particularly family size was fairly strong.

Adams and Cohen (1976b) also published data from the previous study concerning the teachers' predictions of the child's "(a) creative ability, (b) level of intellectual ability, (c) vocational training ultimately obtained, (d) educational grouping or placement, and (e) quality of teacher-student interaction." It was found that physical attractiveness had a significant effect on the first four judgment scales, with the percentage values for omega-square being 2, 12, 26, and 8, respectively. In both publications (1976a and 1976b) few interactions of attractiveness with the other factors were reported.

Is There a Relationship Between Facial Appearance and Behavior?

Adams and LaVoie (1975) noted that finding strong effects of physical attractiveness on expectancies would not necessarily mean that people would actually *behave* differently as a function of the child's appearance. Much more research is needed on this more crucial point. Most of the studies of the effects of facial attractiveness on teachers have been very artificial in nature. However, a study by Adams and Cohen (1974) had much more ecological validity. The teacher-pupil interactions of three experienced female teachers of kindergarten, fourth-, and seventh-grade classes were observed during the third and fourth days of a new school year. These days were chosen because at this time the teachers would not yet know their pupils well. After the classroom observations had been completed the teachers were asked to rate each of their pupils for (a) facial attractiveness (b) disruptiveness, (c) verbal fluency, and (d) "physical appearance." The verbatim records of the observed teacher-pupil interactions were classified "blind" as being from the teacher (a) support statements, or (b) controlling statements, or (c) neutral statements. None of the individual teachers' ratings of their pupils were found to be related to the nature of their interactive statements, except for facial attractiveness, where for the seventh-grade pupils (only) more teacher-pupil interaction took place for the attractive pupils. However, since only one teacher was observed for each age group of pupil, no generalization of this finding to other teachers should be made. More generalization would be significant findings across all three teachers. Although the raw data suggested a tendency for the attractive children to receive more support statements and fewer control statements, the only significant finding was that the pupils rated by their teachers as below average in facial attractiveness experienced more neutral statements than did those of above-average attractiveness.

This study of Adams and Cohen is much more the kind of research that one would like to see psychologists conducting. These authors pointed out that even their study was in some ways rather limited, and one hopes that someone will conduct a similar yet wide-ranging study.

Does Appearance Modify the Effects of Other Factors?

Like Adams and LaVoie, J. Rich (1975) examined whether the effects of a child's conduct on teachers would be affected by the physical attractiveness of the child. He cited Dion's (1972) finding that facial appearance influenced judgments of misbehavior but noted that "her subject population consisted of undergraduate college women most of whom had probably never assumed a position of responsibility for the socialization of children. Parents, or teachers, however, may be less influenced by a child's physical attractiveness than were Dion's subjects." Rich also made the valid point that

> Even if it were definitely demonstrated that teachers have differential expectations for attractive and unattractive children, and they treat such children differently on a first-impression basis, it would be important to determine the effects of the stereotype when new information describing the child is available. What value is there in knowing that teachers' expectations of the attractive child are positive and those of the unattractive child negative if these expectations are immediately discounted when new information is provided? For the physical attractiveness variable to be of real significance to educators, it must be shown that a child's physical appearance affects teachers' evaluations beyond first impressions.

In his own study (which along with that of Dion [1972], is reported more fully in Chapter 6) Rich found that although "attractive children generally receive more desirable personality ratings than unattractive children, a misbehavior was deemed less undesirable" by experienced schoolteachers "if attributed to unattractive rather than attractive children."

M. Ross and Salvia (1975) in their study failed to vary along with physical attractiveness the kinds of factors that Rich would have wished. They gave to teachers a child's report file "which presented evidence of below average academic functioning, low IQ, some evidence of immaturity, and no significant behavior problems."

Attached to the file was a photograph of an attractive or unattractive boy or girl. The teachers were asked to indicate their strength of agreement with each of four statements that were concerned with whether (a) placement in a special class for educable mentally retarded students would be appropriate for the child, (b) further psychological evaluation of the child would probably reveal a lower level of functioning than was indicated in the report, (c) the child would experience future difficulties in peer relationships, and (d) further academic difficulty could be expected from the child. For each statement a significant effect of attractiveness was found. Ross and Salvia concluded that, "The fact that relatively unattractive children were rated more negatively presents potential problems for educators. There is a great deal of subjective judgment in educational decisions and unattractive children seem to be at a distinct disadvantage simply because they are unattractive."

In 1982 Salvia came to a similar conclusion regarding the effects of pupils' facial attractiveness upon another group of educational professionals, this time school psychologists (Elovitz & Salvia, 1982). A "psychological report" was sent to over 1,000 school psychologists and 324 returns met various criteria so that the data could be analyzed. The report concerned "a third grade child referred by his/her teacher for poor school achievement and behavioral problems." A variety of test data was presented that clearly supported the teacher's referral. One of several attractive or unattractive facial photographs was attached to the report. The psychologists were required to rate the child on a variety of dimensions and an overall effect of attractiveness was found.

The judgment most responsible for the attractiveness effect was the amount of agreement with the statement that. "A program for the mentally retarded would probably be most appropriate for this child." Other judgments that revealed a fairly strong attractiveness effect were (a) "A program for the social-emotionally disturbed," and "A program for the learning disabled would probably be most appropriate for this child," and (b) "The percentage of this child's school day that could probably be successfully integrated into regular fourth grade classes next September is. . . ." Weak, but statistically significant effects were found for "This child will experience future difficulties in peer relationships," and for "Further psychological evaluation of this child would probably reveal a lower level of functioning than was indicated in the report." No effects of attractiveness were found for (a) "Placement in a special class would be appropriate for this child," (b) "A recommendation should be made to return this child to the same grade for the next year," and (c) "Future academic difficulty can be expected for this child." These null effects may have been due partly to the report indicating such a low level of achievement that no other factor could redeem judgments on these scales. (This points to the need to vary more than just the facial appearance factor in studies of this sort.) The data on the dimensions for which there was an attractiveness effect reveal that whereas a program for mentally retarded children was not deemed so appropriate for the attractive stimuli (who were expected to have fewer difficulties in peer relationships, and who would not reveal a lower level of functioning upon further psychological evaluation), a program for social-emotionally disturbed children and one for learning disabled children was deemed more appropriate for them.

Elovitz and Salvia (1982) noted that the greatest effect of facial attractiveness was on "classifications carrying the least stigma," which were "acceptable for attractive pupils, while the most stigmatizing classification was far more acceptable for unattractive pupils." They concluded that

> The direction of bias suggests these results are not due only to more positive expectations held for attractive children in general. The negative expectations held for unattractive students implies an association between the mental retardation (MR) label and unattractiveness. . . . School psychologists may be reacting to a realistic expectancy that unattractive children are more likely to be mentally retarded, as individuals with MR often have discriminable physical traits . . . that are considered unattractive.

Whatever the validity of this last statement may be (and various parts of this book mention this topic), we should note (as for other studies mentioned in this chapter) that facial attractiveness was found to have an effect when the person/material being reacted to was in some way of poor quality. Whether attractiveness would have had similar, or any, effects if Elovitz and Salvia has employed a "good" psychological report or had varied any other relevant factors is not possible to say.

Therefore we would like to emphasize that the true implications of the findings of studies that simply vary physical attractiveness and no other ecologically valid variables cannot be determined. One needs to determine the effect of physical appearance when it is in competition with other relevant factors. This was done by Boor and Zeis (1975), who asked students to judge from facial photographs the IQ of other students whom they had never met. Although the stimulus persons' assigned grade point average, college year, and college major significantly influenced the students' judgments of IQ, facial attractiveness did not. It is unlikely that the lack of an attractiveness effect found in this study was due to its use of students as judges rather than teachers, who are typically used in studies in this area. A similar null effect of physical attractiveness on student teachers' ratings of academic attributes of schoolboys (whom they had never met) was found by Tompkins and Boor (1980), although attractiveness was found to affect ratings of social attributes (e.g., "popularity with peers").

Experienced teachers were used by Demeis and Turner (1978) in a study in which photographs of attractive and unattractive fifth-grade boys accompanied tape-recorded responses (of 90 to 120 seconds' duration) to the question "What happened on your favorite T.V. show the last time you watched it?" Each of the 68 female teachers responded to 12 pupils on a measurement scale used to rate speakers' (a) personalities, (b) current and (c) future academic abilities, and (d) quality of response. Each of the independent variables (i.e., race of face and black versus standard spoken English, as well as facial attractiveness) had a significant main effect on all four types of rating. However, whereas the effect of the three levels of attractiveness for the four types of rating was as predicted for white faces (i.e., the higher the attractiveness the more positive the ratings), for the black faces those of medium attractiveness occasioned the most positive ratings. (It is possible that this unpredicted effect is due to all the teachers being white.) For the black faces, those of high attractiveness did lead to more positive ratings than those of low attractiveness, but the use by Demeis and Turner of the third level of attractiveness (i.e., medium) underlines the need for studies of attractiveness not to use merely two (usually arbitrary, although different) levels of attractiveness.

Adams (1978) also varied race of face as well as physical attractiveness, but he failed to vary any other factor (apart from sex) that might affect teachers' expectations. A total of 240 female preschool teachers (112 of whom were black) in four midwest states were interviewed in private by a white male interviewer. Each teacher read the same "folder statement" about a child, but the sex, race, and attractiveness of the accompanying photograph varied across teachers. The teachers then rated the child on intellectual potential, academic achievement, classroom behavior, social behavior, and athletic ability. The effect of attractiveness (only two levels were used) was significant for intellectual potential, academic achievement, social behavior, and athletic ability, but not for classroom behavior (where the difference between the two means was in the predicted direction). Few meaningful interactions of attractiveness with the other independent variables were found. Adams concluded that, "A child's degree of attractiveness . . . had a strong influential effect upon preschool teachers' initial expectations for the child's behavior and likely school success." However, research needs to closely examine whether, in fact, such expectations have any subsequent effects. Given the time and effect that Adams must have put into the contacting and interviewing of the 240 teachers (and retesting 32 of them 1 month later in a praiseworthy and successful reliability check), it is a pity that he did not take up the suggestion made by Adams and LaVoie (1975) that studies examining the effects of physical attractiveness in the educational setting should concomitantly vary the nature of other scholastically relevant information (e.g., the "folder statement").

Facial Appearance Versus "Subnormality"

Aloia (1975) did vary along with facial attractiveness a factor that he hypothesized would influence trainee teachers' expectations concerning a child's "subnormality." In response to each child's photograph the subjects in this study were required to rate the child along 5-point scales for (a) clumsy-skilled, (b) strange-ordinary, (c) unintelligent-bright, (d) helpless-capable, and (e) timid-confident. Thus, "The rating of perceived subnormality for each photograph could range from 5 to 25." Unlike previous studies that had varied attractiveness by employing "normal"-looking children, in Aloia's study one set of photographs (deemed unattractive) was of children in an institution for mentally retarded persons "who possessed obvious signs of physical deformity or stigmata, e.g. Down's Syndrome." The other photographs (deemed attractive) were of children "attending regular classes who possessed no signs of physical deformity." (Chapter 7 contains details of much more research on the various effects of facial deformity.) The photographs were accompanied by one of the following statements: "(i) this child is ten years old and mentally retarded, (ii) this child is ten years old and normal, (iii) this child is ten years old." Each student took part in only one of the study's six conditions. Although no check seems to have been carried out to determine whether the faces deemed attractive or unattractive did in fact differ in attractiveness, it was found that "the presence of physical stigmata in the unattractive photographs influenced judgments of subnormality," whereas the nature of the accompanying labeling statement did not have a significant effect. The effect of attractiveness was similar across all three levels of label, thus suggesting that attractiveness had a powerful effect. However, one should ask whether Aloia's method of varying the other factor in his study (i.e., the label) was a worthwhile one.

W. Shaw and Humphreys (1982) also examined the effects of children's facial appearance on teachers' expectations. They hypothesized that photographs of children with a normal dental appearance, in contrast to those with a visible dental anomaly, would, when attached to a school record card, favorably bias teachers' questionnaire replies regarding academic, social, and personality expectations. It was also predicted that the teachers' judgments would be influenced by "background" facial attractiveness. The record card employed was of a type commonly used in Wales, and it presented the educational history of an "average" child. Each of 320 experienced teachers rated the child whose card they received on 16 scales, and they were led to believe that the study was concerned with "the validity and usefulness of the information contained in school record cards." The facial photograph on the card varied in a number of ways. It was either male or female, and high or low in "background" attractiveness. In addition there were five variants of each child's dental appearance: "normal," cleft lip, missing incisor, crowded incisors, and prominent incisors. (As reported in Chapter 7, Richman [1976, 1978] noted that among children with a cleft lip, despite their IQs being in the normal range, reduced educational achievement was observed.)

Shaw and Humphreys found that the variable of dental appearance had no effects upon the teachers' responses. Furthermore, "background" attractiveness of the face had an effect on only 1 of the 16 scales (likeability), and on 7 scales it was the unattractive face that occasioned (nonsignificantly) more positive ratings. Although Shaw and Humphreys did not check in their study that the faces they deemed attractive were in fact so, they report that the same faces' attractiveness had significantly influenced children's and adults' judgments in a previous study. They concluded that "this may suggest that teachers, more familiar with the presence of children, are less susceptible to variations in physical appearance, or perhaps more likely that the provision of additional information (the report card) and the naturalistic setting of the experiment, overrides the effects of the physical appearance stereotype." Shaw and Humphreys wisely asked the teachers to rate their confidence on a 5-point scale after making each of their 16 judgments. They noted that, "An examination of the mean confidence rating for each of the 16 questions revealed that in no instances were high mean values obtained." Thus in this, and therefore perhaps other similar studies, the teachers were making evaluative judgments but with little confidence. Future studies should address the issue of how confident people (including teachers) are when asked to rate a person on the basis of physical appearance alone, especially when that person is a stranger.

Is the Research Poor?

Morrow and McElroy (1984) similarly found that students' physical attractiveness had minimal effects on teachers' evaluations. With regard to previous research on the effects of facial appearance in the educational setting they made the very worthwhile points that "the research procedures followed . . . are often quite limited and may contribute to such overwhelming transparency concerning the research objectives as to jeopardize the results," and that "the absence of data on explained variation suggests that one explanation for the number of mixed findings in past studies is that the magnitude of the attractiveness bias is relatively small and is highly sensitive to sample size in determination of statistical significance."

In their own study Morrow and McElroy varied the to-be-evaluated students' previous academic performance as well as their physical attractiveness. In addition, a repeated measures design was employed (which has rarely been used in this area of research). Each of 55 male faculty who taught business courses at a Midwestern university evaluated information regarding eight male and female students who were studying business. The statements (in folders) describing each student's course work to date were varied (i.e., well above or below class average), as was the accompanying photograph (attractive or unattractive). The subjects were required to indicate their willingness to assign a high or a low final course grade to the student, to advise continuing study of business courses, to write a favorable recommendation for the student, to serve as the student's advisor, to provide an opportunity for the student to earn extra credit, and to indicate the extent to which they would like to have the student in an additional course that they taught.

No main effects of attractiveness on any of the judgments were found, and therefore Morrow and McElroy concluded that this variable has minimal effects when other ecologically valid independent variables are manipulated. However, a possible criticism of their study is that the subjects may not have bothered to look at the photographs. Although Morrow and McElroy seem unaware of this possibility, the finding of a significant interaction between attractiveness and previous academic performance suggests that the subjects may well have processed the photographs. This interaction (which occurred for only two of the response scales) led Morrow and McElroy to state that "a pro-attractiveness bias may be achieved only when competency is low or in question." However, they noted that even here "the magnitude of the bias is quite small (i.e. omega-square $< 1\%$)." Thus they concluded that "the importance attributed to physical attractiveness should be reassessed."

Martinek (1981) did not ask teachers to evaluate pupils whom they did not know; rather he asked two physical education teachers to rate students in classes that they taught for 30 minutes per week for several months on 7-point scales for "(a) overall performance in physical skill; (b) social relations with peers; (c) cooperative behavior during class; (d) ability to reason." Photographs of the pupils were rated for attractiveness by adults who did not know the pupils. In addition two trained observers noted many details of actual class interactions between the teachers and the pupils. The data revealed a significant effect of attractiveness on teachers' expectations concerning physical skill performance, social relations with peers, and (for only one of the two teachers) cooperative behavior during class. Unfortunately, Martinek reported no data with which to determine whether these teacher expectations bore any relationship to actual behavior along these dimensions. However, he does state that the teachers were unaware that physical appearance was involved in the study. Martinek's behavioral data regarding teacher-pupil interactions mostly revealed nonsignificant effects of physical attractiveness on teacher/pupil behavior. Only for one of the several class groups did the teachers show more "acceptance and use of student ideas" for the more attractive students.

Conclusion

Overall, it can be concluded from the studies reported in this section concerning the effects of facial appearance on teachers' expectations that there is very limited evidence of such effects, and this evidence has been found largely with teachers' reactions to the faces of pupils whom they have never met. The question of whether such expectations actually do influence pupil performance is much more difficult to investigate than is the mere existence of such expectations. Studies of the relationship between facial appearance and academic performance will be examined below once we have looked at studies of the effects of facial appearance upon the evaluation of academic work.

The Effects of Facial Appearance on Academic Work

Landy and Sigall (1974) asked male college students to evaluate an essay (on the effects of television on society) supposedly written by a female college student. The students were told that the essays were to be entered in a contest run by a television station and because of this some background about the author of each essay was provided. By means of a photograph attached to each essay some of the evaluators were led to believe that the essay writer was physically attractive and others that she was unattractive. In addition, one half of the students read an essay that was "well written, grammatically correct, organized and clear in its presentation of ideas," whereas the other subjects read the essay that was poorly written, disorganized, and simplistic. Subjects' evaluations of the essay were significantly affected by attractiveness for the poor essay but not for the good essay. Landy and Sigall made an "interesting speculation" concerning this statistical interaction effect when they put forward the idea that if a person's work is competent then personal appearance may be less likely to influence evaluations of that work than when the quality of work is poor. They suggested that "if you are ugly you are not discriminated against a great deal as long as your performance is impressive. However, should your performance be below par, attractiveness matters: you may be able to get away with inferior work if you are beautiful. . . . Perhaps this expectancy leads evaluators to give physically attractive persons the benefit of the doubt when performance is sub-standard." This interactional effect in which physical attractiveness is much more important in poor than in good circumstances is somewhat of a recurrent theme in the present book.

The subjects in Landy and Sigall's study were also asked to evaluate the essay writer on intelligence, sensitivity, talent, and overall ability. A physical attractiveness main effect was found both for overall ability and for the other three measures combined. Again, whereas for the poor essay there were significant effects of author appearance, this factor had no effect when the essay was good in quality. Landy and Sigall concluded that "physical appearance not only affects the way in which others react to a person, it also affects the way in which they react to a person's accomplishments." These researchers made the further point that the effects they discovered could lead to "efforts to alter this tendency and the inequalities it must produce," although they noted that they had used only females as essay authors and only male evaluators.

Is Facial Appearance More Important in the Evaluation of Females' Work?

Since some studies of physical appearance (and common parlance) suggest that reactions to females and therefore possibly their work may be more affected by their physical attractiveness than are those to males, Bull and Stevens (1979) varied the physical attractiveness of both sexes of essay writers. Also, instead of using a semirandom sample of students as essay evaluators, most of the evaluators in Bull and Stevens' study were experienced teachers. In our study the subjects were told that they were taking part (during their in-service training) in a study of interassessor agreement in the evaluation of essays. In fact all the subjects read the same essay in terms of its content. However, for some it was written in a handwriting found in a pretest to be "good" and for others in a handwriting found to be "poor." The remaining third of the subjects read the essay in typed form. To the essay was attached a school report card that gave the writer's initials, surname, and address together with details of past educational achievement. This report card was the same for all evaluators and they were told that they were provided with it so as to give them some idea of the academic standard of the writer. A photograph, supposedly of the essay writer, was stapled on the report card and a paper clip attached the card to the essay. The paper clip, which it was necessary to remove in order to gain access to the essay, was placed across the photograph and in this way it was hoped that the markers would notice the photograph which was either of a male or a female (age approximately 20 years) who, by prior determination, was either attractive or unattractive. The evaluators were asked to read the essay and then to rate it on four dimensions (style, ideas, creativeness, and general quality). They were also asked to rate the writer for intelligence, sensitivity, talent, and general ability.

For the male author no significant effects were found for any of the judgments. For the female author no significant main effects of attractiveness were found. However, for the female author significant interactions were found between attractiveness and the factor of typed versus good versus poor handwriting for judgments of intelligence, talent, ideas, and general quality. If Bull and Stevens' study had used only the two handwritten forms of the essay then main effects of attractiveness would have been found on these four dimensions, attractiveness occasioning higher marks. However, it was found for the typed version of the essay that physical attractiveness led to lower scores being awarded. In 1979 we were unable to offer an explanation of why the expected effect of attractiveness was reversed when the essay was typed and we are still at a loss to do so, save for suggesting the possibility that when an unattractive person is seen to try very hard (the typed essay?) then positive evaluation may occur. However, at least for the female authors' handwritten versions of the essay the Bull and Stevens study does replicate the outcome of the study by Landy and Sigall (1974). That we found no effects of male author physical attractiveness could possibly be attributed to Landy and Sigall's notion that author attractiveness may not affect essay evaluation unless the essay content is poor, since for our male author condition the ratings tended to be slightly above rather than below the midpoint of the rating scales. However, this was also the case for our female authors' ratings.

Kaplan (1978) also designed a study to see if Landy and Sigall's outcome could be replicated. Like Bull and Stevens he used female and male authors but in addition he purposely varied the sex of essay evaluator. In his first experiment Kaplan had male and female undergraduates evaluate a female's essay employing a similar procedure to that employed by Landy and Sigall (1974), but purposely using an essay of poor quality for the reasons Landy and Sigall suggested (see above). Since Kaplan hypothesized that people may discriminate against the most attractive members of their own sex, he considered that it was important to examine how females might judge an essay written by an attractive female. Kaplan reported that few main effects were occasioned by author attractiveness and that only ratings of sensitivity and ability were affected by this factor. However, examination of the statistical interactions revealed that whereas evaluations by females seemed not to be affected by female author attractiveness, the males' ratings of female author sensitivity, talent, and style were affected. In his second experiment Kaplan (1978) used male instead of female authors and he found no effects of attractiveness on either female or male evaluators. Thus his second study replicates the outcome of Bull and Stevens (1979) regarding male authors. Kaplan concluded that his "results have practical significance. In most situations the work of women is evaluated by men. In comparison to male evaluators, females are less likely to be biased by external factors when evaluating other women. In addition, female judges tend to give more favorable evaluations in general. Thus women should demand that their work be evaluated by other women."

Like Kaplan, Anderson and Nida (1978) varied both sex of evaluator and sex of author. In addition they employed three levels of physical attractiveness of author and three levels of essay quality. Again a procedure similar to that of Landy and Sigall (1974) was used. A main effect of physical attractiveness was found only for ratings of "composite essay quality," and further analysis revealed that this was due to a significant difference between two extreme levels of attractiveness. The only other significant effects were three-way interactions between physical attractiveness, sex of rater, and sex of author for ratings of "composite essay quality" and "overall ability." Anderson and Nida noted that from same-sex raters, authors of medium level of attractiveness received the highest evaluations (thus partly supporting Kaplan's notion), whereas from opposite-sex raters authors of high attractiveness received the highest ratings. Authors of low attractiveness uniformly received low evaluations. In connection with Landy and Sigall's (1974) suggestion of a possible interactive effect of physical attractiveness and essay quality, no interactive effects at all of essay quality were found by Anderson and Nida, who concluded that high physical attractiveness only leads to more positive evaluations from raters of the opposite sex.

Holahan and Stephan (1981) also examined whether sex of evaluator would be important in the evaluation of a female author's essay. In addition they obtained subjects' scores on an Attitude Towards Women Scale since they hypothesized that an individual's sex-role attitudes may be associated with the degree to which he or she is influenced by a physical attractiveness stereotype. They pointed out that "the joint influence of physical attractiveness, sex-role attitudes, and competence is unknown." Male and female undergraduates saw a facially attractive or unattractive female author of an essay which was either of high or low quality on the topic of "The Consequence of No Longer Watching Television." No effects of attractiveness were found upon subjects' evaluations of the essays. For the rating scales concerning evaluation of the writer's talent there was for male subjects only an interaction effect of attractiveness. For the low-quality essay the attractive author was rated as having more talent; however, for the high-quality essay it was the unattractive author who received the higher talent rating. On ratings of author likability it was again only the male subjects who were affected by her attractiveness. For them there was a significant main effect of attractiveness occasioning more liking, but significant interactions revealed that the unattractive author was more likeable for males with more positive attitudes toward women and who read the high-quality essay, and for males with medium attitudes and who read the low-quality essay.

Holahan and Stephan concluded from their findings that the lack of effect of attractiveness on essay evaluation "probably reflects both the fact that physical attractiveness is more relevant to judgments about a person than to judgments about an essay and that assessments of an essay are more subject to objective verification (and thus are less likely to be distorted) than are assessments of the person." That attractiveness had no effect on females' ratings of author attributes was taken in 1981 to suggest that "because of changing opportunities and aspirations of females in our society . . . women are not now using physical attractiveness in their judgments of other females." Thus not only subject sex differences but differences in males' attitudes toward women are of importance. Holahan and Stephan argued that, "Previous studies in which physical attractiveness main effects have been found and in which individual differences among subjects have not been examined may have overestimated the importance of this variable." To this we might add that few, if any, studies have also purposely varied the social context (Bem, 1974) in which data are gathered on the social psychological effects of facial appearance.

In a study by Cash and Trimer (1984) some attempt was made to vary the "context" in which an essay was written (i.e., its topic). They asked female college students to assess a poor-quality essay written by a facially attractive or unattractive author who was supposed to have entered an essay competition at another university. They found facial attractiveness to significantly influence the mark given to the essay, and ratings of essay quality and author ability. In addition the effects of attractiveness were found to be greater when author sex was the same as the sex-typing of the essay title (e.g., a female title—"How to Make a Quilt"; a male title—"How to Buy a Used Motorcycle"), this being especially so for female authors. Thus Cash and Trimer suggested that when women evaluate the performance of other women facial appearance has a much greater effect for "in-role" than for "out-of-role" performances. This finding bears some similarity to the interaction of facial appearance and sex-role effects found in studies in the employment setting, which are discussed in Chapter 3, and it may account for the interactive effects of sex of author and facial appearance found in several of the studies cited above involving essay assessment.

Race of Face

Maruyama and Miller (1980) attempted not only to replicate Landy and Sigall's findings but also to examine the effect of race of face. In their first study male students evaluated an essay of good or average standard supposedly written by a fairly attractive or unattractive black or white female student. Their procedure was similar to that used by Landy and Sigall, and after the picture and essay had been seen the folder was removed before the subjects began filling in the response questionnaire. For each subject Maruyama and Miller combined the ratings into a single composite score and they found significant main effects of attractiveness of writer and of essay quality (but no interaction between these two factors). In their second study Maruyama and Miller attempted to induce the subjects to scrutinize more thoroughly the photograph by changing the essay topic to "How This Picture Is Me." Essays good and poor in content were used. Male students evaluated the essays and although no main effects were found, there was a marginal interaction ($p < .06$) between race and attractiveness that revealed that whereas attractiveness led to higher evaluations for the white author, it had the reverse effect for the black author. In their third study Maruyama and Miller used photographs more toward the extemes of the attractiveness dimension, and here again the male raters' evaluations were significantly affected by female author attractiveness.

Good Versus Poor Work

Fugita, Panek, Balascoe, and Newman (1977) asked both male and female undergraduates to evaluate a female's essay (on either city planning or dietetics) on a number of scales rather different from those used by Landy and Sigall. The supposed author's photograph accompanying her short biograhical statement was either attractive or unattractive. A significant main effect of attractiveness was found (there being no interaction between attractiveness and sex of rater) and further analysis revealed that this was entirely due to attractiveness significantly affecting evaluations of the essay on city planning, with no effects of attractiveness for evaluations of the essay on dietetics. Fugita, Panek, Balascoe, and Newman suggested that one possible reason for this interactive effect of essay topic could be that of essay quality. However, contrary to the suggestion of Landy and Sigall (that attractiveness may be more likely to have an effect when an essay is poor in quality) it was the dietetics essay that was overall rated somewhat below average, whereas the essay on city planning (which occasioned an attractiveness effect) was found to be rated somewhat above average in quality.

Conclusion

What these studies on the effects upon essay and writer evaluation of physical attractiveness suggest is that author attractiveness often seems to have a significant effect, particularly if the essay is believed to have been written by a female. The nature of the physical attractiveness effect may be influenced by essay quality, although whether attractiveness has a greater effect for poor- than for good-quality essays is not clear.

Whatever the mediating effects of essay quality may be, what studies on this topic should do is to compare the relative power of the two variables of physical attractiveness and essay quality. Studies in which these two factors are varied should not merely report the levels of significance for the statistical effects of each variable, they should also compare the strength of the physical attractiveness variable with that of the quality factor. If quality were found to have a much more powerful effect than attractiveness then statistical effects of the latter, however "significant" they are, may be ecological trivial. However, if physical attractiveness has a similar or stronger effect than essay quality this would be a finding worthy of note.

Future studies on this topic should also consider whether undergraduates should be used as the evaluators. One valid criticism of psychology is concerned with the possibility that peculiar results may occur when you ask inexperienced people to do strange things. Most undergraduates have little experience of evaluating other people's essays and the study by Bull and

Stevens seems to be the only one that has used experienced teachers. A further criticism of research on this topic is that in reality it is rarely the case that essay evaluators assess work written by strangers yet are provided with a photograph of the author. Most evaluations are made of essays written either (a) by authors known to the evaluators, or (b) by strangers of whom no photographs are provided. In only a few scholastic/academic circumstances (e.g., in applications to join a university, college, or school) are strangers' essays accompained by photographs, but the importance to essay authors of the outcomes of such applications may justify more research being conducted on this topic. Similarly, since some employment (and other) applications may involve the provision of a photograph plus a form of essay, research on the effects of physical appearance in this context seems warranted.

Is There Really a Relationship Between Facial Appearance and Academic Performance?

We have seen above that whereas some studies have found a significant relationship between facial appearance and what people (including teachers) expect academically of children, several others have found no such relationship. The crucial question, of course, is not concerned with mere expectations but with the possibility that facially attractive individuals actually do perform better in academic tasks.

M. Clifford (1975) found, as have some others, that teachers expressed more favorable academic expectations for attractive students. In her first experiment, which was a replication of M. Clifford and Walster (1973), 420 first-grade teachers received a school progress report card that described "a fairly successful pupil." Attached to this card was a photograph of an attractive or unattractive boy or girl. Attractiveness was found to have a very significant effect on judged IQ ($p < .001$), as well as on the rated degree of parental interest in the pupil's achievement, and on the estimated level of education that the child would reach. However, as with the study by M. Clifford and Walster (1973), the apparently strong effect on IQ seems to have resulted in a mean difference of merely 2 IQ points! In her second (1975) experiment Clifford asked teachers to rate for attractiveness the facial photographs of children whom they did not know. The children's mean attractiveness ratings were then correlated with the real performance measures of IQ; standardized achievement scores in reading, spelling, and mathematics; and year-average report card grades. Contrary to Clifford's prediction, physical attractiveness did not significantly correlate with any indices of performance. In fact, nearly half the correlations were negative. Clifford concluded that, "The suspicion that educators may estimate IQ from a student's physical appearance, establish a corresponding academic expectancy of the student, and then affect the self-fulfilling prophecy appears to be unwarranted." Clifford pointed out in her second study that she found "relatively little consensus among teachers on judgment of individual attractiveness" and, although the interteacher agreement was highly significant ($p < .001$), the reader could take this as a suggestion for why Clifford failed to find her predicted relationship between rated attractiveness and academic attainment. However, Clifford made no comment on whether the interjudge agreement concerning attractiveness was higher in her first than her second study (or than in M. Clifford and Walster [1973]). Therefore, it may be wrong to assume that interrater disagreement was the reason for the relationship not turning out as predicted.

In 1938 Holmes and Hatch found not only that observers independently agreed upon the attractiveness ratings ascribed to faces but that the real mean grade point average of "plain and homely" female students was *higher*, than that of "good looking and beautiful" students. Even when Holmes and Hatch took note of the fact that in their data it seemed that the more attractive women ceased their education at an earlier age, this relationship still held. One might have expected this early study to have been mentioned in M. Clifford and Walster's (1973) oft-cited paper, which perhaps more than any other study has suggested to people that there may be a positive relationship between facial attractiveness and educational achievement. Also rarely cited is an early study by Cook (1939), who found not only that people readily assigned intelligence on the basis of facial photographs alone but, more importantly, that there was very little evidence that the intelligence ratings correlated with "true" intelligence (as measured by the Thurstone Intelligence Test IV). It is of interest that when Cook compared the 10 faces rated highest and lowest in intelligence he subjectively noticed that, "In the high group no one feature was out of proportion to the rest of the face," whereas "Only four of those in the low group approached this symmetry." In the low group he noted several individuals with minor facial abnormalities. (The reader is referred to Chapter 7 for a more detailed examination of the effects of facial abnormality.)

In contrast to the findings of Holmes and Hatch (1938) are those of Singer (1964), who had photographs of 192 female first-year undergraduates judged for attractiveness by 40 academic staff at the same university (who presumably did not know the students). The mean attractiveness ratings were correlated with the girl's grade point average and a significantly positive correlation ($+0.19$) was found, this being entirely due to there being a significant correlation for the 92 girls who were "first-borns" ($+.40$). (The data for the "later-borns" did not produce a significant correlation.) In attempting to account for this positive relationship Singer pointed out that, "The grade point averages were achieved in courses" (with very large classes) where it is highly unlikely that "the attractive girls at that time could have been singled out by the instructor for special treatment." Instead Singer suggested that when marking assignments teachers may "give the benefit" of the doubt to students "whose names and faces they associate and remember." He added that "there are none so likely to have their names and faces remembered as the attractive girls in the class. Although we have no evidence directly relating to this point, many of our colleagues acknowledge that they can recall the names of the pretty girls in their classes."

Although Singer's explanations of the relationship between academic performance and attractiveness in female "first-borns" may seem rather far-fetched, as mentioned in Chapter 4, data are now available that suggest that attractive faces may be more memorable. Singer also attempted to explain why he observed a relationship for "first-borns" but not for "later-borns." He found that "first-born girls tend to sit at the front of the class, see the instructor after class, and visit the instructor in his office more often than later-born girls." If this is the case then one can understand why it was only for "first-borns" that Singer found attractiveness to correlate significantly with grade point average. If people react more positively to attractive individuals then the behavior of "first-borns," more so than "later-borns," possibly enabled their instructors to affect their academic performance (and remember them?).

If teachers do expect better performance from attractive pupils (our review above suggests that this by no means is always the case), and *if* such expectations do, in fact, affect the pupils (in positive rather than negative ways) then this could be one of several explanations of positive relationships (when they exist) between student attractiveness and performance. R. Lerner and Lerner (1977) found not only that teachers gave higher ratings for the academic ability of children in their classes who were independently rated as attractive, but also that students' actual academic performance correlated significantly ($+0.2$) with attractiveness. Although our review of the literature suggests that Lerner and Lerner were rather overstating the case in their introduction when they claimed that, "In sum, the evidence suggests that, compared to the physically attractive child, the physically unattractive child experiences . . . the perception of maladjustment by both teachers and peers, and the belief by teachers of less educational ability," their finding of a significant appearance-performance relationship is worthy of note. However, as Lerner and Lerner pointed out, the percentage of variance in academic performance accounted for by attractiveness in their study was small. Nevertheless, they stated that there exist "theoretical implications of the present findings. Children differing in physical attractiveness, evoked differing reactions in their peers and adult supervisors. On the basis of such differential reactivity to child individuality, it is argued that a child will experience differential feedback and, as a consequence of the progression of such a circular function, further lawful, individual development will proceed." Lerner and Lerner suggested that the consistency between "teacher perception ratings and physical attractiveness, on the one hand, and the measures of actual behavior/personality and physical attractiveness on the other, is congruent with such a circular function. This function would involve a linking of appraisals of ability based on physical attractiveness stereotypes with differential treatment based on such appraisals, and would eventually lead to behavior channeling and hence stereotype consistent performance." Again Lerner and Lerner could be accused of overstating their case. However, they did make the point that "it must be noted that although the present study's findings are consistent with the organismic circular function feedback notion, they in no way provide unequivocal support of this construct."

Facial Appearance and School Referral

The findings of Barocas and Black (1974) suggest that to ignore the possibility of there actually being a relationship between academic factors and physical appearance may be unwise. Photographs of 100 children from four classes in the same school were judged by undergraduates for physical attractiveness and the school records of these children "were examined for any referral to a supplemental service. A total of 21 referrals were observed and they were arrayed as follows: 1 psychological, 14 speech, 5 hearing and 1 learning disability." It was found that unattractive children received significantly *fewer* referrals. In trying to account for this finding Barocas and Black noted that

> There is little reason to believe that attractive children would have more problems than unattractive children. If anything, the hypothesis might well be in the opposite direction. . . . At least two social mechanisms may account for the data reported here. Appearance has been shown to generate expectations which, in turn, influence assumptions about a child's work. Those experience-linked expectations may also cause the teacher more easily to exploit supplemental services for those children already defined as having a greater likelihood of success in life. In addition . . . teachers may be more attracted to handsome children and, as a result, spend more time with them. They would then be in a better position to note the presence of problems in need of remedy and be more likely to initiate referrals.

In support of this notion Barocas and Black pointed out that the nature of the referrals in their study were educationally helpful to the child rather than concerned with classroom behavior. They suggested that more research be done on the topic of referrals and that such research should differentiate between remedial problems and control problems, with the possibility that attractive children receive more of the former but fewer of the latter.

Data from a study by Salvia, Algozzine, and Sheare (1977) corroborated Singer's (1964) finding (for female "first-borns"). The school record cards and scores on the Iowa Test of Basic Skills (ITBS) were collated for schoolchildren of high (top 10%) and low (bottom 10%) physical attractiveness. For the ITBS (which involved vocabulary, reading comprehension, language skills, study skills, and arithmetic) there was no main effect of attractiveness. A significant interaction between pupil age and attractiveness revealed that for the fourth grade (but not for the third or fifth grade) the attractive pupils achieved a significantly higher total ITBS score. The end-of-year school record card grades (for reading, language, spelling, arithmetic, science, social studies, and scholarship) were examined for the 84 children in this study. A main effect of attractiveness was found and the effect of attractiveness did not interact with age or school record category. The attractive children received significantly better school record card scores. In order to determine whether this effect merely could have been the result of differing ITBS scores an analysis of covariance was performed and this found the effect of attractiveness on school record card scores to be independent of ITBS scores. This independence could suggest either that the record card scores more accurately reflected the children's ability than did the ITBS scores, or that the record card scores reflect teachers' biases in favor of attractive children (which some studies reveal that they possess). Whatever the explanation, physical attractiveness seems to be involved. If the effect of attractiveness on record card scores is due, at least in part, to teachers' biases then it should be noted that whereas most studies of teacher expectations have examined teachers' reactions to the attractiveness of children whom they had never met, in this study the teachers who put the scores on the record cards had taught the children for a whole school year. Salvia et al. pointed out that the results of their study do not necessarily offer support for a teacher bias effect. They suggested that any number of factors not limited to the school environment (e.g., health, nutrition, social class, personality) could account for the relationship between attractiveness and school record card grades.

Facial Appearance Versus Other Factors

A number of these possible factors were studied by Sparacino and Hansell (1979), who related them to undergraduate students' grade point averages. In their first study Sparacino and Hansell, using stepwise multiple regression analysis, found that for males their IQ, father's education, and father's occupation were significantly associated with grade point average, whereas physical attractiveness was not. Similarly for females, attractiveness had no effect but IQ, father's occupation, need for approval, locus of control, and Type A behavior did. Thus attractiveness was unrelated to grade point average and this was confirmed by further analysis involving analyses of variance and correlations. In their second study (which drew subjects from the same population as the first) Sparacino and Hansell collected the same types of data and they added information concerning the students' high school graduating average grade. For females, their university grade point average was found to be related to their IQ, father's education and occupation, need for approval, Type A behavior, high school graduating average grade, and number of hours per week spent studying, but not to attractiveness. For males, grade point average was found to be related to their IQ, father's education and occupation, family size, and physical attractiveness. However, the relationship between males' attractiveness and grade point average was *negative*. (Further correlational analysis revealed that this negative association held for first-, second-, and later-borns).

Sparacino and Hansell noted that in their first two studies the students "were frequently enrolled in large, introductory lecture classes and, we believe, relatively unlikely to have extended personal contact with all (or even most) of their instructors. In addition, grading in such classes is often determined on the basis of objective (i.e. multiple-choice) exams which are comparatively free of evaluative bias. It may therefore be argued that our samples provided an overly conservative test of possible bias due to attractiveness." As a consequence of this, in their third study Sparacino and Hansell collected data from pupils in a small private school that encouraged student-teacher academic interaction. For males physical attractiveness was found to be unrelated to academic achievement and for females there was a weak *negative* relationship.

Overall, then, in none of Sparacino and Hansell's three studies was a positive relationship found between academic performance and physical attractiveness. When a relationship was noted between these two factors it was found to be negative, as it was by Holmes and Hatch (1938). Sparacino and Hansell tentatively suggested that perhaps unattractive students "may evoke some sort of sympathy response" or that there exists "a negative evaluation bias toward more attractive students." Whatever the explanation, they may have been right when they concluded that "the relationship between physical attractiveness and academic performance might seem elusive and obscure," and they pointed out that the studies that have most strongly led people to believe that there is such a relationship have been concerned not with actual academic *performance* but merely with expectations about such performance.

This problem was examined by Felson (1980), who in his first experiment asked teachers for each child in their class to "Rate the child's ability" on a 3-point scale. Strangers' ratings of the attractiveness of the 416 children involved in the study were found to correlate significantly with teachers' ability ratings both for girls ($r = +.16$) and for boys ($r = +.22$). One explanation of this finding is that the teachers' ratings of ability were biased by the children's attractiveness, and if this were so, then in the light of the studies mentioned above it would not necessarily be the case that the children's actual academic performance should relate to attractiveness. However, Felson found that there was a significant, if weak ($r = +.20$), association between attractiveness and "actual" academic performance (grade point average) for boys, although not for girls. He suggested that "stereotyping against unattractive children in the past may have resulted in less actual achievement on their part. Genetics could also play a role in producing this relationship. If attractive persons are more likely to marry intelligent persons and if intelligence and appearance have a genetic component, then the children of these marriages may be more likely to be intelligent and attractive."

In his second experiment Felson (1980) examined some of the data collected from a national sample 2,213 10th-grade boys. During a lengthy interview the boys provided information on many factors, of which Felson was interested in grade point average, vocabulary test score, father's education, and time spent on homework. In addition, "At the conclusion of the interview, interviewers were asked to 'Rate respondent's general appearance (take into account his physical appearance, grooming and dress)', as either 'excellent (unusually good), good, fair, or poor'." Felson found that, "The results are almost identical to the results in the first study for boys. There is a small, positive correlation between attractiveness and grades ($r = .22$), but also between attractiveness and test scores ($r = .21$)." (No effect of birth order on these relationships was found.) Felson realized that these data could be explained by the possibility "that interviewers rate a child as better looking if the child has more favorable grades," but in denying this his recourse to the fact that "these are trained interviewers rating the child" seems inadequate. Nevertheless, in his first study it was strangers' ratings of attractiveness that were found to correlate with actual academic performance. Felson concluded that, "While the relationships are small, the inherent difficulties in the measurement of attractiveness suggest that the actual relationship may not be trivial."

Feingold (1982b) also made the point that studies of attractiveness typically assume that the physical attractiveness scores attributed to individuals during the studies are accurate estimates of their general, ongoing level of attractiveness. This, of course, may or may not be the case and this is something that should be examined (see Chapter 9). Feingold found that strangers' ratings of adults' physical attractiveness (based on photographs) did not significantly correlate with intelligence test scores. (In fact, the correlations for males and females were both negative.)

Similarly, Murphy, Nelson, and Cheap (1981) found no significant relationship between high school seniors' grade point average and their rated attractiveness, even though students unacquainted with the stimuli indicated that they expected the more attractive ones to receive higher grades. However, the size of Murphy et al.'s correlation of $+0.2$ (nonsignificant for their sample size) is very similar to that found between grade point average and attractiveness by Singer (1964) (i.e., $+0.19$), by Lerner and Lerner (1977) (i.e., $+0.2$) and by Felson (1980) (i.e., $+0.2$). That these surprisingly similar correlations have occurred by chance may be rather difficult to believe. However, as pointed out by Lerner and Lerner, the amount of variance in grade point average that these correlations suggest can be accounted for by facial appearance is small.

Maruyama and Miller (1981) also found only small correlations between children's facial appearance and their educational performance. As part of a large study designed to assess the effects of school desegregation in California, data on several hundred children's school performance were gathered. Photographs of the children were also available and these were rated by undergraduates for their attractiveness. The vast majority of the correlations between attractiveness and many measures of school achievement and IQ were below 0.15. Maruyama and Miller concluded from this ecologically valid study that, "Perhaps the failure of attractiveness to affect classroom outcomes should not be too surprising." Although attractiveness may influence expectations, they held the view that "research argues that expectations often do not carry over to influence outcomes."

Conclusion

At the present time we feel that it must be concluded that the case for a meaningful relationship between facial appearance and actual academic performance is not proven. Although a number of studies seem to have consistently observed significant, if rather weak, effects, others have found no relationship.

The Effects of Teachers' Facial Appearance

Earlier we surveyed studies of the effects of student's facial appearance on teachers' expectations and we now turn to studies of the effects of teachers' facial appearance on pupils. Irilli (1978) asked third-grade students to rate from photographs teachers whom they had never met. It was found that whereas teachers' age and sex had no effects, their physical attractiveness did. Attractive teachers were rated as superior teachers and the pupils indicated that the attractive teachers would be more fun, more interesting, more comfortable to be with, and more willing to play games with them. A similar effect was noted by Lombardi and Tocci (1979), who found that photographic facial attractiveness influenced college students' ratings of a professor (whom they had never met) for "warmth, sensitivity, ability to communicate, knowledge of subject matter and superiority," with neither sex of stimulus nor sex of subject having any interactive effects with attractiveness. However, the unattractive stimuli were rated as significantly "hard working."

Goebel and Cashen (1979) made the points that in the evaluation of teachers "the use of student ratings appears to be proliferating. Perhaps the basic reason for this is that ratings do yield quantifiable data, thereby simplifying the important decisions to be made with regard to teaching quality. . . . Yet a perusal of the literature reveals a lack of rigorous investigation of bias effects." Thirty pupils in each of grades 2, 5, 8, 11, and 13 were shown photographs of six attractive and six unattractive adults whom they did not know and they were asked to rate on 5-point scales these "teachers" for interaction, evaluation, overload, structure, skill, rapport, and overall (global) assessment. It was found that attractiveness had a significant effect for each age group on the pupils' ratings for rapport (i.e., "This teacher is friendly to the students"), for interaction (i.e., "This teacher encourages students to ask questions and give their own ideas"), and for global assessment (i.e., "This person would be a good teacher"). For all age groups attractiveness also had a significant effect (a) on skill (i.e., "This teacher explains things so that the student can understand them"), except for those in the 2nd grade; (b) on structure (i.e., "This teacher has things well organized"), except for those in the 11th grade; and (c) on overload (i.e., "This teacher gives students too much work to do"), except for those in the 8th and 13th grades. Attractiveness had an effect on evaluation (i.e., "This teacher expects students to do good work") only for the 8th and 13th grades.

Goebel and Cashen noted that these biases in favor of attractive "teachers" were found when no other information was provided concerning "teacher characteristics and/or performance." They continued that, "It would be comforting to assume that there would be a diminution of these biases as the students' knowledge of teacher characteristics expanded, but there is no basis for such an assumption." They suggested that the first impression a "teacher makes on students influences their future observations in a biased direction. Having formed a belief about the teacher at first sight, the student is less likely to attend to new and contradictory evidence." There is, in fact, no real evidence from the realm of teaching to support this assertion, although the psychology of information processing suggests that it is a worthwhile suggestion. Furthermore, there is no guarantee that in the real world pupils form the strength of first impressions found in Goebel and Cashen's study, which required the children to make first impression evaluative responses that they may well not bother to do in real life. Nevertheless, Goebel and Cashen made the useful point that their study may call into question the use of student evaluations in judging the professional competence of teachers.

Saxe and Bar-Tal (1977) also examined the effect of teacher attractiveness on pupils' initial reactions. They introduced to four eighth-grade classes in Israel a new "teacher" who was that day visiting their school. For two of the classes the confederate was made up to appear very attractive and for the other two classes she appeared unattractive. The "teacher" remained in the classroom for a few minutes "without interacting very much with the students" while several routine announcements were made. After she left the pupils were asked to rate her on a number of scales. When in the attractive condition she was rated as significantly more sociable, less strict, more pleasant, teaching more interesting classes, giving less homework, giving higher grades, and being more preferred as a teacher. Saxe and Bar-Tal noted that "the scales on which physical attractiveness effects were obtained were scales which assessed the likeableness of the teacher or scales which assessed student perceptions of the teacher's kindness. On the four scales on which there were no attractiveness effects, the scales measured skills directly related to teaching (e.g. knowledge of the material)."

Facial Appearance and Teaching Skill

Hore (1971) examined the teaching skills of attractive and unattractive trainee teachers. Hore stated that, "An educational psychologist observing the teaching performance of borderline pass-fail students noticed their consistent unattractiveness" and that "no direct evidence in the literature could be found on the relationship between attractiveness and teaching ability." The teaching assessments of 68 male and female attractive trainees were compared with those of 57 male and female unattractive trainees. A significant difference was found for female but not for male trainees, in that the attractive trainees had received significantly better assessments. Hore pointed out that this result has several implications, for example, "Unconscious bias in the tutor's assessment of a lesson taught by an attractive student teacher may have been a factor." To Hore's suggestion we could add the possibility that the attractive female teachers may have been more interpersonally skilled (see Chapter 8). Hore also felt that the finding for females "may help to explain why lesson-destroying blunders by attractive student teachers are sometimes treated leniently by classes who would normally take advantage of the mishap."

Hore's notion that teachers' attractiveness may bias ratings of competence was examined by Chaikin, Gillen, Derlega, Heinen, and Wilson (1978), although they did not cite Hore's paper. They noted that "no published study has examined . . . the effects of a teachers' attractiveness on students' evaluations of the teacher or on student academic performance." Their findings regarding students' evaluations were similar to those of Goebel and Cashen (1979) (see above) in that a female teacher when made to look attractive was rated by children as a better teacher, more kind and understanding, more likeable, friendlier, happier, more enjoyable to have as a teacher, and more interesting than when she was made to look unattractive. (No effect was found for how easy it would be to talk to the teacher.) In addition, the pupils who saw an attractive teacher conducting a lesson indicated that it was easier to concentrate on the lesson, that the lesson was more enjoyable and more interesting to listen to, and that the teacher tried harder. Since each group of children saw only one of the two different versions of a 10-minute videotaped lesson (one version involving the teacher looking attractive, the other version unattractive) these findings could possibly be due to the teacher somehow behaving differently on the two tapes. However, Chaikin et al. made an attempt to control for this not only by instruction to the teacher but also by checking that (a) verbal behavior and (b) smiling and eye contact did not differ across the two recordings (other behaviors were not checked).

Chaikin et al. also compared how effective upon learning had been the two teacher versions. The children were warned prior to their exposure to the recording that they should pay attention to it because afterward they would be given a short test on its contents. Even though their (above) findings "clearly indicate that a physical attractiveness stereotype exists in students' ratings of a teacher," the attractiveness of the teacher did not influence performance on the test. From the study by Chaikin et al. it can once again be concluded that although there is evidence that facial attractiveness can affect expectations, there is little evidence that these expectations have any important effect.

Conclusion

The overview provided in this chapter of research in the educational setting suggests that rather basic and easy to conduct studies of mere expectations, which are usually based solely on the use of photographs, have often found evidence that such expectations can be influenced by facial appearance. However, the evidence that such expectations have any meaningful resulting effects is much weaker, several studies having found rather limited or no such effects.

Chapter 6

The Effects of Children's Facial Appearance on Adults and the Effects of Facial Appearance on Children

In this chapter we shall survey studies of the effects of children's facial appearance on their disciplining by adults. Then we will look at research on adults' reactions to infants' facial appearance. Finally, we shall examine the questions of at what age children (a) can discriminate based on facial appearance and (b) demonstrate stereotyping based on facial appearance.

Langlois and Stephan (1981) put forward a model that attempted to explain the (possible) effects of physical attractiveness in peer relations and social behavior, and that suggested that facial appearance may influence the way in which information is selected and processed by a perceiver. They made a worthwhile attempt to bring cognitive psychology into the study of the social psychology of facial appearance, as did Warr and Knapper (1968). However, they pointed out that, "Compared to the rather extensive literature on differential expectations associated with physical attractiveness, there are few data relevant to the issue of differential treatment of attractive and unattractive children."

Children's Facial Appearance and Their Disciplining

Dion (1972) suggested that children's physical characteristics may influence adults' evaluations of their behavior. She argued that in striving for cognitive consistency

> . . . people may interpret an individual's actions in a manner consistent with their knowledge about his personal dispositions. Thus, if adults believe that children differing in attractiveness typically display different personal characteristics, these expectations may affect their evaluation of an attractive versus an unattractive child's behavior . . . [Dion assumed] that adults hold a physical attractiveness stereotype of children similar to that held for other adults. If so, adults should expect that physically attractive children typically engage in more socially desirable behavior than do unattractive children. The knowledge that an attractive child has committed a harmful act is obviously inconsistent with these expectations.

Dion hypothesized that an attractive child who commits a harmful act will be judged as less likely to habitually exhibit antisocial behavior than an unattractive child. (Research described in Chapter 4 could be taken to support this hypothesis.) In her study female undergraduates read a brief description of a child's misbehavior and saw a photograph of the child. The unattractive photographs led to significantly more inferences implying a chronic antisocial behavioral disposition than did the attractive photographs when the misbehavior was severe rather than mild (which occasioned no significant attractiveness effects). Furthermore, for the severe misbehavior, the unattractive children were seen as more likely to commit a similar transgression in the future. In addition, the unattractive children were rated as more dishonest and more unpleasant than the attractive children. No support, however, was found for the hypothesis that the intensity of advocated punishment would vary as a function of attractiveness, and so here again we have an example of attractiveness affecting people's expectancies but not their intended behavior.

Disciplining Boys and Girls

An effect of attractiveness on punishing behavior (albeit a very minor form) was, however, found by Dion in 1974. Undergraduates watched an ostensibly live videotape of an interaction between an adult and a child who appeared to be physically attractive or unattractive. They were then asked to monitor the child's performance on a picture-making task and to administer a penalty (withdrawing between one and five pennies) whenever the child made an incorrect response as shown to the subject (who could no longer see the child) by a light. The subjects' final task was to fill in a questionnaire concerning the child. It was found that female subjects who believed that they were withdrawing pennies from an unattractive boy withdrew significantly more regarding the same task performance than did other subjects who saw the boy looking attractive. However, the significant effect of attractiveness was reversed for the girl in that when attractive she had more pennies withdrawn. No effect of attractiveness of boy or girl was found for the withdrawal behavior of male subjects. Rather surprisingly, attractiveness of boy or girl had no effects on female or male subjects' trait ratings of the child. Dion suggested that attractiveness may have had a significant effect (on females) only for the boy because "the image of the ideal male still stresses individual achievement and competence while the ideal female is expected to be interpersonally oriented." Whatever the explanation of the sex of stimulus effect, one should bear in mind that in this study the subjects who saw the child appearing attractive saw a different, although similar, videotape from those who saw the child appearing unattractive. Even though Dion attempted to have as similar behavior as possible shown in the videotapes (and she pointed to the null differences found for the questionnaire), it is still possible that the boy's differential behavior, rather than his appearance, could have caused the observed effect.

Instead of undergraduates J. Rich (1975) used as subjects experienced female schoolteachers who were given written details of an incident involving a misbehavior at school. The teachers were asked to imagine that they had seen a child falling down the stairs who had been tripped by one of the children at the top of the stairs, all of whom denied being the cause but several of whom were glancing toward one child who had a slight grin. Attached to the description of the misbehavior was a facial photograph supposedly of the grinning child, which was either attractive or unattractive. The teachers were asked (a) to state how strongly they felt that the photographed child had tripped the other child, (b) to rate the child on seven personality scales, and (c) to state, assuming that the child had committed the misbehavior, the extent to which they agreed that the child should be punished, and what severity of punishment would be appropriate.

Rich found that unattractive boys received more blame than did attractive boys, but that this effect was reversed for girls. The attractive children received higher ratings (but for "intelligence" this was reversed for girls). Unattractiveness led to stronger punishment being advocated for the boys, whereas the reverse was found for the girls. These significant interactive effects of attractiveness and sex are similar to that found by Dion (1974), and Rich suggested that if unattractive girls are judged as having less internal locus of control then their misbehavior may be excused as being caused by their environment. He also suggested that attractiveness may be thought to relate to two different aspects of personality, virtue and social desirability. He noted, that, "If it is conceded that virtue and social desirability are not synonymous in Western societies, this line of speculation may help explain why unattractive females receive very favorable evaluations under certain conditions." This notion could be used to explain why, as stated in Chapter 5, Bull and Stevens (1979) found an unattractive female who had apparently taken the trouble to type her essay to receive high marks.

Disciplining by Men and Women

Whereas Rich and Dion used only female subjects, K. Marwit, Marwit, and Walker (1978) used both female and male, black and white, experienced and trainee teachers who read a description of one of two misbehaviors (either throwing a tantrum in class or stealing lunch money from a teacher's desk). They saw a photograph of an attractive or unattractive boy who was black or white and they were asked to indicate their strength of agreement with statements regarding the severity of the incident, the disciplinary action they would recommend, and character evaluation. Attractiveness was found to have no effect on student teachers but the experienced teachers rated the transgressions as more severe when committed by an attractive boy. Marwit et al. noted that this finding may appear initially to refute the "what is beautiful is good" hypothesis; however, they stated that, "If it is true that what (or who) is attractive is generally judged to be 'good' then misbehaviors by attractive children would present the greatest possible discrepancy between what is expected and what is observed, and therefore would present the greatest threat to a teacher's self-esteem and to classroom decorum. The result would be more severe action to reduce that threat."

It is worthy of note that the findings for the female subjects used by both J. Rich (1975) and Dion (1974) seem to refute the "what is beautiful is good" hypothesis for stimuli of the opposite sex. One third of Marwit et al.'s experienced teachers were male, and perhaps it was these who caused the apparent refutation of the "what is beautiful is good" hypothesis for the female stimuli. However, Marwit et al. reported no data analysis regarding sex of subject.

In 1982 S. Marwit repeated the K. Marwit et al. study using 32 of the original 1978 student teacher subjects, who had by that time become teachers with a few years experience. In the light of his 1978 finding that attractiveness (of boys) influenced practicing teachers but not student teachers, S. Marwit hypothesized that an increasing bias toward attractive children would accompany these subjects' shift in role from student to practicing teacher. A significant effect of attractiveness was found, but only for black pupils, and this effect was in the opposite direction to the effect of attractiveness found by Marwit et al. However, S. Marwit (1982) reported that, "Re-examination of Marwit et al.'s earlier data indicated a strong tendency among student teachers toward the same interaction of race × attractiveness, which had unfortunately not been reported because the $p < .06$, but not $p < .05$." The transgressions of unattractive black students were judged more severely than those of attractive black students. The lack of effect of attractiveness on white pupils was not discussed (nor was the discrepancy between the 1982 and the 1978 significant attractiveness effects), and perhaps S. Marwit could also have included in his analysis a race of teacher factor.

Support for the notion that the unattractive child is reacted to more severely comes from a study by Berkowitz and Frodi (1979), who asked female students to administer a loud sound punishment whenever a child made a mistake in a learning task. Berkowitz and Frodi found, as had Dion (1974), that attractiveness had no effect on subjects' trait ratings of the child. Even so, when unattractive both the boy and the girl were given more intense punishment. These authors suggested that this was because "undesirable physical characteristics evoke aggression-facilitating reactions because they are aversive to potential aggressors."

Ecological Validity

However, no support for a relationship between children's facial appearance and their disciplining was found by Felson (1981), who pointed out that several previous studies had lacked ecological validity, particularly in the sense that the subjects and stimulus persons had never interacted. His study examined, using a correlational design, the relationship between physical attractiveness and data on school conduct/disciplining and on peer ratings of aggression. In his first sample the school conduct grades of over 400 boys and girls were correlated with strangers' photographic ratings of their attractiveness, and with classmates "sociometric" judgments (i.e., "Name the three boys/girls in this classroom who you think are the most good-looking"). Very small and clearly nonsignificant correlations were found. Felson also correlated attractiveness with classmates' judgments of aggression (i.e., "Name two students in the class who fight the most"). Again no significant relationships were found to support the notion that unattractive children are the more deviant.

Felson's second sample included over 2,000 boys who were asked by interviewers how often they had been suspended/expelled from school, how often they were kept after school, and how much teachers seemed to take an interest in them. The "experienced interviewers rated the physical appearance of the respondents at the conclusion of the interview as either excellent, good, fair or poor." For this sample, even though various sorts of bias seem possible, again the correlations were small, and there was no evidence that even extreme unattractiveness/attractiveness had any effects. Felson concluded that, "Experimental studies may exaggerate the importance of appearance in judgments of deviance because they focus on strangers and because they restrict the availability of other informations."

Overall, we again find contrary findings concerning the social psychology of facial appearance. It seems that there is little agreement in the literature concerning the effects of children's facial attractiveness on adults' disciplinary/ punishing behavior, and it is interesting to note that in several of these studies (which lack ecological validity) the trait ratings were not influenced by children's attractiveness when other information about the children (i.e., their behavior) was made available.

A much more realistic study of the effects of children's facial attractiveness was conducted by Langlois and Downs (1979), who had noted Waldrop and Halverson's (1971) finding that children who were found to have minor physical anomalies of the face and head at age 2½ years displayed behavior problems not only at that age but also 5 years later. (For more information on Waldrop and Halverson's finding see Chapter 4, plus Waldrop, Pedersen, and Bell [1968], Waldrop and Goering [1971], Waldrop, Bell, and Goering [1976], and Halverson and Waldrop [1976]). Langlois and Downs (1979) stated that there has been a lack of research concerning the influence of children's physical appearance on their behavior. They were of the opinion that "the processes which mediate the relationship between *perceptions* of behavior of attractive and unattractive children and the *actual behavior* emitted by these children remains largely unexplored." They posed the questions, "[D]o adults and children react differently to attractive and unattractive children because these children in fact behave differently? That is, are unattractive children aggressive and antisocial while attractive children are friendly and behave prosocially?" (Chapter 8 examines research on facial appearance and interpersonal skill.) Alternatively they asked whether "both children and adults have assimilated cultural stereotypes based on physical attractiveness which distort the perception of the behavior of others to fit these stereo-types."

Of course, these two processes may possibly interact in that people may expect children with certain types of facial appearance to behave in certain ways, and these expectations may be part of the reason why physically attrac-tive children behave differently from unattractive children, if, indeed, this behavioral difference exists.

Langlois and Downs (1979) attempted to investigate whether such be-havioral differences are displayed by young children. The subjects in their study were well-acquainted classmates whom adults who were unacquainted with the children rated from photographs as facially attractive or unattractive. The children's behavior was observed in their nursery school, and they were from two groups (mean ages 3 years 4 months and 5 years 1 month). Dyads of the same sex and similar age were observed interacting in a play area. One observer per child recorded the frequency of a variety of "affiliative, aggres-sive, high-activity play, and low-activity play" behaviors. In each dyad one of the children was facially attractive and the other unattractive. It was found that for affiliative behaviors there was a significant statistical interaction effect in the sense that individuals paired with children of their own level of attrac-tiveness exhibited more affiliative behaviors (such as smiling and touching) than did those paired with children of the contrary level of attractiveness. For aggressive behavior, only a four-way interaction involving attractiveness was significant, this being that whereas attractiveness had no effect for the 3-year-olds, for the 5-year-olds when one (in the male dyads) or both (in the female dyads) members were unattractive more aggression was observed. High-activity play also failed to reveal a main effect of attractiveness, and a three-way interaction revealed that boys and unattractive girls displayed more high-activity play behavior than did attractive girls. Low-activity play be-havior did have a main effect of attractiveness in that attractive children dis-played more low-activity play (e.g., sitting, playing with doll or puzzle, grooming) than did unattractive children. This main effect was qualified by a four-way interaction that showed that the 3-year-old attractive boys displayed the lowest amount of low-activity play.

Langlois and Downs concluded that "behavioral differences between attractive and unattractive children were found among aggressive behaviors, activity level and sex-stereotyped behaviors but not in affiliative behaviors." Although we would not entirely agree that such a conclusion is totally war-ranted by their findings (i.e., affiliation in both age groups did seem to be affected by attractiveness, whereas aggression only had an effect for 5-year-olds), we believe to be important Langlois and Downs' view that negative evaluations of unattractive children seem to be a reflection of the actual tendency of these children to behave in certain ways. However, even though the observers were "naive as to the purpose of the study," the possibility that the children's facial attractiveness may have biased the behavioral recordings cannot be ruled out, although the results of Langlois and Downs' interobserver reliability checks may argue against this somewhat. Nevertheless, we may be unwise to ignore their concluding comment that, "Although many interesting questions remain, it now seems clear that differences between attractive and unattractive children are indeed behavioral realities and do not merely exist in the eye of the beholder."

Physically Abused Children

If there are differences in the actual behavior of attractive and unattractive children, as suggested by the findings of Waldrop and Halverson (1971) and of Langlois and Downs (1979), then this could explain why McCabe (1984) found physically abused children to have atypical cranial/facial proportions. In her first study she compared 3- to 6-year-old physically abused children who had been placed in a "California residential facility by the court" with a similarly aged control group from a nursery school. Additionally she compared a group of physically abused children "who were referred to a university research project by the Massachusetts Department of Social Services" with a control group. The "cranial/facial proportions of these children were measured by trained research assistants who were naive to the purpose of the project." (The cranial/facial proportion was calculated by dividing the forehead height by the distance between chin and brow minus half the nose width.) It was found that the abused children in both samples had smaller cranial/facial proportions. (There was also a significant relationship between the children's height and abuse in one of the two groups, with the control group children being the taller.) In her second study McCabe (1984) used photographs of physically abused children aged 2 to 7 years and 12 to 15 years randomly chosen from police files and compared these with control groups of photographs. (The cranial/facial proportion was calculated by dividing forehead height by the distance between chin and brow.) For both age levels the abused groups had significantly smaller cranial/facial proportions.

McCabe pointed out that the cranial/facial proportion decreases as children grow older and therefore the abused children had proportions that could have been taken to indicate that these children were older than their true age. This being the case, McCabe argued that "this may lead to caregivers' unrealistic expectations" of them, which might contribute to the abuse. However, no persuasive argument is made to support this hypothesis, and even if it were true, for abuse to follow one would need to presume that the abusive "caregivers" (who would normally be the child's parents) were unaware of the child's true age. More parsimonious hypotheses would be based on the notions (a) that abused children who have the atypical cranial/facial proportion found by McCabe actually behave in ways that lead to punishment or abuse (note the above findings of Waldrop and Halverson [1971] and of Langlois and Downs [1979]), and/or (b) that such children are less facially attractive and this contributes of their punishment or abuse, as many studies reviewed in this chapter might suggest, including those now to be reviewed concerning adults' reactions to infants' facial appearance.

Adults Reactions to Infants' Facial Appearance

Above we noted McCabe's (1984) finding that physically abused children (aged from 2 years) had atypical cranial/facial proportions. If the facial appearance of such children can occasion abuse, then we should examine the extent to which infants' facial appearance may affect adults.

Sternglatz, Gray, and Murakami (1977) noted that ethological theories suggest that infant facial appearance should affect adult caretaking responses, and inhibit responses such as aggression that might normally be made by one adult to another. They suggested that the absence of "cute facial features . . . may partially account for the battered child syndrome." They pointed out that, "The available field literature seems to indicate that the end of intensive mothering and social immunity are determined by the disappearance of the infantile physical characteristics rather than by the choice of the infants." Sternglatz et al. showed to adult students schematic line drawings of infant faces in which they varied the vertical positioning of the eyes, nose, and mouth; the size of the iris; and the width of the eyes. The adults were required to rate the faces' attractiveness. The highest attractiveness ratings were for the face characterized by a relatively large forehead and large eyes. In general, faces were rated as attractive when feature positioning and size were toward the middle of the range employed, with attractiveness decreasing the more the facial features deviated from the midrange.

Brooks and Hochberg (1960) varied the eye height in drawings of an infant's face, and their subjects were required to rate the faces they saw for cuteness. Data similar to those of Sternglatz et al. were found. In noting the findings of Brooks and Hochberg and of Sternglatz et al. we should be aware that the variations they employed for the infant facial features may have exceeded those found in real life. Nevertheless, their findings do bear some resemblance to those of Secord (1958) (whom they do not cite), who gave a brief personality account of an individual to subjects who were required to give an indication of the physical appearance they expected this man to have by rating 32 facial and hair characteristics. These subjects who were told that the man was "warmhearted and honest" rated most of his features as likely to be average, but those told that he was "ruthless and brutal" rated his appearance on 25 of the scales as likely to be significantly toward the extremes.

Hildebrandt and Fitzgerald (1983) also suggested that infant facial attractiveness may influence caregivers' responses. As yet, however, no studies seem to exist that have directly examined this question. In 1978 Hildebrandt and Fitzgerald showed to adult students photographs of 4- and 8-month-old infants. These subjects were found to look longer at the faces of children they ranked (as their last task) as the cutest, but there was no effect of cuteness on skin conductance or facial muscle activity. (Unfortunately, in this study facial expression was confounded with "static" cuteness; however, a 1983 study by Hildebrandt found that, "General facial configuration appeared to be more important than facial expression in determining adults' perceptions of infants' cuteness.") Hildebrandt and Fitzgerald suggested that "if parents do not perceive their infant as physically attractive . . . the quality of the caregiver-infant relationship may be affected." However, they stated that "conclusions regarding the relationship between perceived cuteness and actual caregiver-infant interaction must be advanced cautiously given the relative lack of empirical research directed toward an analysis of the behavioral consequences of 'babyishness' or perceived 'cuteness'."

Some research on this point is available. Parke and Sawin (1975; cited in Langlois, 1986) noted that mothers of attractive babies seemed to maintain more eye contact and kiss them more often. Parke, Hymel, Power, and Tinsley (1977; cited in Langlois, 1986) found that the more attractive their infant the higher were the fathers' expectations for involvement with their baby. Langlois (1986) also cited an unpublished study by Langlois and Casey (1984) in which significant (but moderate) correlations between infant attractiveness and maternal behavior were found (for "affect and interest in the baby" but not for "routine feeding and play"). In particular it was noted that mothers of 3-month-old girls "more often kissed, cooed, and smiled at their daughters while holding them close and cuddling them."

Infant Facial Appearance and Nursing

We would suggest that one reason for caution in the evaluation of results such as those cited above is concerned with the question of whether some parents of "objectively" unattractive infants react to them as such. Elsewhere in this book we have suggested that the possible relationship between facial appearance and other aspects of an individual need not be only that the former influence ratings of the latter, but that the latter may affect the former. Given this, then parenting or other such experiences with infants who may be unattractive (to strangers) may result in such children not being reacted to as if they were attractive. Corter et al. (1978) found that although nurses consensually rated the facial attractiveness of premature infants, those nurses who had cared for particular premature infants rated their attractiveness higher. However, many infants and young children are at least on some occasions away from their main caregivers and in the hands of strangers. For example, Corter et al. suggested that in many hospitals infant-nurse interaction may not go much beyond the initial stages of a relationship. They reported that "in the Hospital for Sick Children [in which the study was conducted] it was found that premature infants were attended to by an average of 71 different nurses during an average stay of 48 days." Consequently, "it is reasonable to assume that the amount of non-medical attention nurses pay to infants might vary partly as a function of how 'pleasant looking' a particular infant is . . . it may be that 'first impressions' based on physical attractiveness have some weight in determining the social environment experienced by premature infants." In a similar vein Hildebrandt and Fitzgerald (1983) suggested that "infant cuteness may be especially influential in group care settings, where caregivers must make choices about which of several equally familiar infants to attend to at any given moment," and that "settings in which infants are exposed to high caregiver turnover of supplemental caregiving may be those in which the stereotype 'what is beautiful is good' is most likely to surface." When citing Waldrop and Halverson's (1971) finding that hyperactive boys had more craniofacial abnormalities, Hildebrandt and Fitzgerald noted that "suboptimal caregiving may be the key factor underlying the correlation between newborn physical anomalies and two-year-old personality characteristics."

Facial Appearance of "Good" Babies

Although, as we have said, there is no direct evidence on this issue, there is evidence that adults do expect facially unattractive infants to cause their parents problems. Stephan and Langlois (1984) showed to undergraduates facial color photographs of newborn infants and of infants aged 3 and 9 months. The subjects rated the faces for attractiveness and then on a number of individual difference dimensions. Factor analysis of the individual difference ratings reduced these to four indices: (a) "good baby" (ratings on good, healthy, cheerful, attached to mother, responsive to other people, cute); (b) "active baby" (active, persistent, masculine); (c) "smart-likeable" (smart, likeable); and (d) "causes parents problems" (the ratings for causes parents few/many problems did not intercorrelate with any other factors). Overall, these indices were found to be similarly related to facial attractiveness in that attractive infants were rated more smart-likeable, good, less active, and as causing parents few problems. However, only for "smart-likeable" and "active" was the relationship with attractiveness significant for newborns. The race of infant (black, Caucasian, or Mexican-American) had few effects, and only for Mexican-American faces were some relationships with attractiveness (e.g., on "good-baby" and "smart-likeable") in the reverse direction. Stephan and Langlois compared the strength of the relationship between the four indices and attractiveness on the one hand, and ethnicity on the other. They found that, "On 10 of the 12 dependent measures (four dimensions × three time periods), the babies' attractiveness accounted for more variance than race." Stephan and Langlois concluded that "attractive infants were typically rated as 'better' than unattractive infants," but we believe some comment should be made concerning their study's methodology in the sense that the ratings of attractiveness were not made independently of the other judgments. Nevertheless, this study by Stephan and Langlois is one of the very few that has examined stereotypical reactions to infants' and newborns' facial appearance, and worthy of further study is their contention that "strong and consistent expectations for the behavior of attractive and unattractive individuals soon after birth . . . imply the possibility of differential treatment of attractive and un-attractive infants beginning immediately after birth."

Another worthwhile topic for research is concerned with the age at which children come to show the stereotyping based on facial appearance often shown by adults. This question can be subdivided into two parts: (a) the age at which children produce evidence of being able to discriminate or process attributes of facial appearance such as attractiveness, and (b) the age at which they show stereotyping based upon such attributes.

At What Age Can Children Discriminate Facial Attractiveness?

Adams and Crossman (1978) pointed out that, "Binet in his early construction of the Stanford-Binet intelligence test used an item which required 6 year olds to discriminate between a beautiful and an ugly person." Binet's use of this item may have been based more on intuition than research since it seems that only fairly recently have studies been published examining the age at which children can discriminate facial attractiveness.

The youngest age groups employed in Cross and Cross' (1971) study were 7-year-olds, and it was found that their attractiveness judgments of facial photographs did not differ from those of the 12- and 17-year-old subjects. N. Cavior and Lombardi (1973) also found that by age 7 years children rated the attractiveness of full-length photographs (of 7-, 12-, and 17-year-olds and adults) very similarly to older children and to adults. However, the data for their 5- and 6-year-olds did not reveal an overall significant effect for ratings of attractiveness. Cavior and Lombardi also found that whereas the within-age group interrater agreement reached the significant level of consensus shown by 11- and 17-year-olds by age 7, the interrater agreement was smaller, although significant, for 6-year-olds but was not significant for 5-year-olds. Cavior and Lombardi concluded that "children begin to use similar or common criteria in judging physical attractiveness at age 6 and increase thereafter until the age of 8, when they use the same criteria as older subjects. . . . the cultural criteria used by older persons begin to be acquired at age 6," and they suggest that a Piagetian explanation may be appropriate for their findings. Thus Binet may have been wise not to require children below age 6 years to discriminate among faces based on attractiveness. More recent research has, however, cast doubt on the assumption that very young children are unaffected by facial appearance.

Infants' Reactions to Facial Appearance

Even though Bradshaw and McKenzie (1971) (see below) believed that it may be difficult to assess the reactions to faces of very young children, they were aware of work in the 1960s that had examined "the tendency of young infants to attend to visual patterned stimuli having face-like characteristics."

Kagan, Henker, Hen-Tov, Levine, and Lewis (1966) measured the reactions of 4- and 8-month-old infants to three-dimensional models of "faces." Four different stimuli were used, these being a "regular" face, one with the facial features "scrambled," one with no eyes, and one with all the inner features (e.g., eyes, nose, and mouth) missing. Each of these four stimuli retained a normal facial and hair outline. The infants' gaze fixation time, smiling, and vocalization to each stimulus were noted. Fixation time scores "were essentially equivalent for the regular and scrambled face. If fixation time alone had been measured, the data would have suggested that the 4-month-old infants were not differentiating between the regular and scrambled facial patterns." Similarly, "the vocalization scores failed to differentiate between regular and scrambled faces." However, since "smiles were markedly more frequent to the regular than to the other three faces," the null hypothesis was rejected by Kagan et al.

M. Lewis (1969) also concluded that young infants could discriminate between regular and distorted faces. He found that 3-month-old infants had longer gaze fixation times to a photograph of a regular (and of a "cyclops") face than to a drawing of a normal schematic face or of a scrambled schematic face. Six-month-old infants had longer fixation times to the regular photograph and to the regular schematic face than to the cyclops photograph or to the scrambled schematic face. The fixation times of 9- and 13-month-old infants showed no significant effects of stimulus type. With regard to the infants' smiling, the regular photographic and schematic faces occasioned significantly more smiling than the cyclops or scrambled schematic face for each age group of infants. Similarly, there was no interaction effect for vocalization between age and stimulus type, with more vocalization occurring to the regular photographic face than to the other three stimuli. No stimulus effects were found for "fret/cry" behavior.

In discussing these findings Lewis concluded that even 3-month-old infants can discriminate between various types of "facial" stimuli, and that the fixation time interaction between age and stimulus type may be explained by the infants' development of relevant schema. He suggested that aspects of his stimuli other than their "faceness" (e.g., their complexity) may have occasioned his data, but we could take his finding of no stimulus effects on fixation time for the older infants as arguing against this notion.

Haaf and Bell (1967) and Haaf (1977) found that 3½- to 5-month-old infants fixated a regular face more than a scrambled face. Haaf, like Lewis, suggested that stimulus complexity may have been a contributing factor to these findings. Using even younger infants of 5 and 10 weeks old, Haaf (1974) found no evidence for a preference.

Jones-Molfese (1975) criticized studies such as those by Haaf and by Lewis in the sense that "there is the difficulty of distinguishing blank stare looking from meaningful perceptual-cognitive interactions with the stimulus." Instead of measuring the infants' fixation time upon facial stimuli presented to them, she noted which stimulus from pairs of stimuli (two from the following three—a photograph or drawing of a normal face, or a drawing of a scrambled face) each infant "preferred." Preference was determined by fixation time, but the infants were required to make the operant response of gazing at the screen concealing a stimulus for 2 seconds before the screen was removed. As soon as the infant looked away from the stimulus the screen was replaced. Jones-Molfese found that by no means all the 40 infants preferred the regular face to the scrambled face, and that infants' age (4, 8, and 12 months) had no effect. She suggested that since the regular and scrambled faces were equal in terms of complexity, this could explain the lack of a consensual preference if the infants were responding to stimulus complexity rather than facial feature configuration.

So far we have reviewed studies of infants' reactions. Let us now examine studies of the reactions of newborns.

Neonates' Reactions to Facial Appearance

Goren, Sarty, and Wu (1975) noted newborn babies' (i.e., 9 minutes old) looking behavior at a moving stimulus that was either a schematic face, or a scrambled face, or just a face outline. They found the newborns to display greater travel of head and eye movements to the schematic face. However, Maurer and Barrera (1981) found 1-month-old babies to display no differentiation, based on visual preferences and habituation, between schematic and scrambled faces. The apparant discrepancy between these two sets of findings may be resolved by the fact that the study by Goren et al. employed moving stimuli whereas that of Maurer and Barrera (and those of other researchers) used static stimuli.

Employing moving stimuli Dziurawiec and Ellis (1986) recently replicated Goren et al.'s findings. They found that the eye- and head-turning behavior of babies less than 1 hour old was significantly greater to a moving schematic face than to a scrambled face (and to a blank face). Dziurawiec and Ellis concluded that future research should examine the question of whether "those neonates who show a strong preference for looking at faces develop into babies and children measurably more socially able than those who are less responsive to faces?" (Chapter 8 focuses on the possible relationship between facial appearance and social skill.)

Infants' Responses to Facial Attractiveness

Another question that future research could examine is whether newborns respond more to attractive than to unattractive faces. Dion (1977) studied young children's operant responding to facial photographs of 5-year-olds deemed (by preschool children not used in this study) to be attractive or unattractive. One face was available for each child to view, but in order to illuminate the photographic slide (for 5 seconds) the child was required to press a lever. It was found that those children who had available an attractive face made (significantly) twice as many presses before indicating that they wished to leave the test room than did those who had available an unattractive face. Age of subject (between 2 years 9 months and 6 years) did not interact with attractiveness and so Dion concluded that "physical attractiveness has incentive value for young children." Since Dion did not report the mean age (or standard deviation) of her sample we cannot tell from her study at what age facial attractiveness begins to have an incentive value.

However, a recent study by Samuels and Ewy (1985) does suggest that young infants may be responsive to facial attractiveness. The infants were shown pairs of adult faces, one attractive and one unattractive (deemed by adult raters) in each pair. The fixation time to each face was noted. It was found for both the 3- and 6-month-old infants that there was a very significant effect of attractiveness in that for all but 1 of the 11 pairs of faces the attractive stimulus had a greater fixation time than the unattractive stimulus. Since Wilcox (1969) had concluded that the complexity of facial stimuli may affect infants' visual preferences, Samuels and Ewy examined whether their attractive facial stimuli were more complex than their unattractive stimuli. They found that their low spatial frequency analysis of the stimuli did not predict infant preference as well as did attractiveness. However, since it did so predict for 8 of the 12 stimulus pairs, and attractiveness did so for 11, Samuels and Ewy's conclusion that "infants, even at three and six months of age have visual preferences for attractive faces" should be qualified by the findings concerning their stimuli's "informational content." Indeed, Samuels and Ewy did suggest that research should be directed toward determining what constitutes an attractive face (see Chapter 9) so that it may be more clearly determined whether their infants were merely responding to physical rather than aesthetic aspects of the stimuli (if, in fact, such a dichotomy is justified).

From the above studies of young children's and infants' reactions to facial appearance it is not at all clear at what age they come to discriminate between regular and scrambled faces, or prefer attractive or unattractive faces. The weight of the present evidence suggests that perhaps infants may be able to make these discriminations, but more research on this topic is required before a firm conclusion can be made. There is certainly no evidence that infants make stereotypic judgments based on facial appearance, but in stating this one has to bear in mind the question of how evidence for such judgments could be found with infants.

Let us now turn to studies that have sought to determine at what age children make stereotypic judgments based on facial appearance.

At What Age Do Children Demonstrate Stereotyping Based on Facial Appearance?

Studies that Have Employed Children of Varying Ages

Richardson (1970) showed 5- to 12-year-old children drawings of youngsters with or without different handicaps. In addition to a general liking for the nonhandicapped over the handicapped child, Richardson found for younger subjects that the more the stimulus child differed in overall appearance from the child without a handicap, the less the handicapped child was liked. For older subjects, Richardson found increased liking for the stimulus child as the disability became more distant from the face. Furthermore, the dislike of the cosmetic (i.e., not impeding any function) as opposed to the functional form of handicap increased with age.

Chigier and Chigier (1968), using a methodology similar to that of Richardson, found that groups of 10- and 11-year-old Israeli children, although showing a slightly different overall order, still produced a relatively high level of agreement when ranking handicaps. It should be noted, however, that Richardson's interpretation of the children's consistent preferences against handicaps, although supported by Matthews and Westie (1966) using different techniques, was criticized by Alessi and Anthony (1969), who maintained that Richardson's results were due to a statistical artifact. However, Alessi and Anthony's own results supported the general tenor of Richardson's conclusions.

In 1971 Bradshaw and McKenzie followed the rather ecologically invalid Brunswikian approach of showing to subjects very simple drawings of schematic faces. Children of ages 5, 8, and 12 years and young adults were required to indicate which face in each of many pairs of faces was the more "happy or wise or generous or trustworthy or young or male." Bradshaw did not use as subjects children of less than 5 years of age because these "S's are unlikely to be able to give meaningful responses, to understand the nature of the problem, or even to be able to maintain attention sufficiently long." The schematic outline faces were constructed with systematically varied features such that the eyes were placed far apart or close together, and high or low on the face. The nose was short or long, and the mouth wide or narrow. Each of these 16 variants was then paired for presentation to the subjects with a "standard" face "all of whose features were exactly intermediate between the two extremes in the comparison stimuli."

The adult subjects' judgments of which of each pair of faces was the more "male" were influenced by high eyes and wide mouths, as were those of the 12-year-olds, and a long nose had the same effect for all subjects save the 5-year-olds. For judgments of "young" a short nose had a significant effect on all groups except the 5-year-olds. There were very few, if any, nonchance effects on judgments of "wise and trustworthy." Judgments of "generous" were affected by a short nose for all subjects save the 5- and 8-year-olds. By far the highest number of significant effects was found for judgments of "happiness" in that all age groups were similarly affected by a wide mouth and by a short nose, and all but the 5-year-olds were affected by high eyes. Thus, whereas the 12-year-olds, and very often the 8-year-olds, were influenced by the faces in a manner similar to the adults, the 5-year-olds demonstrated far fewer effects of the facial variants upon their judgments.

Bradshaw and McKenzie did not provide an adequate explanation of the developmental effects found in their data, and no argument or evidence (except for the data reported previously) is offered by them as support for their statement that, "Any differrences seem to be largely attentional." It could be that Bradshaw and McKenzie's task was not appropriate to 5-year-olds. However, data from more recent studies (e.g., Dion, 1973; see below) would not support this conjecture. However, Bradshaw and McKenzie did fail (unlike Elliott, Bull, James, & Lansdown, 1986, and Rumsey, Bull, & Gahagan, 1986; see below) to determine whether his youngest subjects had understood the task.

From the work of Cross and Cross (1971), of N. Cavior and Lombardi (1973) (which was described earlier in this chapter), and of Bradshaw and McKenzie (1971) it seemed in 1971 to be the case that 5-year-old children did not react to certain aspects of facial appearance as did older children, and therefore it could have been concluded that they had not yet acquired the kinds of stereotypical reactions sometimes found, as the present book describes, in adults. However, in 1973 Dion reported a study that suggested that children aged 3 years were, in fact, consensually affected by facial attractiveness. Dion noted that N. Cavior and Lombardi's (1973) conclusion that children aged under 6 do not appear to have a reliable concept of physical attractiveness was based upon a study that had "several methodological ambiguities" that "make this conclusion somewhat tenuous." Dion pointed out that Cavior and Lombardi had used full-length, not facial, photographs, but she does not suggest why this could have prevented facial appearance from consensually affecting the 5-year-olds. Second, she noted that Cavior and Lombardi had employed photographs of 10- and 17-year-olds and that they had suggested that future research use photographs of people of the same age as the subjects.

Children's reactions to children of their own age.   In her own study Dion (1973) showed to children aged 5 to 6 years and 3 to 4 years 12 facial photographs of 6-year-olds that had been rated by adults as attractive or unattractive. From a small array of such faces each child was asked to "pick two children he would like as friends and two children whom he would not like as friends." Then each child was asked to indicate which child from the entire array of 12 faces might be likely to exhibit certain antisocial and prosocial behaviors. The children were asked to "Find someone you think fights a lot," then "hits even without good reason," "might hurt you," "says angry things," and "scares you." After these antisocial behaviors, some prosocial behavioral descriptions were used ("very friendly to other children," "helps children when they are hurt or sad," "doesn't like fighting or shouting," "doesn't hit even if someone else hits first"). Third, the children were shown six pairs of photographs and were asked to indicate which in each pair was the prettier (for girls) or cuter (for boys).

Dion found that both age groups separately chose the more attractive face in each pair as the more pretty/cute, and she stated that, "The general absence of significant associations between subjects' age and their judgments of relative attractiveness of the photographs indicates that even children as young as 3 years discriminate differences in facial attractiveness." She suggested that N. Cavior and Lombardi's (1973) failure to find an effect with their 5-year-olds may also have been due (a) to the fact that in their study the children seem to have been required to rank order sets of five photographs (rather than respond to pairs as in Dion's study), and (b) to their using a range of attractiveness rather than just the two extremes she employed.

With regard to friendship choice Dion found an overall effect of attractiveness, but she does not report whether this effect applied equally to both her age groups of subjects. However, she does so for the judgments of social behavior where attractiveness was found to affect five of the nine judgments of the prosocial and antisocial behaviors (listed above) for the older subjects, and four of these five for the younger subjects. Since Dion does not state what the mean age (or standard deviation) was for her younger age group ($n = 27$, "aged 3 years 2 months to 4 years 11 months"), one cannot precisely be sure at what age her observed effects began to manifest themselves.

Massimo (1978) also examined the reactions of children of various ages (5, 8, and 10 years) to the attractiveness (decided by adults' ratings) of facial photographs of children of these ages. In her doctoral dissertation abstract she reported that subjects were asked (a) to indicate which person (from the high-, medium-, or low-attractiveness levels used) they most preferred, and (b) to select stimulus persons who would be likely to exhibit each of five prosocial and five antisocial behaviors. Massimo concluded that her "Results showed strong support for the hypotheses of increased consistency and use of an attractiveness concept with age. Five-year-olds manifested significantly lower consistency of judgments than did eight- or ten-year-olds. . . . No real difference between eight- and ten-year-olds on both the development and consistency of the concept indicates that the attractiveness concept is relatively stable by age eight." Massimo suggested that children's preferences for attractive individuals may be stronger when merely looking at photographs of children not known to them rather than when being asked to select the stimulus person most likely to reciprocate their preference choice.

Faces known to the children. A similar point was made by Langlois and Styczynski (1979), who used as stimuli faces known and not known to the subjects. Children aged 3, 5, 8, and 10 years acted as subjects, and they were shown photographs of their classmates (with whom they had been in class for at least 8 months). The photographs were rated for attractiveness by 20 adults who were unacquainted with the children. Photographs of 12 of each child's classmates were displayed on a board and the children were asked to indicate three they liked a lot and three they did not like very much. In addition each child was asked to indicate for a range of prosocial and antisocial, competent and incompetent, behaviors which child was likely to exhibit such behavior. Finally, photographs of a child's classmates "were formed into same sex pairs with the two levels of attractiveness represented within each pair," and the child was asked to indicate which was the prettier/cuter, more handsome. This "paired comparison task was utilized to minimize cognitive demands which might interfere in assessing the youngest children's ability to judge attractiveness."

With regard to the children's judgments of attractiveness, "A t-test was performed to compare the children's choices on the picture pairs to the number of times they would have agreed with adult choices by chance. When asked to select the more attractive child, the children's judgments agreed with adult rankings beyond a chance level . . . $p < 0.05$ for the nursery school children and . . . $p < 0.01$ for the grade school children." Thus both the younger (i.e., 3- and 5-year-olds) and the older (8- and 10-year-olds) revealed an attractiveness effect, and the somewhat lower significance effect for the younger ones might be taken as revealing a developmental effect. However, Langlois and Styczynski statistically analyzed the attractiveness data for age of subject effects and found none. They therefore concluded that "the younger children were as consistent as the older children in their agreement with adult ratings of physical attractiveness."

For the "liking" data there was no main effect across age of attractiveness on which children were chosen as "liked a lot." Subjects aged 8 and 10 years did significantly choose attractive classmates, whereas the younger girls and the boys aged 5 seemed, if anything, to have chosen their unattractive classmates. Regarding the "dislike" data there was a main effect of attractiveness (caused solely by the male stimuli) but this was in the opposite direction to that suggested by prior research. The male attractive classmates were significantly more frequently chosen as disliked, this effect increasing with age. No significant effects of female attractiveness were found for "dislike" choices.

The effect of attractiveness on behavioral expectation was more in line with the findings of previous research, with the attractive children being perceived by their peers as likely to behave more prosocially than their unattractive classmates. This main effect was due largely to the male subjects age 3 and 10 years (the 5- and 8-year-olds showed a nonsignificant reversed effect). Regarding antisocial behavior the results were similar to the "dislike" data (and, of course, not independent of such data) in the sense that attractive boys were selected as more likely to exhibit antisocial behavior, especially with increasing age.

With regard to competence, attractive boys were chosen as competent more frequently by the 10-year-old children. There was also a significant main effect of attractiveness on incompetence choices in that attractive children were again most often chosen in response to questions this time about incompetent behavior (e.g., "clumsy, not smart, can't draw/color well, always forgets, loses things"). This effect was due largely to the older male stimuli (only the data for reactions to the 3-year-old boys—that is, the data provided by their 3-year-old classmates—were in line with the "what is beautiful is good" notion. However, unattractive girls were for all ages rated as slightly, but not significantly, more incompetent.

We can conclude from the results of Langlois and Styczynski's (1979) analyses of their data (which are not clearly reported by them) that whereas the outcomes of parts of their study are in line with the findings of previous research, others are not. They found evidence that children as young as 3 years of age can choose which of a pair of facial photographs of classmates is the more attractive (by adult standards). Some evidence for the "what is beautiful is good" hypothesis was found using subjects acquainted with the stimuli in that (a) children aged 8 and 10 years (but not 3 and 5 years) indicated that they liked their attractive classmates, (b) children aged 10 years (but not younger than that) selected attractive peers as more competent, and (c) there was a qualified main effect of attractiveness leading to more choices of prosocial behavior. However, for the "dislike," "antisocial," and "incompetence" data there were opposite effects in that attractive males were chosen more frequently, especially with increasing age. Langlois and Styczynski pointed out that these findings contrary to the "what is beautiful is good" hypothesis are similar to those found in their previous study of acquainted nursery level schoolchildren (Styczynski & Langlois, 1977), which found that whereas the effects of attractiveness on estimated behavior for unacquainted children were in line with Dion's (1973) findings, those for acquainted peers were not. In trying to account for their replicated findings regarding the effects of boys' attractiveness upon their classmates Langlois and Styczynski (1979) suggested that "the behavior of attractive boys may be more salient than that of unattractive boys: attractive boys are attended to and noticed more readily whether they are behaving in a positive or negative manner. This is consistent with recent data showing that attractive children receive more visual attention than do unattractive children." Why this explanation should not equally apply to girls they do not say.

Langlois and Styczynski concluded that

> At or by age eight, children's perceptions changed such that either attractive children were evaluated more positively than unattractive children when the converse had been the case at earlier stages, or substantial increases or decreases occurred in the positive evaluations of attractive and unattractive peers. Thus, although there does not appear to be a consistent linear relationship between age and the influence of appearance on peer relations, it does seem that important shifts in peer perception take place between five and eight years of age.

They suggested that a child's eighth year may often be the one in which increased role-taking and decentering skills occur, and that, "The age-related shifts in cognitions of peers combined with the lack of straightforward linear relationships between appearance and peer relations suggest that a cognitive-developmental rather than a learning theory model best accounts for the obtained data."

Does facial attractiveness have a greater effect for girls than for boys? With regard to the main theme of the present book we should also note Langlois and Styczynski's (1979) conclusion that our results suggest that in the context of the child's natural environment in-volving interactions with known peers, being physically attractive provides social advantages for girls. Attractive girls are generally better liked than unattractive girls and are liked more as age increases. By age 10 they are also perceived as more competent. Further, these girls are seen as being less anti-social and incompetent than their unattractive female peers. However, our results across two separate studies indicate that a high level of attractiveness may be a disadvantage for boys in their day-to-day interactions with familiar peers. It thus appears for boys, familiarity and beauty may breed contempt.

Children's reactions to deformed faces.   So far in our review of studies that have employed age of child as an independent variable we have been con-cerned with their reactions to facial attractiveness. Many of the previous studies specifically mentioned that none of their unattractive faces were dis-figured or deformed. However, since (as shown in Chapter 7) adults often do appear to react to facial deformity, it would seem worthwhile to determine at what age children demonstrate stereotyping in response to facial disfigurement.

Elliott et al. (1986) showed to subjects of various ages (6 to 7 years, 9 to 11 years, 13 to 15 years, 25 to 35 years) facial photographs of adults taken before and after fairly minor oral/plastic surgery to the lower part of the face that had resulted in noticeable (but not necessarily considerable) apparent improve-ment in appearance (as judged by the surgeons). Each subject saw nine before- and nine after-operation photographs each of a different person (i.e., no subject saw the "before" and "after" photographs of the same person), and they were required to judge these for friendliness, happiness, intelli-gence, social skill, and attractiveness. Since it was believed that "it would be asking too much of the observers below eleven years to understand how to rate a face along a seven-point scale" the youngest age groups used bipolar, 2-point scales. Once each subject had judged all 18 photographs, one of the first five faces that they had seen was (without warning) re-presented and their judgments to it were again noted. This was done in order to see how reliable the subjects were in their reactions. Such a procedure seems necessary in studies using young children in order to demonstrate, if no evidence of stereotyping is found, that the instructions were nevertheless understood and that the procedure was appropriate for children of their age.

Elliott et al. found that even the youngest subject's reactions demon-strated significant reliability. However, neither the 6- to 7-year-olds', nor the 9- to 11-year-olds' data revealed any effect of the "before" versus "after" operation variable on their reactions, whereas the older children and the adults rated the "after" faces as more attractive, intelligent, and happy. Therefore, we concluded that the reactions of children aged less than 11 years may not be affected by minor facial deformity, and that, "This being the case, if surgery to reduce facial deformity can be performed on children before their peers start to demonstrate negative attitudes towards deformed faces, then (other factors being considered) this should be done."

A study by Rumsey et al. (1986) came to a similar conclusion regarding the age at which children's reactions came to be affected by facial deformity. They showed to children aged 5, 6, 7, 8, 9, 10, and 11 years photographs of adults taken before and after oral surgery. These photographs were different from those employed by Elliott et al. in that no plastic surgery was involved, the oral surgery merely moving "forward" or "back" the mandible (by up to ½ inch), sometimes with slight rotation. Each subject was shown simultaneously both the "before" and "after" operation photographs of a person and was asked to choose one in response to either a "positive" question (e.g., "Which one would help you?") or a "negative" question (e.g. "Which one would tell you off?"). It was found that the 11-year-olds significantly more so than the younger children chose "before" photographs in response to "negative" questions and "after" photographs in response to "positive" questions. In order to check that our study's methodology had been suitable for the younger children we also asked the children which of each pair of faces (i.e., one "before" and one "after") was the more pretty/handsome. We found that although for the children aged below 10 years there was no significant relationship between "before"/"after" and their attractiveness choices, when their choices of faces in response to the "positive" and "negative" questions were compared with their own choices for pretty/handsome, the data for the children aged 6 years and above differed significantly from the chance relationship demonstrated by the 5-year-olds' data. From these findings we concluded that children aged below 11 years were not influenced by minor facial deformity, but that they did, however idiosyncratically, stereotype on the basis of how pretty or handsome they personally considered the "before" or "after" operation faces to be.

Thus from the studies by Rumsey et al. (1986) and by Elliott et al. (1986) it can be concluded that the young children not only understood the instructions but also that they did demonstrate stereotypical reactions to facial appearance. However, their reactions, unlike those of the older children, were not influenced by the small reductions in facial deformity occasioned by the facial surgery.

Conclusion. From the studies reviewed above that have each employed children of various ages in order to determine at what age they demonstrate stereotyping based on facial appearance it can be concluded that there is limited evidence that by age 5 years some children demonstrate some aspects of the stereotyping based on facial appearance found in older children and in adults. By age 8 years it seems that although such stereotyping based on attractive and unattractive (but not deformed) facial appearance is fairly well established, that concerning facial disfigurement is not, in that children aged less than 11 years do not consistently demonstrate stereotyping based on facial deformity.

In an attempt possibly to clarify this issue we shall now turn studies of young children's stereotyping based on facial appearance in which the age of the subjects has not been an independent variable.

Studies that Do Not Have Child's Age as an Independent Variable

In 1944 Young and Cooper published one of the first studies examining the relationship between facial appearance and children's sociometric choices. They found that children's and adults' (live) ratings of the facial attractiveness of children whom they did not know were significantly related to these children's classmates' friendship choices. Although they did not cite Young and Cooper's finding, in 1974 Dion and Berscheid pointed out, concerning research on the social psychology of facial appearance, that, "Studies to date have focused primarily on young adults' reactions to attractive versus unattractive peers," and they argued that younger persons' possible reactions to facial attractiveness were worthy of study. They showed to children aged 4 years 4 months to 6 years 10 months photographs of their classmates. Each subject was asked to indicate three classmates whom he or she especially liked and three that he or she disliked. In addition, 33 statements (from 14 categories) describing various social behaviors were read aloud to the child, and for each he or she was asked to indicate who exhibited that behavior (e.g., "Find someone who fights a lot"). Adults unacquainted with the children rated their photographs (of face plus body) for attractiveness. No main effect of attractiveness on liked/disliked was found, but a significant three-way interaction revealed that whereas for boys of both age groups attractiveness was significantly and positively related to popularity, it was only numerically (and not significantly) so related for the older girls, and was significantly negatively related to popularity in the younger girls.

For the social behavior statements, those concerning aggression were found to be related to boys' attractiveness in that unattractive boys were nominated by their peers "as engaging in more antisocial aggressive acts" than attractive boys. However, no effects of attractiveness were found for statements concerned with "friendly approach," "total conformity," "adult dependency," or "child dependency." A nearly significant ($p < .06$) main effect of attractiveness was found for "independence," with the attractive children receiving rather more independence nominations. Attractiveness had a significant effect for females regarding "Find someone who is afraid of lots of things" in that unattractive girls received more nominations. Unattractive boys and girls were nominated more frequently for "Find someone who scares you." No further effects were found. From these findings Dion and Berscheid concluded that "young children's physical attractiveness is related both to popularity in their peer group and to peers' perception of their social behavior. It appears, therefore, that the relevance of physical attractiveness as a social cue is not limited to young adults nor to first impression situations." (Unfortunately Dion and Berscheid did not state for how long the subjects had been acquainted.)

Children's first impressions.   Langlois and Stephan (1977) examined children's first impressions concerning the facial appearance of 8-year-olds whom they had never met. In addition to investigating possible effects of attractiveness, Langlois and Stephan examined the effects of the ethnicity of the facial stimuli and of the subjects in order to determine (a) the relative contributions of attractiveness and ethnicity to children's preferences and behavioral attributions, and (b) whether physical attractiveness effects generalized to nonwhite populations. Six- and 10-year-old "Anglo, Black and Mexican-American" children were shown photographs of 8-year-old children from all three ethnic groups that had been selected by adults (from all three ethnic groups) as attractive or unattractive. (No further details of interrater agreement across the three ethnic groups were given.) Each child saw an 'attractive' and an 'unattractive' photograph from the three ethnic groups, and they were required to indicate (using "three squares of increasing size") "How much do you like this child? How much does this child share his (her) toys? How friendly and nice is this child? How handsome/pretty is this child? How much does this child hit others? How much does this child need help from others? How smart is this child? How mean is this child?" The data concerning the second and third questions significantly intercorrelated, as did that for the fifth and eighth, and so "Each of these pairs of questions was combined to yield a composite index."

A significant main effect was found for attractiveness (i.e., as deemed by adults) in that the children rated as more handsome/pretty the faces so deemed by adults. (A significant four-way interaction revealed that the 6-year-old males failed to differentiate between 'attractive' and 'unattractive' black and Anglo faces.) Similarly, there was a main effect of attractiveness on "liking," on "smartness," on "friendly and nice" (and therefore on "sharing"), and on "mean" (and therefore "hitting"), in that attractiveness occasioned more "positive" ratings. No effect of attractiveness was found for "needs help."

Langlois and Stephan (1977) concluded that, "The consistent significant main effects for physical attractiveness on the behavioral expectation measures, and the lack of such main effects for ethnicity suggest that physical attractiveness is more influential than ethnicity in determining children's attributions and peer preferences." They reported that few age effects (i.e., 6 versus 10 years of age) were found, which is in line with the notion that by around age 6 years children display some of the adult stereotyping based on ("normal") unattractiveness and attractiveness. (By normal is meant the absence of facial abnormality, which several of these studies specifically excluded from their samples of faces.)

Adams and Crane (1980) also found an effect of facial attractiveness on young children's choice of who was "the nicest person," which did not interact with race of face. However, in their study, although the 4-year-olds did demonstrate this form of social attribution, there was no effect of facial appearance upon their "social play preference" in terms of whose photograph, or how near to it, they placed a photograph of themselves. Although Adams and Crane seem not to have checked that their subjects had understood the requirements of the social play preference task, they did make the worthwhile point that at age 4 years children may display only some of the more rudimentary aspects of the "beauty-is-good" stereotype.

The effects of acquaintance.   Styczynski and Langlois (1977) also examined the reactions of young children to children's attractiveness. They pointed out that in the study by Dion and Berscheid (1974) the children's attractiveness had been determined by adult raters and that "it is not known if their [own] ratings would have agreed with adults or unfamiliar peers." (As our previous review of studies on this topic reveals, it is not yet absolutely clear at which age children come to differentiate facial attractiveness in the same way as do adults.) Styczynski and Langlois decided to investigate whether young children who had been acquainted with the stimulus children for at least 8 months would rate and react to their attractiveness as would children who were not acquainted with them. (Note that previously we pointed out that Dion and Berscheid did not state for how long their subjects had been acquainted.) Children aged 3 to 4 years, and 5 to 7 years (overall mean age 4 years 3 months) were shown facial photographs of some of their classmates that adults had rated as high or low in attractiveness. The children were asked to indicate which three children they especially liked, and three they did not like very much. They were then asked to indicate which child they considered most likely to exhibit each of a variety of prosocial, antisocial, and competence behaviors. Some other young children of a similar age also acted as subjects. These were unacquainted with the stimuli and they were asked to "find someone you might especially like" (or dislike) from the photographic array before answering the questions concerning the various behaviors. As a final task all the subjects were presented with six pairs of the stimulus faces (in each pair there being one attractive and one unattractive face as determined by the adults' ratings), and they were asked to indicate which of each pair was the more pretty/cute/handsome.

It was found that the children acquainted with the stimuli and those who were not chose as the more attractive faces those so deemed by the adults, and that there was no difference between the two age groups of child subjects. Therefore Styczynski and Langlois (1977) concluded that "children perceived facial attractiveness using the same criteria as adults even after extensive interaction with the children being rated." However, no effects of attractiveness were found on either group of children's choices of which stimuli they liked/ disliked. When the like and dislike data were compiled into a single "popularity index" then a not quite significant interaction ($p < .06$) revealed that whereas boys unacquainted with the stimulus children indicated that the attractive ones would be more popular, those boys acquainted with the stimulus children indicated that the unattractive stimuli were the more popular.

For the behavioral expectation data a main effect of attractive children being selected as more prosocial was found (with no effect of acquaintance). No main effect of attractiveness for antisocial behavior was found, but significant two-way interactions revealed that whereas unacquainted children viewed the stimulus children with unattractive faces as more likely to behave antisocially, the reverse was true for acquainted children (as was found by Langlois and Styczynski, 1979; see above). Styczynski and Langlois suggested that "it may be that classmates take more notice of the behaviors, both positive and negative, exhibited by their attractive peers. . . . It was also possible that attractive children assert themselves more in social situations because they are more confident of a positive response, thus behaving in more extreme pro-social and antisocial ways."

No effects of attractiveness on competence were found, and a four-way interaction for incompetence revealed that whereas girls acquainted with unattractive boys nominated them as incompetent, acquainted boys so nominated attractive boys. Styczynski and Langlois stated that "attractiveness is not a consistent variable in children's assessments of peers' capabilities." Overall they concluded that although "acquaintance does not affect attractiveness judgments of pre-school children," it has "a significant effect on pre-school children's popularity ratings and behavioral expectations in relation to attractiveness." They therefore stated that, "Past conclusions regarding the influence of physical attractiveness based on research with unacquainted children must be seriously questioned. Evidence suggests that when the effects of physical appearance are explored within actual social situations, attractiveness may indeed be a social disadvantage, especially with boys."

Are unattractive children at risk?   Vaughn and Langlois (1983) suggested that, "Children whose relationships with peers are inadequate, either because interactions occur at low frequencies or because the quality of such interactions is inappropriate, are considered 'at risk' for later problems with adjustment," and that, "Children whose sociometric status is low are more likely than their peers to be identified as deviant (e.g. school dropout, mental health problems) during adolescence and adulthood." They suggested that this at-risk diagnosis could be used to justify interventions aimed at training in social skills. (Chapter 8 contains more information on this notion.) In their study children aged 4 and 5 years were asked to indicate which classmates they liked. In addition, the amount of visual attention each child received from classmates when in class was noted. Adults unacquainted with the children rated their physical attractiveness (head and torso), and a significant positive relationship was found between attractiveness and degree of liking (as indicated by a "paired comparison task," but not by a "picture board task"), this being more so for the female than the male stimuli. No significant relationships between attractiveness and visual attention were found.

Vaughn and Langlois' findings suggest that more research on children's social competence needs to be carried out in order to help define those socially "at risk." They argued that merely children's physical attractiveness or their rated popularity may not be valid guides to their social competence, and they concluded that, "Although we do not doubt that physical attractiveness influences some aspects of children's relationships with peers, it would be most unfortunate if children were identified as socially incompetent on the basis of an attribute that is not itself a component of social competence." Whether there is a relationship between facial appearance and social competence is discussed in Chapter 8. Suffice it to say here that the strength of evidence for such a relationship is not strong, nor may it be the case that facial appearance bears a meaningful relationship to other forms of competence.

Felson and Bohrnstedt (1979) found, as did Styczynski and Langlois (1977), that children's physical attractiveness by no means always displayed positive relationships with classmates' judgments of performance. In their study 12- and 14-year-old children were asked to name the three most physically attractive, the three "smartest" (i.e., most intelligent), and the three most athletic children in their class. In addition children unacquainted with these children rated their photographs for attractiveness. These data together with the children's actual grade point average for the school term, and the boys' basketball proficiency, were analyzed using Felson and Bohrnstedt's LISREL model ("a general maximum likelihood method for estimating a system of linear structural equations"). Felson and Bohrnstedt found that

> In none of the models do perceptions of physical attractiveness significantly affect perceptions of either type of ability. On the other hand . . . the effect of perceived academic ability on perceptions of attractiveness is strong for both the males and females, and the effect of perceived athletic ability (for males) is even stronger. It is interesting that in all the analyses, perceptions of physical attractiveness are more closely related to perceptions of ability than to objective indicators of physical attractiveness

(i.e., to the ratings given for attractiveness by the unacquainted children). From these findings they concluded that "persons who are attributed academic or athletic ability are perceived as good-looking."

What is good is beautiful.   Felson and Bohrnstedt (1979) saw their data as supporting the conclusion arrived at by Gross and Crofton (1977) that "what is good is beautiful." Gross and Crofton (1977) found that people perceived female students as more physically attractive if they had received a favorable description of their personality. Felson and Bohrnstedt took "The fact that perceptions of ability affect perceptions of physical attractiveness more than the objective indicators of attractiveness" as not commenting

> . . . favorably upon the external validity of experimental research supporting the physical attractiveness stereotype. In that research, subjects usually evaluate strangers on the basis of a short description of the person, or perhaps a report card, accompanied by a photograph. Given this limited amount of information, perhaps it should not be surprising that a photograph plays a role in the subjects' impressions of the person's personality or ability. However, in more natural settings, such as the one in which the present research was conducted, persons are likely to have much more information and therefore are less likely to rely upon appearance in their personality or ability judgment.

Felson and Bohrnstedt concluded that "it is children's perceived performances (academic, athletic, social, etc.) that determine who is defined as
physically attractive and who is not, i.e., performances appear to generate
local standards of beauty within the classroom," and that, "Clearly, all the
analyses suggest that it is the good who are seen as attractive, and not the
other way round."

Conclusion. Felson and Bohrnstedt's (1979) conclusion notwithstanding, we
should ask what can be concluded from the studies reviewed previously regarding the age at which children demonstrate stereotyping based on facial
appearance. Dion and Berscheid (1974) found some limited evidence that
children aged between 4 years 4 months and 6 years 10 months do display
such stereotyping, as did Adams and Crane (1980) for 4-year-olds, and Langlois and Stephan (1977) found such stereotyping in 6-year-olds. Vaughn and
Langlois (1983) found 4- and 5-year-olds' popularity to relate to their attractiveness. Styczynski and Langlois (1977), however, found that although children aged 3 to 4 years could discriminate between attractive and unattractive
faces (as deemed by adult raters), no significant effect of attractiveness on
liking/popularity was found, although a significant effect on expectations of
prosocial behavior was noted, and the effect of attractiveness on expected
antisocial behavior was qualified by acquaintance. Felson and Bohrnstedt
(1979) found for 12-year-olds that there existed a stereotyping relationship
(although reversed in direction) between facial attractiveness and evaluations
of the stimuli, but like Styczynski and Langlois they argued that acquaintance
of the subjects with the stimuli is an important factor regarding research on
the social effects of facial appearance.

   Overall, from these studies of stereotyping that have not had subjects' age
as an independent variable it is not clear at which age children come to
demonstrate stereotyping based on facial appearance, although it seems to be
fairly well established that by age 6 years children not only discriminate
between (normal) unattractive and attractive faces, they also display some
stereotyping based on this.

Overall Conclusion

In the light of the research that was then available Adams (1977a) suggested a
developmental perspective for examining the "Social Psychology of Beauty."
He argued that "four central assumptions about the developmental relationship between outer attractiveness and inner behavioral processes and outcomes can be extracted from the current research literature. The first and
most central assumption is that physical attractiveness stimulates differential
expectations toward another." The second assumption was that "an individual's attractiveness appears to elicit differential social exchanges from
others." The third was that "an important developmental outcome results

from this social exchange. As a consequence of receiving relatively constant positive or negative social reactions from others, physically attractive or unattractive persons are likely to internalize differing social images, self-expectations and interpersonal personality styles." (See Chapter 8 for a review of some of the literature on the possible effects of facial appearance on the self.) The fourth assumption was that "because of their greater experience with positive social interactions, attractive people will be more likely to manifest confident interpersonal behavior patterns than lesser attractive individuals."

When this perspective of Adams was published the literature did not overwhelmingly support his assumptions. For some of the assumptions the literature was contradictory, and for others it was sparse. Unfortunately, today the picture is not much clearer, and it is still true to say, as did Adams (1977a), that, "Little has been done in the way of investigating the relationship between physical attractiveness and individual development in the traditional context of longitudinal or cross-sectional designs."

A further criticism of research in this area came from Sorell and Nowak (1981), who stated that "the lack of research regarding the appearance-related social interactions of children outside school settings seems unfortunate." They correctly pointed out that research now needs to focus on "the extent to which stereotyped attributions are actually manifested in measurements of personality and behavior. . . . The dearth of research designed from this perspective may be seen as fundamental weakness in the appearance literature."

Hildebrandt (1982) employed Adams' perspective, and she argued that "some physically atypical children encounter difficulties in social interaction due at least in part to their physical appearance." Although the evidence for this is still not strong, partly because of the lack of research on the questions of (a) under what conditions facial appearance is most likely to be influential, and (b) to what extent children's behavior enhances or reduces any effects of facial appearance, we agree with Hildebrandt that "awareness of the potential biasing effect of children's appearance on adults' expectations and behavior is an important first step in assuring fair treatment and optimal development of all children."

Chapter 7

The Social Psychology of Facial Disfigurement

The importance of facial appearance in many aspects of social functioning was discussed at length earlier in this book. However, little attention has been paid to the psychological and social problems experienced by people who are considered by others to be ugly, or those who are disfigured or deformed. Despite indications that the possession of an aesthetically unattractive appearance may impair the social functioning of many, there has been little recognition from either society or psychologists of the problems encountered by those whose deviations from society's norms are primarily in terms of appearance, and not necessarily associated with a loss of body functioning. Macgregor (1974) went so far as to state that of all the concerns within the field of physical disability and rehabilitation, for her the greatest was the large number of people with facial deviations who seem to be classified as "marginal" or "forgotten" people. Yet the profound social significance of the face, taken together with society's prejudices toward those who have an atypical appearance, can mean that an unattractive facial appearance could be a severe social handicap.

This chapter represents a review of research concerning the problems encountered by those with atypical faces. Although the emphasis of the chapter is primarily on those disadvantaged by their facial appearance, the lack of research pertaining specifically to these people has led to the inclusion, where relevant, of research concerning those with physical abnormalities of other parts of the body (e.g., the physically disabled).

The Birth and Development of Facially Disadvantaged Children

The Birth of a Facially Disfigured Child

Parents will have expectations and hopes for their child even before it is born, with many prospective parents feeling slightly nervous about whether the child will be "whole." At the time of the birth, the two most common questions are "Is it a boy or a girl?" and "Is it alright?" (Shakespeare, 1975). The reaction to having produced a child who is in some way disfigured begins at this point. Some researchers have tried to document the pattern of the reactions that follow. Shakespeare (1975) stated that parents of an abnormal child initially experience shock, a feeling of disbelief, and a desire to be left alone while coming to terms with the situation. These feelings are followed by a mourning reaction—a kind of grief for the perfect child the parents had hoped for.

Lansdown (1981) stated that the birth of a congenitally disfigured child is a shock to the family system, and he also put forward the view that the anger and despair experienced take the form of a bereavement reaction. Lansdown believed that parents experience a variety of emotions, including "grief, anxiety, confusion, depression, disappointment, disbelief, frustration, guilt, hurt, inadequacy, rejection, resentment, shock, stigmatisation and withdrawal." Easson (1966) stated that the initial repugnance experienced by parents following the birth of a child with a congenital defect is followed by overprotectiveness, with the child becoming reliant on a sheltered existence (see below). Easson believed that similar reactions are often experienced by parents of children with handicaps that were not immediately evident at birth. In such cases the process of realization is more gradual. Nevertheless, many still experience shock, depression, frustration, anger, guilt, and feelings of isolation.

Several authors have observed the parents of children born with a cleft lip/palate. McWilliams (1982) commented that parents of a newborn baby with a cleft lip/palate face a crisis that they handle according to their own strengths and weaknesses, previous background, stress mechanisms, and personal philosophies of living. Spriestersbach (1963) noted that parents initially worry about the survival of their child, later experiencing anxieties about the child's speech, dentition, and social development. Brantley and Clifford (1980) found that mothers of cleft lip/palate children expressed significantly more concern and anxiety about their babies than did mothers of non-disfigured babies.

Reactions of parents following the birth of babies with craniofacial disfigurements are also negative. In addition, parents typically have many fears concerning the care of their children. Clifford (reported in Kapp, 1979) noted that such parents showed less pride in their child. He added that the negative ratings the mothers made of their offspring's appearance tended to carry over to the evaluation of the child's personality and level of intellectual functioning.

Hildebrandt (1982) noted that premature infants are more likely to be victims of abuse in later life, and speculated that premature babies fail to elicit the same positive caregiving response as full-term infants because the former possess fewer "babyish" characteristics and a less attractive appearance than the latter. In support of this, Hildebrandt cited Frodi et al. (1978), who stated that the aversiveness of the cry of a premature infant has been found to be compounded by the facial configuration of the premature baby.

An examination of the literature leaves no doubt that action is required in order to alleviate the problems experienced by parents of congenitally disfigured children. At present, the facilities for helping parents in many institutions leave much to be desired, with physicians and hospitals yet to establish acceptable procedures for managing the problems facing parents in the first crucial hours and days. In the case of babies with cleft lip/palate, for example, there is evidence that after the initial shock, parents want and need detailed information about the possibility and timing of repair, how to sort out feeding procedures, and so on (see, for example, E. Clifford, 1973).

Macgregor's work (1982) has painted a rosier picture of facilities in the United States than is apparent in Britain. She pointed out that in addition to improving surgical corrective techniques, attention has now been directed toward the study of "peripheral," but equally important, matters. The medical community now recognizes the necessity for a holistic approach to disfigurement and rehabilitation, including aspects such as parents' reactions, feelings, and attitudes and the development of satisfactory parent-child interaction—all essential components in the adjustment and adaptation of an anomalous child. Macgregor highlighted parents' need for professional attention if they are to be able to help both the child and themselves, together with long-term follow-up, as worries, needs, and concerns change over time.

The Development of Disfigured Children

A child's experiences during his or her early years contribute to his or her self-knowledge. The foundations of the self-concept are laid as early as the first few months, as the baby begins to distinguish what is "self" and "not self" (R. Burns, 1979). As children get older, they meet others outside the family, and encounter images from books, radio, and television concerning what children of their age are doing. Many of these experiences are potentially negative for children who are visibly different from the norm. From an early age they are less likely to receive positive communication ("Oh what a lovely boy/girl!"), and thus may become less responsive, learning less about themselves from other people (Adams, 1977a, 1977b). It may also be the case that less is expected from a disfigured child. For example, N. Bernstein (1982) suggested that many people consider children with cleft lip/palate to be less intelligent than "normals." He went on to suggest that a child's degree of disfiguration may determine more than anything else how the child feels about his or her handicap, even though the functional level of handicap may be relatively minor (as in the case of cleft lip/palate). Longacre (1973) has noted the difficulty in finding adoptive parents for children with a facial deformity, despite the fact that the disfigurement may not be in any way a physical handicap.

Some researchers have attempted to document the behavior patterns of children with specific anomalies. N. Peterson (1982), for example, looked at the social interactions and playmate preferences of four mild or moderately retarded children with Down's syndrome, and four normal 4- to 5-year-olds in the classroom and during play. Subjects were found to prefer to interact with peers who were like themselves in all of the situations. However, the normal children interacted more frequently with other children than did the children with Down's syndrome, who engaged in more isolated play.

Kapp (1979) investigated the behavior patterns of children age 5 to 8 years with cleft lip/palate. She found that children of both sexes exhibited disturbances in the emotional and social aspects of their self-concepts, and more often identified with a stimulus child who was unhappy or crying than with a stimulus child who was depicted as being happy. The children with cleft lip/palate played alone more often than nondisfigured children in a control group, and were often teased and chased away from play groups. Kapp noted a common wish of the children with cleft lip/palate to be able to blend in and not be noticed. She suggested that some of these children lacked the skills necessary for reciprocal play. Many saw themselves as more consistently "receiving from" than "giving to" their playmates. Kapp further suggested that as a result of overprotective parenting, the children may come to overidentify with the idea of being the one needing to be taken care of, and may lack belief in their ability to be happy. Starr (1978) compared 72 children with cleft lip/palate with 48 matched controls. He found no significant differences on a behavioral checklist, a self-esteem scale and an "Attitudes towards Clefting" scale, with the exception that the children with cleft lip/palate were physically more aggressive than the control children. Starr (1980) also looked at the behavior of "unattractive" and "attractive" children with cleft lip/palate, and once again found no significant differences in behavioral ratings, self-esteem, or attitude scales.

D. Harper and Richman (1978) examined MMPI profiles of forty-six 15- to 19-year-olds with orthopedic disabilities, and of fifty-two 14- to 19-year-olds with cleft lip/palate, and found greater behavioral inhibition in both groups compared with nondisfigured controls. Those with orthopedic disabilities showed a more isolated and passive orientation to interpersonal interactions, and a more generalized feeling of alienation than did the subjects with cleft lip/palate. The latter showed greater self-concern and ruminative self-doubt regarding interpersonal interaction than did those with orthopedic disabilities.

Richman and Harper (1978) reported a study of two groups of visibly disfigured subjects—one group with cleft/lip palate and one with cerebral palsy—with both groups compared to normal controls. They found that the subjects with visible disfigurements displayed significantly more inhibition of impulse and lower educational achievement than did controls. D. Harper and Richman (1978) also reported teachers' ratings of the school behavior of one hundred twenty-four 10- to 18-year-olds with either a cleft lip/palate or cerebral palsy. The children with cleft lip/palate were rated as showing significantly more impulsivity than controls. As an additional observation, Harper and Richman noted that those subjects who were rated as having mild physical impairment displayed greater behavioral inhibition than the more severely physically impaired.

The Effects of Children's Facial Disfigurement on Teachers

Richman and Harper (1978) reported a study of teachers' perceptions of the academic ability of a group of children with cleft lip/palate. The teachers accurately assessed the ability of a sample of nondisfigured children, but for those with cleft lip/palate they underestimated the ability of the high-ability group, and overestimated the ability of the low-ability group. They speculated that this effect may have been due to the operation of a stereotypical expectancy of a certain ability level for disfigured children, together with a sympathetic response to low-ability disfigured children. This study, together with others cited elsewhere (see Chapter 5 for a discussion of the effects of childrens' appearance in the educational setting), highlights the fact that the role of the teacher in the adjustment of the disfigured child is likely to be an important one. It seems that teachers could do much to influence the quality of life for disfigured children—at least in the classroom. Teachers could be made more aware, for example, of the tendency for the disfigured child to be left out in play sessions, and of the possibilities of manipulating the classroom environment to prevent this. The teacher is also in a position to influence by example the acquisition and maintenance of stereotypes that work to the detriment of the disfigured, thus influencing the opinions children may form of a disfigured peer.

The Family Environment

The family environment is obviously an important factor in the development of a disfigured child. The attitudes, expectations, and degree of support  shown by the people closest to the child are likely to have an enormous influence on the child's perception of his or her own disfigurement. It may even be that the family can influence the child's perception of the degree of handicap (N. Bernstein, 1982). Shakespeare (1975), for example, has suggested that it may be that a mildly intellectually handicapped person may be unnoticed in a "low intelligence" family with few academic interests, and that physical weakness may be less important in a family uninterested in sports and active pursuits. On the other hand, parents may be overly ambitious for their handicapped child, and a failure to reach the desired standard may make the child's limitations hard to accept, leading the family to consider requesting residential care for the child. In a similar way, a facially disfigured child may fare better in a family that shows little concern for the role of physical appearance in successful social and professional life.

Lansdown (1981) maintained that if the family is supportive and positive, the handicapped or disfigured child will be able to develop a self-image that is essentially positive. Thus in long-term relations, peers will be able to react more to the child's personality than to his or her disfigurement. However, this sort of positive atmosphere may be difficult for many families to achieve or maintain, especially if little support or encouragement exists outside the family. Hewett (1970) highlighted this problem when asking a group of mothers of children with palsy whether they felt isolated. Twenty-one percent said they did, with most believing it was a feeling rather than a real isolation. Many mothers wondered whether they were dealing with things in the right way and whether other families were going through the same problems. These families would be ideal candidates for support groups (see below).

Other common dilemmas for the family include the issue of hospitalization, which is frequently necessary for the cosmetic or functional repair of a disfigurement. Here a balance must be struck between increasing the child's chances of physical and social adaptation (by having the operation) and the emotional reaction the child may experience on being away from home and on having to cope with the pain and discomfort associated with surgery and treatment. A hospitalized child is separated from his or her peers at a time when those peers are needed most. He or she is also vulnerable to falling behind with school work, N. Bernstein (1976) suggested that if extra tutoring can be provided in the hospital setting, the pride the child may be able to take at outclassing his or her peers at reading, writing, and the like may in some way compensate for the problems associated with the disfigurement and the attendant surgical intervention. The level of interference from doctors, hospitals, and the like is potentially very high, and for many families there may be a tightrope of trying to develop normally despite the professionals, while still taking advantage of the services they provide. (See below for a discussion of health care provision for disfigured persons.)

What of the disfigured child's own perceptions of the family environment? Richman and Harper (1978) looked at the perceptions that children with cleft lip/palate had of their mothers. They found that the children (especially males) saw their mothers as exerting psychological control and as being more intrusive than did children with cerebral palsy or nondisfigured children. The mothers of children with cleft lip/palate seemed to have a tendency to nurture their offspring and to foster a dependency that may be more acceptable to girls than boys.

E. Clifford (1974) discovered that some facially disfigured children do perceive their parents as having predominently negative reactions to them since their birth, but many thought that despite their parents' apprehensions and worries the parents were able to nurture them and to take pride in them. It seems that for many parents it is possible to overcome negative feelings and to create at least a perception of acceptance.

Common Problems Associated with the Later Development
of Disfigured Children

Lansdown (1981) commented in relation to subjects with cleft lip/palate that in adulthood such people are conditioned to seek others outside the family, and in so doing, inevitably encounter stares and misconceptions. (see below for a discussion of the problems encountered in social interaction). Peter, Chinsky, and Fisher (1975) reported that many of their 195 patients with cleft lip/palate had more difficulty in meeting new people than did their 190 sibling controls. In addition, the sample with cleft lip/palate married at a lower rate and tended to have fewer children than the controls. Van Denmark and Van Denmark (1970) suggested that the level of achievement of those with cleft lip/palate in the world of work is less than ideal. Also, the social contacts of these people may be limited somewhat by their disfigurement, and there are closer ties with the immediate family. Van Denmark and Van Denmark also stated that marriage had occurred at a lower rate for their sample with cleft lip/palate compared with the nondisfigured sample. They did add, however, that there were no compelling studies that supported the assumption that people with cleft lip/palate are seriously disturbed or that they differ in major ways from nondisfigured peers.

A Historical Perspective on Disfigurement and Society

What of the influence exerted on disfigured people and their families by the society in which they live? Human societies have always had in their midst the physically maimed/deformed/ugly. Reactions to such people have varied, but have in general been that of abhorrence. The occurrence of deformity has at various times been thought to be due to gods, evil spirits, fairies, elves, or subhuman beings (Macgregor, 1974). From the first cave paintings to the present, all cultures have been involved in representing and interpreting the human form, with the majority endorsing the value of youth and beauty, and many associating distortions of the human form with evil and terror.

Ballantyne (reported in W. Shaw, 1981c) reported the existence of one tablet dating to 2000 years BC, which forecast that the infant "that had no tongue, the house of the man will be ruined—that has an upper lip overriding the lower, people of the world will rejoice." In ancient Greece, blemishes were inflicted as a form of punishment. The Greeks used the term *stigma* to refer to signs cut or burned into the body to signify something unusual or bad about the moral status of the person. Infanticide was even resorted to in some cases of children whose appearance was unacceptable. Artistotle, who is credited with one of the earliest objective studies of the face, concluded among other things that, "Men with small foreheads are fickle, whereas if they are round or bulging out, the owners are quick tempered. . . . The staring eye indicates impudence, the winking, indecision. Large and outstanding ears indicate a tendency to irrelevant talk and chattering" (cited by Burr, 1935). Somewhat later, Frederick of Denmark ruled in 1708 that no person with a facial deformity should show himself or herself to a pregnant woman.

Historically, facial deformity has also been associated with mental retardation. Hogarth's 18th-century paintings of depravity and inmates of mental institutions are notorious for portraying ugly or deformed faces (Munro, 1981). In more recent times, in Nazi Germany the handicapped, insane, and deformed were included in death camps along with Jews, gypsies, and homosexuals. Even now, in societies such as ours that use the criterion of normality as a measure of acceptance and affiliation, the imperfections and irregularities that occur in nature are a source of intrigue and revulsion (Macgregor, 1974). Many still assume that a person with a congenital deformity (whether facial or otherwise) it also mentally retarded (see below).

The Importance of Societal Values

Society exerts an influence on the disfigured person from the moment of birth, when friends and relations may not send the customary cards and gifts, and subsequently, when parents have to cope with the curiosity of those who have noticed that the child does not look "normal" (Shakespeare, 1975). Society defines what is and what is not a handicap, whether it is being a woman, a homosexual, or a member of a religious minority, or having a physical deformity. Society also dictates the acceptability or unacceptability of aberrations in appearance, labeling with devaluative connotations those who are considered deviant in any way. Society's norms and values will to some extent affect the degree of acceptance or rejection of a disfigured person. For example, whether a disfigured person lives in a community where such factors as tolerance and good neighborliness are prized, and whether it is considered appropriate to provide support for the family of a disfigured person, will dictate to some degree whether or not the person will be included or excluded from the mainstream of society.

Previous chapters in this book have revealed that there is a high premium placed on physical appearance in our society. Media advertisements for beauty aids endorse the idea that beautiful people have better prospects for happy professional and social lives. The boom in the cosmetic industry, in plastic surgery, in diet foods, and in the fashion business are all indicators of the major economic investment made in appearance. This in many cases intensifies the effects of a physical deviation. Most people have the desire to conform to the standards of the society in which they live, and a failure to do so (whether temporary or permanent) sets people apart both in their own estimation and in the opinions of others.

The bias that many societies have toward the physically perfect may make the plight of those who are deviant desperate, and many may feel under pressure to reestablish a "normal" appearance in order to get back into the realms of what is acceptable. E. Clifford (1973) maintained that the person who is disfigured "is marked, not because he fails to achieve the ideal state of being beautiful, but because he has failed to achieve a minimum standard of acceptability." This failure may be caused by even relatively minor disfigurements. For example, in several societies a small chin is taken to denote weakness, and a large nose alcoholism and self-indulgence. Thus even people with minor disfigurements may feel enormous pressure to try to change their appearance in order to escape from stereotypic judgments of their personality. Facial beauty is especially prized in our society (Rumsey, 1983), and this creates particular pressures for people with facial disfigurements. The face is particularly difficult to conceal, and heavy makeup may create an effect that is worse than the disfigurement itself. Trust (1977) stated that the visibility of a facial abnormality means "walking around as a permanently branded second class citizen." Hirschenfang, Goldberg, and Benton (1969) have also noted that facially disfigured persons are at a particular disadvantage. As we shall discuss below, they are regarded as social inferiors, and many are conscious of the lowly status they are assigned in society. Clifford (1973) maintained that the existence of an orofacial anomaly affects family, friends, acquaintances, and strangers. Furthermore, these effects are reciprocal, because all these groups provide feedback to the disfigured person, forming in effect a social mirror whose reflections are interpreted by the anomalous person.

The natural tendency of humans to form groups within society may also work to the disadvantage of disfigured persons. Strauss (1980) noted that the formation of homogenous in-crowds depends on the existence of outsiders— rejects or deviants. Physical characteristics provide an easy and reliable means of defining group membership since these are characteristics that are readily evident to anyone who cares to look. Indeed Goffman (1963) included facially disfigured persons in his remarks concerning stigmatized individuals. He saw such people as being disqualified from full social acceptance, and set apart from "normals," who impute a wide range of imperfections on the basis of the original stigmatizing attribute. Strauss maintained that the dominant group usually forms myths and fantasies about deviant persons, and disfigured individuals may be placed in a stigmatized subgroup, independently of their personal qualities.

Negative Stereotyping and Negative Attitudes Toward Disfigured Persons—Do They Exist?

Eliciting the true nature of peoples' feelings toward disfigured persons is a difficult task. Many people find it hard to admit (both to themselves and to others) that they do submit visibly disfigured individuals to any sort of rejection. However, there is some evidence (albeit predominantly circumstantial) that a form of rejection does occur. There is little doubt in the minds of many disfigured people that members of the general public hold negative attitudes toward them (Rumsey, 1983). Although there are many speculative theories and opinions concerning the nature of attitudes toward the visibly handicapped, systematic research is meager—the bulk of information comes from classicial and modern literature, religious writings, folklore, popular humor, and the personal accounts of the visually stigmatized. In the absence of a well-developed body of research concerning attitudes toward disfigured and handicapped persons, much reliance has been made on the descriptions given by these people of their encounters with others. In a host of written and oral accounts, the theme of being pitied, subordinated, and ignored appears (Barker, 1948; Goffman, 1963; Wright, 1960).

Macgregor (1951) pointed out that even a slight anomaly can cause a negative reaction ("I wouldn't trust a man with a low forehead"). She quoted examples given to her by her sample of facially disfigured people. A man with an enlarged red nose caused by angioma, for example, complained that people frequently took him for a drunk. Another, with facial paralysis, reported that others dubbed him as a wise guy, because he talked out of the side of his mouth. I. Katz (1981) cited Carling (1962), who stated that a "cripple must be careful not to act differently from what people expect him do to. . . . they must expect a cripple to be crippled, to be disabled and helpless; to be inferior to themselves, and they will become suspicious and insecure if the cripple falls short of these expectations."

Where does this negative stereotyping of disfigured people come from? Some maintain that the explanations of the origins of congenital disfigurement are remnants of folklore and mythology passed on from generation to generation. Macgregor (1951) reported that a common reaction to harelip was the belief that the mother of the deformed offspring had touched a rabbit when pregnant, and that someone born without an ear encountered explanations such as the mother having been unfaithful to her husband. W. Shaw's (1981c) observations and survey in Wales of current-day beliefs relating to congenital birthmarks (known colloquially as "port wine stains") showed evidence of remnants of medieval folklore. Many of his sample attributed port wine stains to various causes, notably the consumption of strawberries or red cabbage (or to an unsatisfied craving for these during pregnancy). Less frequently, mothers of disfigured children were thought to have been frightened by an animal, to have had contact with blood during pregnancy, or to have suffered an extra-abdominal injury. A few people considered that the mother had probably been frightened by a hare or rabbit.

Other researchers have found evidence for stereotyping stemming from sources other than folklore or mythology. Rumsey (1983), for example, reported that stories written about photographs of facially disfigured people by a sample of eighty-four 7-year-olds reflected prejudices and stereotypes that appeared to emanate directly from popular literature (such as comic books), and from the television.

Developmental Studies of Stereotyping of Disfigured Persons

There is no doubt that children do express negative attitudes toward disfigured and handicapped persons. Centers and Centers (1963) found that even after a long period of exposure, children with amputations were more likely to be named by nonhandicapped classmates as the saddest, least liked, least nice looking, and least fun children in the class. W. Shaw (1981c) has noted that children's disapproval of deviant physical features is openly voiced, and that children with disfigurements such as cleft lip/palate or burns report frequent teasing and harassment. Jansen and Esser (1971—reported in N. Bernstein, 1976) canvassed thousands of subjects, including children. Few reported wanting to be friendly with a deformed person. Almost two-thirds of the sample actually thought that disfigured persons should be kept out of sight. The question arises of at what age such stereotypical reactions develop. Even though, as Adams and Crossman (1978) pointed out, "Binet in his early construction of the Stanford-Binet intelligence test used an item which required 6 year olds to discriminate between a beautiful and an ugly person," to the authors' knowledge, there has been minimal attention paid by researchers to the development in children of stereotyping of facially disfigured persons. (Chapter 6 focuses on children's reactions to nondisfigured faces.)

However, some developmental studies have been carried out to shed light on the age at which stereotypical judgments of handicaps and disability have become apparent. Weinberg (1978) addressed the question of whether 3- to 5-year-olds have an understanding of disability, and whether their attitudes toward disabled children differ from their attitudes toward able-bodied youngsters. Weinberg's results, using twenty-five 3-year-old, fifty-three 4-year-old, and twenty-three 5-year-old able-bodied subjects, suggested a shift from a lack of understanding to comprehension occurring between 3 and 4 years of age, with negative attitudes developing at the age of approximately 5 years. In a second study, using eleven 3-year-olds, forty-two 4-year-olds, and ten 5-year-olds, Weinberg used a forced choice method to reexamine when negative attitudes develop. Her results indicated that by the age of 4 to 5 years, subjects significantly favored able-bodied over disabled children. Kleck and Strenta (1985a) have also stated that by the age of 4 years, not only are children capable of discriminating between handicapped and nonhandicapped people, but they are already likely to reject the former as friends.

Richardson (1970) showed 5- to 12-year-old children drawings of youngsters with different visible handicaps (e.g., a child with crutches and a leg brace, a child with a missing hand, a child in a wheelchair, and a child with a facial disfigurement). He reported a general liking for the nonhandicapped over the handicapped child, and noted that whereas dislike of a functional handicap (e.g., leg brace) decreased with the increasing age of the child rater, dislike for a facial disfigurement increased. Older subjects showed an increased liking for the stimulus child as the abnormality became more distant from the face. Richardson concluded that by the age of 5 to 6, the children had developed consistent attitudes toward different forms of handicap.

Siperstein and Gottlieb (1977) compared fourth- and fifth-grade children's ratings of peers with "normal" appearance to their ratings of those with Down's syndrome. Despite providing subjects with information about the level of competence of each stimulus child, they found that the physical stigmata of Down's syndrome were sufficiently salient in the children's perceptions that they could not easily dismiss them in their evaluations. They concluded that the physical appearance variable was sufficiently potent to diminish the favorableness with which competent children were otherwise judged.

Rumsey, Bull, and Gahagan's (1986) study (see Chapter 6) was specifically designed to examine whether negative reactions to facially disfigured people would be demonstrated by girls and boys aged 5 to 11 years. The children were asked to attribute positive or negative characteristics to photographs in which adults were depicted before and after oral surgery to correct asymmetries of the jaw. Despite the relatively small differences in appearance between each adult's before and after operation photographs, it was found that the 11-year-old subjects attributed significantly more positive attributes to the after-operation photographs than to the pictures of the adult stimuli before their operations. Interestingly, when the children's own judgments of facial attractiveness were used, it was found that they made significantly reliable stereotypical judgments to the detriment of the less attractive stimuli by the age of 6 years. M. Elliott et al. (1986) examined the judgments of subjects drawn from four age groups—6 to 7 years, 9 to 11 years, 13 to 15 years, and 25 to 35 years—to photographs of faces taken before and after relatively minor facial reconstructive surgery. There were no statistically significant effects for judgments of the before and after photographs by subjects of less than 13 years. However, subjects of 13 to 15 years judged the persons in the "after" photographs as significantly more attractive and happier than the "before" photographs, and adults in the 25 to 35 years age group judged the "after" operation faces to be significantly more intelligent than the "before" faces. In addition, the female stimuli were judged to be significantly more attractive in the "after" operation condition, and female subjects rated the "after" photographs of both male and female stimuli as significantly happier than the "before" photographs. Taken together, the results of these two studies suggest that children develop (probably as the result of social learning) stereotypes that work to the detriment of disfigured persons by the age of 11 to 12 years.

Adults' Reactions to Facially Disfigured Persons

Some studies have been carried out to demonstrate the existence of stereotypes held by adults that work to the detriment of facially disfigured persons. Secord (1958) gave subjects a brief verbal "personal" account of two imaginary characters. The accounts were the same except for the words "warmhearted and honest" or "ruthless and brutal." Subjects gave an indication of the appearance they expected the characters to have by rating 32 physical characteristics on 7-point scales. Secord found that 25 out of the 32 characteristics were significantly different as a function of the personality accounts, with subjects using "average" characteristics for the "warmhearted and honest" person (e.g., "average width of nose") but abnormal features (e.g., a "very narrow" or "very wide nose") for the "ruthless and brutal" person.

Some researchers (see I. Katz, 1981; Kleck and Strenta, 1985b) believe that adults' reactions to stigmatized persons are a complex mixture of positive and negative responses, and note that although some studies have assessed reactions to physically stigmatized persons by means of interviews and questionnaires, few have involved observations of overt behavior.

Adults may be socialized to be kind and compassionate to physically disadvantaged persons. As a result of this, *verbalized* attitudes may reflect large-ly positive dispositions toward handicapped individuals. However, some aspects of actual *behavior* are more consistent with the negative affective reactions of children. Heinemann, Pellander, Vogelbusch, and Wojtek (1981) noted that aspects of nonverbal behavior are less intentional than verbal attitudinal statements, and may reflect uneasiness and negative feelings elicited by deviant persons. I. Katz (1981) believes that the social approval afforded to those who treat stigmatized people kindly stems from Judeo-Christian teachings. At the heart of this doctrine is the image of Christ the Healer as a model of devotion to the physical afflicted. Some studies have reflected this positive aspect of attitudes toward the handicapped—for exam-ple, Wright (1960) found that people are inclined to respect those who man-age to cope with adversity. Other studies have shown handicapped people as more intelligent and better adjusted than nonhandicapped people, or as more personally good (Shakespeare, 1975). On the negative side, Katz pointed out that despite evidence for positive verbalized attitudes toward stigmatized per-sons, bodily defects also engender deeper, largely unconscious feelings of rejection. Katz talked of a general tendency to dislike anyone who arouses fear or guilt, and to perceive stigmatized individuals as inferior, perhaps responsible for their own fate. From a historical perspective, Shakespeare (1975) reported that on the whole, public attitudes toward handicaps have shown a change in a positive direction over the years, although a considerable proportion of negative response is still evident. She made the point that a rejecting reaction toward disabled persons is usually found to be part of a generally prejudiced reaction toward any group seen as different, whether in terms of ethnic origin, religion, or handicap. Thus people who are accepting toward one kind of stigma are more likely to be accepting toward all stigma-tizing conditions.

The Relationship Between Societal Values and the Demand for Cosmetic Surgery

The high value placed on physical appearance in society and the powerful pressure that society exerts on disfigured persons can be illustrated by the enormous increase in demand for cosmetic surgery in recent years (Colligan, Sather, & Hollen, 1980). Prior to the advent of plastic surgery in Western culture, the unacceptable/ugly/deformed person was stigmatized or hidden (the latter option pertaining only to a small percentage of people at the bottom end of the continuum of acceptability), and the band of those consid-ered to be within the range of "normality" was broader. However, as plastic surgery techniques have advanced, with surgeons now able to offer "improve-ments" in the appearance of many, our perceptions of the acceptability of physical deviations have altered (Strauss, 1980), with the range of "normal-ity" becoming notably more narrow.

The improvements in surgical techniques coupled with the proliferation of surgeons who are willing to operate have meant that concerns have been reawakened in many people who had formerly accepted their disfigurement and the social role that accompanied it. Western society transmits its criteria for standards of beauty quite explicitly (largely via the media), and also suggests that deformity should be dealt with in a medical context. Medicine has responded by providing a means to alter those characteristics that society deems to be deviant, whether the deviance is of ethnic, traumatic, or congenital origin. In many cases cosmetic surgery may improve matters (Rumsey, 1983). However, the availability of surgery also exacerbates the dilemma of how society should deal with disfigurement. Should we integrate, alter, or reject those whose appearance does not conform to our ever increasingly exacting norms?

Cultural Differences

Although there are common elements in how societies relate to disfigurement, each brings its own special fears, myths, and explanations into the formulation of what is considered to be an appropriate response. Easson (1966) maintained that each society has a built-in set of values of facial appearance to guide behavior (e.g., in many societies a high forehead is often said to denote intelligence). The range of openly displayed disfigurements varies from culture to culture, and although some religions and cultures consider deformity to be a sign of grace or spiritual power, these are in the minority. The segregation of individuals who are disfigured or otherwise stigmatized has been (and still in some cases is) fashionable in many cultures, as witnessed by cloistered settings such as leper colonies, mental institutions, or other asylums to keep deviance hidden from the population of "normals."

In the majority of present-day societies, the impact of wars has done much to increase the prevalence of openly displayed handicaps, with a higher incidence of amputations, burns, and other visible disfigurements in the decades following combat. There is evidence that in Western societies attitudes toward some forms of disfigurement (e.g., physical handicap) are improving, with alterations in terminology (e.g., "Mongolism" has now become "Down's syndrome"), improved access in public buildings, and so on (Shakespeare, 1975). However, open prejudice may still exist in many societies (W. Shaw, 1981c).

Babalola (1978; see Shaw 1981c) noted that in some African tribes, deformed persons are prohibited from elevation to chieftancy. In the Indian subcontinent the family of a deformed child is held in low esteem until certain purifying rituals have been carried out (Dehragoda, 1978; quoted in Shaw, 1981c). In Japan, it has been reported (McGill, 1984) that "dozens" of politicians are treated for "image" problems each year at Tokyo's Cosmetic Surgery Hospital. (Chapter 3 presents an account of research on the role of appearance in politics and persuasion.) In the same newspaper article, it was revealed that the Tokyo Fire and Marine Insurance Company admitted to hiring pretty girls first in preference to plain ones. Similarly, a major Japanese bookseller issues guidelines to personnel instructing them not to hire "ugly" women.

Here then is a summary of the sorts of pressures exerted on disfigured people and their families by the societies in which they live. How do these pressures manifest themselves in the day-to-day lives of disfigured people? One of the most common problems cited by disfigured individuals is that of difficulties in social interaction (Rumsey 1983).

Social Interaction Involving Disfigured Persons

Despite the lack of research concerning problems in social interaction for disfigured persons, some common elements have emerged. Many have referred to problems of initial encounters with strangers. Abel (1952), for example, reported that all of her sample of 74 patients hospitalized for corrective surgery thought that their facial disfigurement was in some way a deterrent to successful living, with many complaining that they were discriminated against in work and social situations. Andreasi and Norris (1972) reported on 9 female and 11 male severely burned subjects aged 18 to 60 years. Their subjects objected to the pity and curiosity they reported seeing in the eyes of strangers. Andreasi and Norris stated that it seemed as if the public singled out disfigured persons as different, even if they did not openly express hostility. The female subjects were especially reluctant to go out in public, because they believed they would have to submit themselves to stares, questions, or even rude remarks.

Bryt (1966) speculated (using only one case history) that a major hurdle took the form of problems associated with interpersonal competence. Hirschenfang et al. (1969) studied 25 in- and outpatients with facial paralysis. They reported that the sample frequently complained of difficulties in making friends, of lack of opportunities for marriage, of the weakening of family constellations, and of problems in obtaining jobs. Hirschenfang et al. noted that staring, remarks, and questions were the most frequent reactions of others, and that this caused their subjects extreme discomfort. Peter et al. (1975) reported that their 195 subjects with cleft palate reported more difficulty in meeting new people than their 190 sibling controls.

Some studies specifically remark on problems encountered by facially disfigured persons with members of the opposite sex. W. Jacobson, Edgerton, Meyer, Canter, and Slaughter (1961) maintained that the majority of their sample of male patients coming in to the John Hopkins Hospital ($n = 33$) in a 2-year period had major problems regarding their heterosexual effectiveness. Knorr, Edgerton, and Hoopes (1967) conducted a survey of 692 plastic surgeons and reported that one of the most frequent complaints made by patients was of difficulty in developing significant long-term relationships. Lefebvre and Munro (1978) studied a sample of male and female craniofacial disfigurement patients aged 6 weeks to 37 years. The teenage boys and girls in the sample reported experiencing "cold treatment" by members of the opposite sex. Peter et al. (1975) found that their sample of persons with cleft palate married at a lower rate and tended to have fewer children than their sibling control group.

Many writers report that in addition to problems in social interaction, facially disfigured persons experience negative reactions from members of the general public. Aamot (1978) reported that his sample of 30 patients persistently claimed that they could sense the negative reactions of others, even if nothing was said, and that they were "rejected" by both sexes. In a study of 34 adolescents with burn injuries, Goldberg, Bernstein, and Crosby (1975) reported that subjects may encounter staring, feelings of pity, and revulsion in others, in addition to teasing and avoidance by peers. Hirschenfang et al. (1969) stated that it is not unusual to see disgust or horror in the expressions of someone who sees a severely facially deformed person.

Kleck and Strenta (1980) conducted a study that, although concerned with reactions to handicapped persons, would also seem to be of relevance to interactions with facially disfigured persons. They examined the nature of behavioral exchange when able-bodied individuals interact for the first time with someone who is handicapped. They recorded differences in emotional arousal, gestural activity, duration of eye contact, use of personal space, and time spent in face-to-face interaction. The results indicated, at least initially, that able-bodied people were negatively aroused, uncertain, and motivated to avoid interactions with handicapped persons.

Davis (1961) reported that interaction between visibly normal and visibly handicapped people can lead to anxiety and a "pronounced stickiness of interactional flow." Davis maintained that the "normal" person experiences embarrassment, and all too obviously conveys the message that he or she is having difficulty in relating to the handicapped person. Marinelli (1974) measured the state anxiety of undergraduates who interacted with a peer who appeared either with a facial disfigurement or nondisfigured. The results indicated that interactions with the facially disfigured peer resulted more frequently in increased anxiety for the subjects.

Here then is evidence of the negative experiences many facially disfigured people experience in interactions with members of the general public. Next we will examine how negative impressions are conveyed to facially disfigured people by others.

How Are the Negative Impressions Conveyed?

Many facially disfigured people complain in a nonspecific way of negative reactions from others. One of the tasks facing psychologists is to shed light onto this. Some researchers (e.g., Goffman, 1963) have offered explanations as to why stigmatized people in general are avoided. Others have noted that different types of stigmata do not always have the same interpersonal consequences. For example, Farina, Sherman, and Allen (1968) looked at the general public's reaction to people labeled as mentally ill versus those confined to a wheelchair, and found that the latter were treated more favorably. Albrecht, Walker, and Levy (1982) collected data from 150 subjects, who expressed preferences for maintaining greater social distances from deviant persons (alcoholics/drug addicts) than from disabled persons (paraplegic/ blind), thus illustrating differential reactions to those with different types of stigma in social interactions.

The little research that has been done relating to the rejection of facially disfigured persons (Rumsey, 1983) indicates that differences even exist in the reactions to various types of facial disfigurement. For example, reactions to congenital disfigurements tend to be more extreme than reactions to traumatic injury (with the possible exception of burn injuries). In addition, reactions to disfigurement involving the communication equipment of the face (primarily the eyes and mouth) may be more aversive than disfigurements of more peripheral facial features (forehead, cheeks, chin).

What is the mechanism of the avoidance of disfigured persons by others? Recent research into the behavior of the general public toward disfigured compared with nondisfigured people suggests that the differences may lie in the subtleties of nonverbal communication. Interest in the role of nonverbal communication has escalated enormously in the last couple of decades, with an increasing realization of its crucial importance and pervasiveness in interpersonal communication. The nonverbal communication literature leaves no doubt of the power of the nonverbal aspects of communication used by both parties in social interactions (see Kleck and Nuessle [1968], Mehrabian [1972], and Wiemann [1974] for eye contact; Matarazzo and Wiens [1972] and Pope, Nudler, Vonkorff, and McGhee [1974] for speech patterns; Hoffman [1968] for gestures). Birdwhistell (1952) endorsed the importance of nonverbal communication by stating that "more than 35% of social meaning is carried by the verbal component of conversation, and 60% or more on the nonverbal band." As Goffman (1971) pointed out, even if participants are not normally conscious of communication in the nonverbal channel, they nevertheless still sense that something is sharply amiss whenever something out of the ordinary is conveyed.

Nonverbal communication is difficult to suppress—verbal exchanges can be avoided, but nonverbal aspects of behavior are conveyed almost automatically. It may perhaps be that members of the public would like to keep private any negative reactions to physical and social handicap, but that they unconsciously convey their feelings through nonverbal behavior. Rumsey (1983) and Rumsey and Bull (1986) have noted, for example, that if facially disfigured people attempt to engage others in brief encounters in the street, many members of the public will try to avoid them if possible, by increasing their pace, averting their gaze, and attempting to ignore the presence of the disfigured person (in much the same way as many of us try to avoid market researchers, opinion pollers, etc.). This avoidance is picked up by the disfigured person, who frequently interprets it as a form of rejection. When, in a few cases, contact is established, deviations from the "normal" pattern of interaction are still often noticed by the disfigured people. Symptoms of avoidance sometimes occur: for example, the other person may perhaps step backward, thus creating more space between themselves and the disfigured person; pauses in speech and action may be followed by compensatory behavior; there may be a lack of eye contact (perhaps because of a desire to avoid being thought to be looking at the facial disfigurement, or because of embarrassment), thus depriving the disfigured person of an important source of communication (Argyle & Dean, 1965; Ekman, 1965). Once again disfigured people seem frequently to interpret these abnormal interaction patterns as symptomatic of negative affect on the behalf of members of the public.

Research in this area is complex, not least because people react to and form impressions of others on the basis of clusters of cues. In their attempts to unravel the complexities of the effects of nonverbal communication, some researchers (e.g., Mehrabian, 1968; Rumsey, Bull, & Gahagan, 1982) have limited themselves to an examination of one aspect of nonverbal behavior, and others have employed stimulus materials and situations that have represented varying degrees of realism (e.g., Goldring, 1967; Kleck et al., 1968). Consequently, research results must be carefully examined in terms of their relevance and generalizability to facially disfigured people.

Many researchers have concentrated on personal space (proxemics) because it is relatively easy to measure objectively, and because, if necessary, it can be measured from a distance without interactants being aware that they are being observed. Two areas of personal space research seem of particular relevance to disfigured and handicapped persons. The first is that of the effect of liking and attraction for the other. Several types of methodology have been used, with varying results. Rosenfeld (1966) found that when subjects were instructed to adopt an "approval seeking" role as opposed to an "approval avoiding" role, they positioned themselves significantly closer to an experimental confederate. Mehrabian (1968) instructed undergraduates to approach a hat rack, while imagining that the hat rack varied in sex, status, and attitude. This, and further studies (e.g., Mehrabian & Friar, 1969) indicated that distances decreased as subjects imagined themselves being more positive toward the hypothetical adressee. Mehrabian (1968) also used undergraduates to judge the attitudes of confederates depicted in sets of static photographs. He found a closer position was interpreted by subjects as communicating a more positive attitude.

Goldring (1967) presented students with cartoon drawings depicting characters at near and far distances. Using adjective checklists, subjects described those at closer distances as more warm, active, excited, and responsive than those depicted at greater distances. Similarly Kleck (1969) found that when subjects were told that another person was "warm and friendly" (as opposed to "cold and unfriendly") they chose seating that was closer to the other person. Barrios and Giesen (1976) reported that a group's positive or negative expectations of forthcoming interaction affected their choice of seating distance from another, with those subjects who were led to expect hostile interaction adopting more distant seats from other members of the group.

The second area of research concerns studies that examine the effects of a social stigma such as a handicap on the proxemic behavior of others. Kleck et al. (1968), using a figure placement task, found that subjects placed an amputee further away from their own self-representation than in other conditions involving representations of a friend, a blind person, or a black person. Epileptic and mental patient stimuli were placed at an even greater distance. This was followed by a study in which Kleck (1970) found that subjects who actually interacted with a confederate who was described as an epileptic chose a significantly greater seating distance than in the control condition.

Tolor and Salafia (1971) used figures about whom a variety of unfavorable personal attributes had been disclosed (i.e., "low intelligence, low prestige, bad personal adjustment"). Subjects placed these at a greater distance than figures to whom positive traits had been assigned. Comer and Piliavin (1972) found that in face-to-face interviews, subjects stayed at a greater distance from a disabled person than from a nondisabled one. Worthington (1974) reported that when she requested directions in an airport while sitting in a wheelchair, subjects stood significantly further away than those who were asked for directions by the experimenter in the nonhandicapped condition. (The methodology of this study is somewhat suspect, because it is not clear whether the increased personal space reported is due to subjects' reactions to the handicap or to the physical constraints of approaching someone in a wheelchair).

N. Bernstein (1976) specifically related his observations of personal space to disfigured people. He used Hall's (1959) typology of proxemics, in which separate personal space "zones" are defined. These consist of "very close" (3–6″), "close" (8–12″), "near" (12–20″), "neutral" (20″–5′), "public distance" (5½–8′) and "across the room" (8–20′). Bernstein maintained that in interaction with a disfigured person, there is a strong tendency for others to avoid "very close," "close," and "near" distances, and to choose instead the "neutral" zone, with "public distance" preferred. Bernstein's comments, however, were speculative and not backed up with experimental evidence.

Rumsey et al. (1982) provided data on the proxemic behavior of 450 members of the general public in encounters with a confederate in three different conditions—with a facial birthmark, with facial scarring and bruising consistent with a road traffic accident, and in a nondisfigured condition. They reported that people stood significantly further away from the confederate in the disfigured conditions than from the nondisfigured confederate. In addition, Rumsey et al. reported that in the disfigured conditions subjects chose to stand significantly more often on the confederate's nondisfigured side (the disfigurement only appeared on one side of the confederate's face). Subjects also stood significantly further away from the confederate in the birthmark condition than in the scarring condition. These results thus given credence to the hypothesis that people react less adversely to a "temporary" type of facial disfigurement than they do to a more permanent congenital one. Wolfgang and Wolfgang (1968) also found that those with temporary disfigurements (in this case, a broken arm) were approached to a closer distance than those with an amputated leg or club foot. (These stimuli were in turn afforded a closer distance than an obese confederate.) Rumsey (1983) commented that this finding has been corroborated by the comments of both genuinely disfigured people and confederates participating in experiments set in a wide range of social situations.

It would seem, then, that disfigured persons are correct in their assertion that they are being avoided, at least to the extent that people stand further away from them than they do from "normals." Two questions remain to be answered, however; first, what are the consequences of this feeling of avoidance, and second, what is the motivation behind the avoidance by the general public?

What Are the Consequences of the Negative Reactions of Others?

Complaints of facially disfigured people regarding social interaction include feelings of powerlessness and lack of control over the environment, especially in interaction with strangers. There seems in many cases to be a discrepancy between how disfigured persons would like social interactions to take place and what actually occurs (Rumsey, 1983). Argyle (1978) used Rotter's concept of locus of control as an analogy for those (such as many disfigured people) who experience difficulties in social interaction, stating that such people tend toward an external locus of control, often experiencing invasions of privacy (e.g., staring) together with feelings of helplessness because of their lack of control over the environment.

Privacy

Westin (1970) defined privacy as the right of an individual to decide what information about himself or herself should be communicated to others, and under what conditions such information exchange should occur. Goffman (1963) stated that a person with a stigma such as a visible disfigurement becomes an "unusual" person. He maintained that the more there is about an individual that deviates in an undesirable direction from what one might expect, the more obliged that person is to volunteer information about himself or herself. In addition, others feel able to strike up abnormal conversations with such people, and pay them an inordinate amount of attention even when involved in seemingly very ordinary events. Furthermore, each time a stigmatized person makes a spectacle of himself or herself, the local community (and sometimes even the media) take special notice, thus further invading the privacy of the visibly stigmatized person.

Researchers (e.g., Macgregor, 1974; Rumsey, 1983) have noted that members of the general public stare quite openly at disfigured people. Although it may be a pleasant feeling to receive flattering attention from a stranger, many disfigured individuals report that they find it distressing to be stared at, and deplore the fact that they are powerless to prevent this. People with visible disfigurements thus lose the "civil inattention" (Goffman, 1971)—the anonimity in a crowd—that the majority of us enjoy. Facially disfigured people, in particular, are deprived of this right since they are unable to hide their abnormality from others. The resulting invasions of privacy may be traumatic experiences. Pennock (1971) and Beardsley (1971) have spoken of invasions of privacy as being especially harmful, since they can destroy individual autonomy, self-respect, and dignity by taking away a measure of the person's control over social interaction.

Loneliness and Isolation

Not only are disfigured people subject to invasions of privacy, but paradoxically, they also frequently experience loneliness and isolation as a result of avoidance by members of the general public. N. Bernstein's (1976) speculations concerning the enlarged personal space zones of disfigured people have been supported by evidence from the study by Rumsey et al. (1982), described above. Feelings of loneliness and isolation in interpersonal situations may have further implications for how disfigured persons react to others. Altman and Haythorn (1967) analyzed the territorial behavior of socially isolated and nonisolated pairs. For 10 days, two individuals lived in a small room, with no outside contact. A matched group did receive contacts. Altman and Haythorn found that the men in the isolated group showed a gradual increase in isolated behavior and in general patterns of social withdrawal, expressing the desire to spend more time alone. Although this represents an extreme case of isolation, it may be that consistently negative experiences may also decrease the disfigured person's desired level of social contact.

In addition, the mere fact of becoming anxious or stressed about a situation may be enough to increase the distance between participants. Dosey and Meisels (1969) used a (somewhat artificial) figure placement task and stressed subjects by telling them that their physical attractiveness was being scrutinized. They found that stressed subjects tended to maintain a greater distance between stimulus figures. Reports that facially disfigured people feel their appearance to be under scrutiny are available in Macgregor (1974) and Trust (1977). In addition Rumsey (1983) recounted the feelings of confederates who, when made up to be facially disfigured, reported being very conscious of being a focus of attention and speculation for the general public. Thus, it is not unreasonable to speculate that facially disfigured people will be on the defensive in social interaction, and may tend to put a greater distance between themselves and other people than would otherwise be the case. This in turn merely serves to increase the loneliness and isolation that many facially disfigured people are prone to experiencing.

Problems of Self-Definition

Few researchers dispute the importance of a positive self-concept for a person's well-being and effective social behavior. Similarly, problems in social interaction can often affect a person's self-definition. If, whether through the medium of personal space or otherwise, a person repeatedly fails to implement a desired level of contact with others, then that person may develop a more negative self-definition than would have resulted from more successful regulation of interaction with others (Argyle, 1978).

There is a wealth of data in social psychology that suggests that the smooth running of social interaction is also of vital importance to the ongoing development of a positive self-concept. Sommer (1969), for example, argued that people acquire and develop their self-concept through interaction. Any change in the normal interaction pattern (e.g., unflattering attention or avoidance) is liable to lead to uncertainty. Festinger's social comparison theory (1957) stated that people who find themselves in ambiguous or uncertain situations will seek the help of others to interpret uncertainties, label feelings, and define perceptions. In this way a set of norms or standards for interpreting both the self and others is built up. A person finding himself or herself to be in a different situation relative to others may undergo a negative change in self-concept. In light of the above discussion of the problems encountered in social interaction by facially disfigured people, Festinger's comments are clearly of relevance to the present discussion.

Symbolic interactionists (e.g., Charon, 1979) have put forward the idea that through interaction, a person comes to hold an internal conception or interpretation of the opinions and attitudes of others. There is a positive relationship between how a person perceives others to respond to him or her and how that person feels about himself or herself. D. Smith and Williamson (1977) have taken the discussion one step further with the view that "our body images are shaped by our communication transactions which in turn shape our future transactions."

Other writers (Macgregor, 1974; Bernstein, 1976) have been more specific in stressing the vital importance of interaction for disfigured persons as a means of them defining their self-concepts. These writers predict that if facially disfigured persons perceive negative reactions from others during the course of social interaction, then their self-concept will become more negative. This more negative view of the self is then carried forward to the next interaction. If Ziller (1973) is correct, those people who experience a lowering of self-esteem in this way will subsequently show less consistent behavior, making successful social interaction even more diffcult. The lack of confidence people with low self-esteem have in their self-perceptions will lead them to become "field dependent" (i.e., they conform to a large extent to the influence and context of the environment), and also to their refusing signs of acceptance and approval from others. (Ziller maintained that those people who are high in self-esteem are not so dependent on the immediate situation because their behavior is governed by a well-ordered set of perceptions.) Thus the image individuals have of themselves plays a part in their interactions with others, providing a perspective for viewing relationships with other people.

Despite many indicators of the likely importance of the self-concept for facially disfigured people, there is as yet little systematic research to study the effects of the self-concept on behavior. Indeed, few scales have been developed that are appropriate for measuring the self-concept of disfigured people. This in itself is hardly surprising, because "self" research is certainly not without its difficulties. Most researchers who have been concerned with the interpersonal consequences of feelings about the self have defined the "self-concept" according to their own theoretical viewpoints, and have developed their own instruments for measurement. These instruments tend to be specific to particular situations, and are consequently unsuitable for use in other studies. However, despite these and other methodological problems, the concept of self should be borne in mind as a major factor in future research on the interaction problems encountered by facially disfigured people.

Why Are Disfigured People Avoided?

The reason disfigured people are avoided is difficult to assess because many factors seem to be involved—however, some researchers have offered explanations. Once again, because of the small amount of research specifically dealing with disfigurement, explanations of avoidance of other visibly stigmatized groups are also included.

Langer, Fiske, Taylor, and Chanowitz (1976), for example, suggested that people with physical handicaps are avoided because they make others feel uncomfortable by their presence. They also postulated that confrontation with a handicapped person constitutes a novel stimulus, and a conflict occurs between the desire to stare and the wish not to be thought rude. This may lead to uncertainty as to how to behave, and a wish to escape or avoid the situation. Novak and Lerner (1968) stated that handicapped people are avoided because they make people aware that the misfortune that has befallen the "victim" might also happen to themselves. Novak and Lerner believed that people do not like to acknowledge the fact that fate can deal anyone (including themselves) a blow. Accordingly, they convince themselves that they live in a "just" world, in which everyone receives their just desserts. Consequently, victims of misfortune are avoided or derogated.

Madan (1962) suggested that the public's behavior reflects deep-rooted attitudes and prejudices that manifest themselves in the allocation of lowered status to those with physical aberrations. Bernstein (1976) thought that the equilibrium of a nondisfigured viewer may be upset, since both normal figure/ground perception and the standard controlled scanning of the environment are interrupted by the unfamiliar sight of a disfigured person. The viewer's eyes are arrested, and the behavior that ensues is no longer subject to normal controls. The immediate reaction is to escape or avoid the situation. Bernstein went on to explain the rejection of disfigured people by stating that we live in a world that is almost wholly oriented by sight. He stated that health and good looks are assumed to be related. Consequently, an individual with an unfavorable physical aspect may be the object of an immediate negative reaction, perhaps because of the feeling that the injury or blemish may be caught or spread. (This may be particularly applicable to the those with congenital facial disfigurements.) In a similar vein, Heider (1958) stated that people may avoid a discredited individual so as not to be polluted or defiled.

Hastorf, Wildfogel, and Cassman (1979) incorporated many of these ideas into their series of reasons as to why physical handicaps can negatively affect social encounters. First, they maintained that the presence of a handicap forces others to realize that they too are vulnerable to similar disabilities. Second, there is the belief or possibility that the handicap is contagious. Third, there may be an uncertainty in the nonhandicapped person as to how to behave, which results from a conflict between norms of sympathy and norms of treating the handicapped person like everyone else. Fourth, there is a desire to explore the handicap as opposed to the norm not to stare. Finally, a handicap is considered by some to be unsightly and to violate the norm of what a "whole" person should be like.

We believe that although elements of all these explanations may be involved in the interaction process, the existing evidence points in favor of Hastorf, Wildfogel, and Cassman's third explanation, that people are generally unsure of how to behave when confronted with a novel stimulus in the form of a facially disfigured person. (Support for this view can also be found in Richardson, Goodman, Hastorf, and Dornbusch [1961] and in Kleck, Ono, and Hastorf [1966], who have noted that "normals" report themselves to be uncomfortable and uncertain when interacting with physically disabled people.) Although many disfigured people complain of avoidance and rejection by others, it seems that in many cases their interpretation of the motivation for this avoidance is overly negative. After all, it is very difficult to behave "normally" when speaking to someone with a facial disfigurement. For a start, few people have had previous experience of interacting with a facially disfigured person, and many are thus uncertain how best to behave in order to minimize embarrassment on either side. Maintaining normal levels of eye contact may be particularly difficult. On the one hand, there is the risk of having one's habitual level of eye contact interpreted as starting at the facial disfigurement; on the other hand, to reduce eye contact is to provide the possibility of being interpreted as unwilling to proceed with the interaction.

Evidence for the overly negative interpretation of the behavior of interactants by facially disfigured persons has been taken from studies of other aspects of social interaction, notably areas involving helping behavior (Rumsey, 1983).

Studies of Helping Behavior Relevant to Facially Disfigured Persons

Researchers have used helping behavior as the dependent variable in studies of the effects of either physical attractiveness or of handicap. The majority of the attractiveness studies have concluded that attractiveness can lead to an increase in helping behavior in a wide variety of situations (Athanasiou & Greene, 1973; Harrell, 1978; Sroufe, Chaiken, Cook & Freeman, 1977; West & Brown, 1975). This would seem to lead to the contrary hypothesis that the handicapped and disfigured would tend to be offered less help than 'normal' people. The results of research on this topic are varied. Bull and Stevens (1980) found that people were no less willing to be interviewed by an interviewer disfigured by unsightly teeth than by the same interviewer without this disfigurement. They noted in addition, that there was a significant difference in the length of time interviewees remained (on average 40% longer when the interviewer had unsightly teeth). Similarly, Walker, Harriman, and Costello (1980) found that subjects were no more likely to answer questions when the requester had a "normal" appearance than when the confederate had an arm in a sling. Thus it can be seen at this stage that research results relating to physical handicap and disfigurement suggest that if differences in helping behavior do exist, the differences are not always necessarily in the direction that work on stigma would suggest.

Kleck et al. (1966) found that subjects terminated interaction sooner with a confederate wearing an eye patch than with the confederate without this disfigurement. However, if the interaction included a helping component, the presence of an eye patch actually increased the degree of helping given. Similarly, Doob and Ecker (1970) found that the presence of any eye patch led to greater helping, providing that the offer of help was not likely to lead to a lengthy interaction. Specifically, the results indicated that the willingness of subjects to fill in a 15-minute questionnaire immediately was unaffected by the confederate wearing an eye patch (32% of subjects agreed to do this in the eye patch condition, compared to 34% in the "normal" condition). However, when the interaction was minimal, with subjects asked to return the questionnaire by post, having completed it at their leisure, 69% of subjects complied in the "eye patch" condition, compared to 40% in the "normal" condition.

Ungar (1979) also used an eye patch as a "handicap," and found that the presence of this handicap led to subjects giving more help in the form of directions, providing the confederate stayed in close proximity to the subject. Soble and Strickland (1974) used a hunchback or "normal" confederate to knock on peoples' doors, asking for interviews either (a) by another person at a later date, or (b) immediately. The results showed that there was little difference in the percentage of subjects agreeing to be interviewed by some-one else at a later date, but when the confederate requested an immediate interview, fewer agreed in the hunchback condition, suggesting an unwilling-ness of subjects to commit themselves to a prolonged interaction with a hand-icapped person. Levitt and Kornhaber (1977) reported that people with a leg brace or crutches were given more money than people without a handicap. However, Bull and Stevens (1981) found that donors gave less to a confeder-ate with a disfigurement in the form of a facial port wine stain than to the same confederate with a nondisfigured appearance.

Piliavin, Piliavin, and Rodin (1975) created a situation in which a confeder-ate fell in a subway, in one of two conditions. In the "disfigured" condition (in which the confederate had a facial port wine stain), 61% of subjects went to the aid of the confederate (mean latency 27 seconds). In the "normal" con-dition, however, 86% of subjects helped the confederate (mean latency 16 seconds). Piliavin et al. suggested that the reduced level of helping offered to the "disfigured" confederate may have been in part due to the fear that the offer to help might necessitate involvement in a prolonged interaction with the disfigured person.

Samerotte and Harris (1976) examined the role of the type and degree of handicap on the helping behavior of subjects. A confederate dropped bundles of envelopes under three conditions: (a) with an arm bandage (mild hand-icap); (b) with an eyepatch and facial scar (disfiguring handicap); and (c) in a normal (no handicap) condition. They found that subjects offered help more often in the "arm bandage" condition than in the "disfigured" and "normal" conditions. Also, the confederate was helped more in the normal condition than in the "disfigured" one. Samerotte and Harris suggested that two com-ponents operate in this sort of helping situation. They postulated that a hand-icapped person is likely to be viewed with more sympathy than a normal person, and that this sympathy will lead to an increase in helping behavior. However, in the case of a disfiguring handicap, the attractiveness of the "vic-tim" will be decreased, and the desire to avoid the person may overcome feelings of sympathy.

Hastorf, Northercraft, and Picciotto (1979) created a situation in which subjects gave evaluative feedback in response to handicapped or nonhandi-capped confederates' low performance on a task (the handicap took the form of leg braces and crutches). They found that the feedback to the handicapped confederate was less critical and more positive. Hastorf, Northercraft, and Picciotto thought that this was a reflection of societal pressure, which pre-vents the administration of very negative feedback to handicapped persons, producing instead a kind of "norm to be kind," with subjects believing that the best way of improving the performance of handicapped subjects was to be rewarding. Alternatively, it may be that the handicapped confederates gave a general aura of diminished competence, and the subjects thus expected a low-er performance level. Hastorf, Northercraft, and Picciotto maintained that their results supported the "norm to be kind" hypothesis. They also noted that if handicapped persons are liable to receive inaccurate and, in general, less critical feedback then this has far-reaching implications, because it may be (from the learning literature) that handicapped people become habituated to (and therefore come to ignore) positive "kind" feedback, and/or only pay attention to negative aspects of feedback.

In a similar vein, Dunn and Herman (1982) discussed the consequences of positive aspects of behavior of nonhandicapped toward handicapped persons. They maintained that when interacting with a handicapped person nonhandicapped person tend to (a) show increased anxiety levels (as measured by galvanic skin response); (b) show more motoric inhibition; (c) express attitudes not consonant with their real beliefs; and (d) say they like the handicapped person and enjoy the interaction, even though they are experiencing high levels of anxiety. Dunn and Herman maintained that the effect of this is to reduce the amount of negative feedback handicapped persons receive, with the amount of noncontingent positive feedback being increased, leading to the risk of patronization and condescension toward handicapped people. Consequently the social world of handicapped persons takes on a facade-like quality in which others do not act naturally, and do not reveal much of their idiosyncratic personalities.

Helping Behavior and Facial Disfigurement

From this summary of research, it can be seen that making predictions from the findings of these studies specifically for facially disfigured persons is far from straightforward. The complex results and conflicting effects are likely to be in part due to the different types of handicap or disfigurement studied, and the particular situation chosen as the setting for the experiment—certainly the results do not seem to generalize from one situation to another with any great consistency. Rumsey and Bull (1986) used the same (facial) disfigurement in situations involving three different levels of social interaction in the hope that more direct comparisons of helping behavior in different situations could be made.

The first study was designed in order that there should be no face-to-face interaction between the confederate and subjects. The method used was an elaboration of the "lost letter technique," which has been widely employed in studies of helping behavior (see Gross, 1975; Hornstein, Fisch, & Holmes, 1968) with varied results. The technique has the advantage of providing an unobtrusive measure of helping behavior in which there is no history of interaction between the helper and the helped, and no likelihood of future interaction occurring (Bihm, Gaudet, & Sale, 1979). The helpers have anonymity in that they are free to make the decision of whether to help (by posting the letter) without the physical presence of the "victim" or bystanders. Using 248 members of the general public, the presence or absence of a facial disfigurement (either a birthmark or trauma scarring consistent with a road traffic accident) was found to have no effect on the helping behavior of subjects.

The second study provided a mininal level of face-to-face contact between the confederate and subjects. The confederate, either with a facial birthmark or nondisfigured, stood in a busy London shopping street holding a collecting tin for a registered children's charity. Although the confederate's facial appearance was clearly visible to members of the public, it was possible for passersby to "help" her by putting money into her charity tin, without the necessity to interact with her socially. The data from 3,310 passersby showed no significant differences in the numbers of people helping the confederate in the disfigured compared with the nondisfigured condition. However, the raw data revealed a notable (but not significant) trend for fewer people to donate money in the disfigured condition, but with those who did donate giving more than donators in the nondisfigured condition.

This pattern of results, reminiscent of those of Bull and Stevens (1980) described above, was also reflected in Rumsey's third study, which was designed to incorporate a controlled level of interaction between the confederate and subjects. The confederate (either with a facial birthmark or nondisfigured) approached a random sample of passersby requesting that they answer some questions relating to television viewing. Using 244 subjects, there was no overall significant difference in the percentages of people agreeing to help the confederate in the disfigured and nondisfigured conditions, but once again the raw data indicated that considerably fewer people agreed to be interviewed in the disfigured condition, but that those who did agree answered more questions, thus engaging in interaction with the disfigured confederate for longer periods of time.

More research is needed in which variations in the age and sex of subjects, the sex and underlying level of attractiveness of the disfigured person, and the level of social interaction are systematically varied in order to elucidate the role of these factors in situations involving facially disfigured persons. A major criticism of helping studies in the past has been the lack of generalizability of results from one situation to another. Cross-cultural differences in results are also likely. Innes and Gilroy (1980) created a situation in which confederates asked for help in mailing bulky letters in Australia, America, and Britain. They found the compliance rate was much higher in Britain (average 81.25%) than in Australia (67.5%) or America (50%). Rumsey (1983) also noted an unusually high rate of return in her British lost letter study (98%) compared with previous lost letter studies carried out in America.

What of theoretical explanations of helping behavior as they relate to disfigured and handicapped subjects? It will be recalled that Doob and Ecker (1970) and Soble and Strickland (1974) postulated that a general desire to help handicapped persons is balanced against a wish not to prolong interaction with the handicapped person. This explanation, however, does not account for the results of studies in which subjects gave less help to disfigured confederates in situations that require minimal interaction, with no expectations of any further interaction (e.g., Bull & Stevens, 1980; Rumsey, 1983).

Samerotte and Harris (1976) and Kleck et al. (1966) have put forward similar two-factor theories to explain the helping behavior of subjects toward physically handicapped persons. In a similar manner to Doob and Ecker, these authors proposed the idea that people feel sympathy toward physically handicapped persons, and this in turn leads to an increase in helping behavior. Unlike Doob and Ecker, however, Kleck et al. considered the second factor to be that if the person is disfigured, their attractiveness is decreased, and the desire to avoid the person is correspondingly increased.

This would seem to be the most adequate explanation to date (bearing in mind methodological problems, sampling difficulties, etc.), and future explanations of the helping processes are likely to involve at least two stages. At the perception stage, some sort of arousal or tension occurs. The decision stage that follows may depend on many factors, but will probably contain elements of variables such as past experiences and expectations of costs and rewards of the current situation (Piliavin, Rodin, & Piliavin, 1969). Whatever the explanation, Rumsey and Bull's (1986) results appear to provide a glimmer of hope. The general public do not seem to be expressing a straightforward desire to avoid facially disfigured persons, and there are certainly indications of a desire on the part of many to offer them help.

Whether nice or nasty, the behavior of others is important. Several researchers believe society acts as a social mirror and that we interpret the reflections society gives us, whether accurate or not. Lansdown (1976) believes that all of us, whether disfigured, disabled, or not, form self-concepts according to our perceptions of the impressions other people form of us. Despite the research results suggesting positive aspects of the behavior of others toward disfigured persons (see above), many disfigured people believe others react negatively toward them. Kleck and Strenta (1980) pointed out the difficulty of disabusing the deviant individual of this perceptual bias, that is, the expectation that the reactions of others will be negative.

Snyder et al. (1977) noted that comparatively little theoretical and empirical attention has been directed toward the fundamental question in cognitive and social psychology—what are the cognitive and behavioral consequences of one's impressions of other people? They posed the idea (adapted from Tversky & Kahneman, 1977) that previously held social stereotypes may influence a person's information processing in ways that bolster, strengthen, and thus confirm the stereotyped intuitions already held. Thus they advanced speculation concerning the ramifications of negative expectations of interaction by putting forward the idea that the way others treat us is in a large measure a reflection of our treatment and expectations of them.

The Behavior of Disfigured Persons Themselves

Additional research findings have added credence to the idea that to some extent it may be the behavior of disfigured persons themselves that plays a role in the problems many say they experience in social interaction. Goffman (1963) has stated that stigmatized individuals can never be sure whether the attitude of a new acquaintance will be accepting or rejecting, so attempts may be made to avoid interaction. Alternatively, the stigmatized individual may approach social interaction with hostile bravado, thus inducing from others a set of troublesome reciprocations, or may vacillate between avoidance and bravado. As discussed above, Goffman's remarks seem to be somewhat applicable to facially disfigured people, many of whom anticipate negative behavior from others in interaction. The inconsistencies evident in the behavior of others and the lack of predictability as to how strangers will react to a disfigured person lead some disfigured people to become preoccupied with themselves and their own behavior.

Zimbardo's (1981) comments concerning shy people are useful here. He maintained that shy people are concerned both with themselves ("I am inadequate, inferior, stupid, ugly, worthless") and with their effect on others ("What do they think about me? What kind of impression am I making? Do they like me? How can I be sure they like me?"). Attempts at interaction are hampered by a fear of failure ("If I'm quiet, people won't notice me. I won't bother to try any more because no-one would want to talk to me anyway."). Shy people often prefer to avoid the responsibility both for starting social encounters and for facilitating the progress of interpersonal contact once established.

It is interesting, in the context of the present book, that Zimbardo used the example of a facially disfigured woman to illustrate his remarks on shyness. He recounted the experiences of Dorothy Holob:

> In 1963, I returned home from a major operation for a serious brain tumor. . . . I kept thinking, "why did this have to happen to me? . . . I tried walking around my block, but I simply could not stand the mocking laughter of children, nor the giggles of some neighbors. When I walked into the shops alone, clerks gave me disdainful glances, and occasionally would toss my purchases at me. Once in a while some crank would telephone me and taunt me. How did I react to the jeers and sarcastic comments? Usually I came home and cried, and sometimes even enjoyed my suffering. For months, I became a recluse.

Kleck and Strenta (1980) carried out an experiment in which amputee subjects, spinal cord-injured subjects, or nonhandicapped controls were shown a videotape of an interaction between a female and a male, who supposedly either had a broken leg or was paraplegic and thus confined to a wheelchair. The videotape had in fact been filmed with the male appearing without any handicap. However, since the camera focused exclusively on the female, subjects were unaware of this fact. The nonhandicapped controls and the spinal cord-injured subjects saw the male confederate's paraplegia as having a strong impact on the dispositions and behavior of the female stranger, whereas with the male in the broken leg condition this effect did not occur. The amputee subjects found no evidence that either the male's paraplegia or his broken leg affected the nature of the interaction, or the female's treatment of the male confederate. In subsequent discussion, the amputee subjects reported positive as well as negative changes in their own interactions with other people, whereas the spinal cord-injured subjects reported primarily negative changes. Some subjects in both groups stated that they focus on the gaze, facial, and verbal behaviors of others in order to ascertain whether their disability is having an impact or not. Kleck and Strenta stated that some subjects "actively scan the behavior of people with whom they interact for evidence to confirm the expectation that their disability is affecting the behavior of others." The expectation that their disability will affect the interaction may well affect the disabled person's own behavior, leading to a self-fulfilling prophecy (see below for a discussion of this possibility), such that a person who expects to be rejected may actively elicit the rejection from others.

Studies Relating Specifically to Facially Disfigured Persons

Some research dealing specifically with the behavior of facially disfigured persons has been carried out. Rumsey (1983) gathered observations of the behavior of facially disfigured people from diverse sources, including health care professionals, the comments of families and friends, self-reports, and previous literature. These sources indicated that facially disfigured persons often experienced difficulties in social situations, detailing behavior reflecting shyness, defensiveness, and depression. Many facially disfigured people were reported as exhibiting lower levels of eye contact, more monotonous tones of voice, lack of body tone, and as initiating conversations less often than other nondisfigured patients, thus appearing withdrawn and depressed. It may be for many disfigured people that the preoccupation with their own plight and the depression experienced as a result of supposedly negative reactions from others manifest themselves in a defensive style of behavior that can be mistakenly interpreted by others as implying that the disfigured person does not want to engage in interaction.

Macgregor (1974) noted three coping strategies among the disfigured patients she saw. The first was the tendency for patients to withdraw or avoid social encounters (the "ostrich" technique), and to efface themselves in order to cushion feelings of inadequacy. The second was to display overt aggression in order to counter expected hostility in others, and the last (for relatively few patients) was to deliberately do something about the problems encountered in interaction by being excessively charming and active in taking the initiative and in sustaining the interaction.

What Are the Potential Consequences of a Preoccupation with One's Own Appearance?

The potential effects of facially disfigured people being preoccupied with their own appearance has been highlighted in two studies by Strenta and Kleck (1985). In the first they showed "normal" subjects slides of themselves appearing (via makeup) to have facial scarring due to burns. Subjects (both males and females) experienced strong autonomic arousal when they viewed themselves with a simulated disfigurement—applying emotional labels such as "shocked" and "distressed." Both males and females reported that such a scar would have a strong effect on their personality and social experiences. They expected that others would avoid them, and any interactions would tend to be strained, especially with members of the opposite sex.

Second, Strenta and Kleck created a situation in which subjects were led to believe that they appeared to others to be physically deviant. Subjects watched themselves in a mirror as makeup was applied to create a facial scar. Subsequently some subjects (unknown to them) then had their "scar" removed under the guise of adding a fixative to the makeup. In interactions that followed, those subjects who thought they were "scarred" (whether or not in fact they were) believed they could sense a strong reactivity to their deviant appearance in the behavior of their nondisfigured cointeractant. Strenta and Kleck reported that those people who thought they were scarred were more likely to focus their gaze behavior on the other interactants. In addition the subjects made links between their own supposedly deviant physical characteristics and the behavior of their cointeractants in that they believed that the gaze behavior of the other participants in interaction reflected their own physical defect.

Individual differences in behavior among facially disfigured persons are, of course, enormous. However, the self-preoccupation that many disfigured people experience may make it difficult for them to realize that other parties to the interaction may also be having problems and experiencing embarrassment. Instead of resenting the tendency for others to avoid interaction with them, it may be more constructive for facially disfigured persons to entertain the possibility that this avoidance is due to the fact that others may be unsure of how best to behave, and do not want to embarrass the disfigured person or themselves by handling the interaction badly. Rumsey and Bull (1986) results, discussed in the preceding section, indicate that many people do in fact feel able to interact with the disfigured. It would therefore be beneficial if disfigured people could be helped to realize that the initial reactions of others are not necessarily a sign of rejection, but may be more those of uncertainty as to how best to behave.

The Reciprocal Nature of Interaction

Research has highlighted the reciprocal nature of interaction. Condon (1966, reported in N. Bernstein, 1976) made careful examinations of interaction patterns using a method of analyzing slowed film segments of human interaction. He found that the body motion and facial patterns of individuals who are emotionally disturbed lack the vitality and rhythmic variability observed in "normal" people. Condon also noted a parallel lack of variability in the speech stream of disturbed subjects, giving a sense of monotony and flatness to the total behavioral presentation. He pointed to the likelihood that other people will pick up these signals automatically, and that they will respond unconsciously in a number of ways. Bernstein hypothesized that the asyn-chronic lack of smooth integration of speech patterns and other behaviors that are observable in physically handicapped and disfigured persons may therefore be the object of immediate negative reactions, even though this initial reaction may be followed by a recognition that sympathy should have been awakened.

As described previously, Snyder et al. (1977) carried out an intruiging ex-periment to examine the cognitive and behavioral consequences of ones's im-pressions of other people. They led male "perceiver" undergraduate subjects participating in short telephone conversations to believe that (as the result of an experimental manipulation) the female undergraduate "targets" with whom they were interacting were physically attractive or unattractive. Snyder et al. found that the initial attribution of "attractiveness" to the female targets (whether or not this attribution was correct) led the male "perceivers" to behave in such a way as to elicit from the female "targets" behavior that was concurrent with this stereotype; that is, those female targets who were per-ceived (unknown to them) to be attractive came to behave in a more sociable, friendly, and likeable way than those "targets" who were unwittingly being perceived as unattractive.

The idea that deficiencies in social skills may affect the impressions people form of disfigured persons is borne out by the literature. Research by Kendon (1967) revealed that subjects whose interviewer did not look at them for part of the interview believed that the interviewer had lost interest in them. Mehrabian (1972) found that a high affiliative style correlated positively with several factors, including the total number of statements, duration of speech, eye contact, head nods, verbal reinforcers, and hand and arm gestures. Wash-burn and Hakel (1973) examined pairs of subjects, one of whom was assigned to be an "interviewer" and the other a "job applicant." The interviewer was instructed either to be enthusiastic or unenthusiastic, and to emit high or low amounts of gestures, eye contact, or smiling. Observer subjects rated the enthusiastic interviewer as being younger, as liking the job better, and as be-ing more easily approachable, more interested, more considerate, and more intelligent. In addition, the applicants, when interviewed by the enthusiastic interviewer, were also rated more favorably by independent observers than applicants in the unenthusiastic condition. Washburn and Hakel believed that this positive behavior in the applicants was a direct result of the more positive behavior of the interviewer.

Rumsey et al.'s (1986) results also support the notion that the behavior of disfigured people during social interaction can have important effects on the reactions of others. They used two factors in the design of their study: first the presence or absence of a large facial port wine stain (produced by makeup), and second, the use of a high or low level of social skill by the "interviewer" confederate. Analysis of the videorecording of the interviews revealed that the social skill variable had a significantly greater effect on the behavior of subjects and on the impressions they formed of the interviewer than did the presence or absence of the disfigurement. The disfigurement factor led to a certain amount of discomfort, that is, more verbal fillers and eyeblinks and a decrease in hand gestures—all of which have been cited as nervous reactions (R. Harper, Wiens, & Matarazzo, 1978; Kanfer, 1960). Subjects also encouraged the disfigured interviewer more, pausing less before responding and nodding and smiling more, thus again giving the impression that they do want to help disfigured people, even though they may be experiencing some degree of discomfort. When instructed to use a high level of social skill (regardless of whether he had a birthmark at the time or not), the interviewer was rated as significantly more friendly, competent, and warm by subjects. In addition, the subjects' behavior showed significant differences in the trials in which a high level of skill was used, with subjects smiling significantly more, and being rated by observers as being significantly more friendly and warm. Although this was a study carried out in laboratory conditions in order to facilitate experimental control, and thus perhaps with limited generalizability to more everyday situations, the results indicate the encouraging nature of the social skill variable. It seems that social skills training could provide a means of helping disfigured persons make use of the idea that the general public are looking to be positive, but that they need help in order to do so (see Chapter 8 for a more comprehensive discussion of the potential benefits of the social skills approach.)

From the studies described here it can be seen that the behavior of facially disfigured persons can affect social interaction with others in two ways. First, the behavior of the disfigured person may in some way be unusual; second, the expectations that the disfigured person has of the behavior of people with whom he or she is interacting may also affect the course of the interaction. We have seen that social skills training seems to provide a promising approach to tackling some of the problems commonly encountered by facially disfigured people. In what other ways can psychologists offer help?

Ways of Helping Facially Disfigured Persons

In Chapter 8 several ways in which psychologists can offer help to those disadvantaged by their appearance are discussed in detail. These include attempting to increase the knowledge we currently have of the mechanism of attitudes toward facially disfigured persons and of how to facilitate changes in these attitudes. Second, a greater awareness of the powerful role the media can play in attitudes toward those disadvantaged by their appearance, both in terms of the negative influence the media (especially television) can have, and also of the positive effects of the media (including its potential as an educational tool), is necessary.

Much can also be done in the provision of health care for those disadvantaged by their appearance. Psychologists could help by promoting an accurate knowledge of the advantages and disadvantages of surgery, of the problems of adopting the surgical model of patient care, and of patients' motivations to seek surgery. Additionally, pychologists need to prove their usefulness in multidisciplinary health care teams concerned with the rehabilitation of surgery and burns patients.

In the face of difficulties associated with changing the behavior of the general public toward disfigured persons what help can be offered directly to those disfigured by their appearance? In Chapter 8 the potential of counseling, self-help groups, and social skills training is discussed.

An additional way in which psychologists can help is to carry out more research into the problems associated with facial disfigurement. There is no doubt that such research could prove invaluable to those experiencing problems associated with their appearance, yet all too few researchers are at present engaged in this work. Why is this? As previous chapters in this book attest, more and more researchers have become involved in studying the effects of physical attractiveness on various aspects of functioning, yet few have tackled the other side of the coin. As indicated above, much of the limited literature on facially disfigured persons has been speculative in nature, consisting on the one hand of reports by surgeons on the physical problems resulting from injury, and on the other hand of scanty anecdotal observations of problems facing handicapped persons in general (Weinberg, 1976; Wright, 1960). Stricker (1970), for example, noted that considerable advancements have been made in the anatomical and functional rehabilitation of malocclusion, cleft lip, craniofacial anomalies, and traumatic disfigurement, and yet despite these advances and the fact that improved surgical techniques are enabling more people to survive road traffic accidents, industrial injuries, terrorist bombings, and the like, the examination of the psychological and social aspects of disfigurement is still in its infancy.

A high proportion of the studies that do exist are subject to sampling bias. (Most studies use samples drawn from those actually attending plastic surgery clinics. This produces a sample of people who are actively seeking treatment, and additionally introduces a bias toward those from middle- and high-income families who can afford to pay for expensive surgery or for related insurance premiums.) Many studies are naive with regard to scientific methodology. Adequate control groups are frequently lacking, and there is a heavy reliance on limited numbers of case histories as a basis for observations and generalisations (see Bryt, 1966; Easson, 1966). Clifford (1973), in reviewing studies of orofacial anomalies maintained that the lack of both theoretical and methodological sophistication must place the conclusions of many studies in doubt.

Issues to Be Considered in Future Research

In addition to providing research with acceptable levels of experimental control, validity and generalizability, several points need to be born in mind. Knapp (1985) has pointed out that in trying to research the effects of appearance in social interaction, the results of previous research using still photographs should be reassessed for their relevance to everyday life. Future research should move from noninteractive situations to interactive ones, and should also include an expanded concern for the context within which the interaction takes place.

The behavior of both interactants is important, as a high degree of interdependence is likely. It is not enough to assess either or both parties' expectations, stereotypes and preferences, we must also examine how they actually behave. Interaction patterns may well affect the participants' perceptions of the attractiveness of each other. For example, the interaction style of an unattractive person may provide compensations for cointeractants, and the behavior of an attractive person may prevent them from achieving success. Even though research which accurately reflects the ongoing, reflexive nature of human communication may be virtually impossible to conduct, we should try to move towards it.

Another problem facing aspiring researchers hoping to undertake an experimental investigation of problems associated with facial disadvantage is that realism and a high degree of experimental control are difficult to achieve concurrently. There is a need to control (or to account for) other aspects of behavior and appearance apart from the facial configuration. The best way to do this is to use the same people in both the attractive and unattractive/ disfigured conditions. This usually necessitates the use of makeup either to produce an unattractive appearance (or disfigurement), or to cover up an existing disfigurement. However, in the case of studies examining the effects of disfigurement, the disfigurement itself is likely to be the tip of the iceberg. Rumsey (1983) made the point that the underlying facial appearance 'beneath' a disfigurement may play a part in the reactions both of the disfigured themselves and of the general public. The type of facial abnormality used, and the location of the disfigurement on the face, have also been shown to play a role in the severity of reactions from others, with congenital disfigurements producing more negative reactions than traumatic injury, and disfigurements located within the 'facial triangle' (bounded by the eyes and the point of the chin) seemingly more aversive than the same disfigurements located on more peripheral areas of the face (Rumsey, 1983).

Research results on hemispheric differences in the processing of information from the facial features indicates that future research should also pay close systematic attention to the side of the face on which disfigurements are located (Rumsey, 1983). It seems from research (see Suben & McKeever, 1977) that the left side of the face (the presented right side) has a greater salience for others, and therefore that a disfigurement on the left side of the face may be considered more aversive than a comparable disfigurement occurring on the right side.

Despite these methodological difficulties, the rewards for continuing to further knowledge of the problems experienced by facially disfigured persons seem many. This is a research area that in time should enable psychologists to offer practical help to many millions of people.

Summary

This chapter presents a review of research relevant to the problems frequently encountered by those disadvantaged due to their facial appearance and by their families. Problems typically encountered following the birth of disfigured children, and during their development and education, are examined. In addition, the types of pressures exerted on facially disfigured people and their families by the society in which they live are described, together with an examination of the manifestations of these pressures (such as problems encountered in social interaction) in the day-to-day lives of disfigured people. The role of the social behavior of the disfigured people themselves is evaluated, and the reciprocal nature of social interaction highlighted. The chapter concludes with a brief look at how psychologists might try to help those disadvantaged by their facial appearance (Chapter 8 examines these possibilities in more detail). In addition, the urgent need to increase the volume of research into the effects of the less palatable side of appearance is emphasized, and several issues that need to be considered in future research are introduced.

Chapter 8

How Can Psychologists Help Those Disadvantaged by Their Facial Appearance?

In the preceding chapters we have presented the evidence concerning the influence that a person's facial appearance can have on his or her life. It seems obvious that there are some disadvantages attached to being at the unattractive or disfigured end of the physical appearance continuum. However, it is one thing to describe and explain the problems facing such people, but another to provide suggestions or insight into how the problems can be eased. Surely this is an issue that should concern contemporary psychologists?

In the past criticism has been leveled at the "relevance" of psychology to real-world problems (see Bull, 1982). Theory, research, and practice in psychology should be intimately related. Yet all too often practice comes a poor third, with practical considerations too frequently ignored. C.S. Myers and Sir Frederick Bartlett each showed that the way to make psychology applicable to a wide range of important but practical questions was to concentrate first on topical problems and then to develop theories, ideas, and solutions, rather than the more familiar alternative of starting with theories and techniques and then seeking to apply them to the world outside (Belbin, 1979). Applicable psychology has yet to make its proper mark, and is in need of important and relevant material to offer society now and in the future. Certainly solutions are difficult to provide—particularly in the simple, straightforward format that the general public would like. The issues involved in the effects of facial appearance are a complex set of interdependent person-situation problems that are difficult to tackle independently of each other. However, we should use this fact to spur us on to greater efforts rather than to discourage us. The knowledge that many people do suffer as a result of their facial appearance should be incentive enough to try to come up with practical help. Psychology is a discipline that has to be capable of making an informed and relevant contribution to issues and problems of the modern world (Middleton & Edwards, 1985). If this means need-driven research, then so be it.

How can psychologists help those disadvantaged by their appearance? This chapter will review a number of promising ways of providing practical help to such people. Specifically, it will examine the factors involved in negative attitudes toward facially disadvantaged persons, and techniques of attitude change. It will look at the role the media play in the perpetuation of stereotypes, and at ways in which the media can be used to help those stigmatized by their appearance. The provision of health care for facial surgery patients will be examined, and suggestions made for improvements in the service offered. Finally, ways of offering help directly to the visibly stigmatized will be discussed.

Attitudes Toward Facially Disfigured Persons

Although to date relatively little research has been published directly concerning attitudes toward ugly or disfigured persons, there is a growing body of literature concerned with attitudes toward disabled persons that is likely to be of relevance to the present discussion. The more we learn about factors involved in the formation and maintenance of such attitudes, the more informed we may become about ways attitudes toward facially disadvantaged persons can be changed (see below).

So, what factors are involved in attitudes that work to the detriment of facially disadvantaged persons? Researchers have offered various classifications of the factors that go to make up attitudes toward disabled persons. Raskin (1956), for example, in discussing attitudes toward blind people, talks of psychodynamic, situational, sociocultural, and historical factors. Gellman (1974) in discussing attitudes toward disabled persons in general put forward the idea that prejudice stems from social customs and norms, child-rearing practices, neurotic childhood fears in anxiety-provoking and frustrating situations, and discrimination-provoking behavior by people with disabilities. Wright (1960) carried out a much-quoted literature review of attitudes toward those with atypical physiques. She highlighted the idea of phenomenal causality between sinful behaviors, punishment and disability, negative reactions to the different and strange, childhood experiences, and prevailing socioeconomic factors.

Livneh (1982) has reviewed those factors that researchers believe make up attitudes toward disabled persons, and has offered a classification system within which to consider the many and varied factors. In order to guide the reader through this myriad of factors, Livneh's classification is presented here, having been revised and extended for the purposes of this book to include extra findings relevant to facially disadvantaged persons.

Livneh's Classification of Factors in Attitudes Toward Disabled Persons

Historical, social, and cultural influences.   I. Katz (1981) has pointed out that the Old Testament enumerates 12 afflictions that disqualified a priest from officiating, including blindness and a variety of facial and bodily disfigurements. Skin disorders were explained in the Bible as punishment for sins—a warning to others of evil within (e.g., to the Hebrews, leprosy was an expression of God's vengeance against sinners, and the clearing of the disease signaled atonement). Until well into modern times, the superstition persisted in Europe that deformed persons were in some way works of the Devil (McDaniel, 1969).

Some maintain that the folklore and mythology that are passed from generation to generation have provided the source of negative attitudes toward disfigured persons (Shaw, 1981c), with evidence of medieval folklore still existing in some countries.

Current sociocultural conditions. Livneh includes in this category the pervasive social and cultural norms, standards, and expectations that lead to the creation of negative attitudes toward disabled persons. An example, is the current Western emphasis on the "body beautiful" and "body whole," youth, health, athletic prowess, personal appearance, and wholeness. Kligman (1985) cites Maxwell and Maxwell (1979), who also mentioned the phenomenon of "ageism." In youth-oriented cultures, deterioration is a potent source of disfavor toward aged people. Wrinkles serve as a reminder of one's own inexorable physical decline, and aged persons "suffer from the same deepseated prejudices that operate towards the unhandsome and physically disfigured." Maxwell and Maxwell even go so far as to speculate that good looks may be associated with longevity. Another example of sociocultural norms is the emphasis on personal productiveness and achievement. Individuals should be socially and economically competitive, and disability is assumed to interfere with these requirements. A third example is the prevailing socioeconomic conditions, including high levels of unemployment, and the importance attached to the nation's welfare and social security systems. Finally, the status degredation attached to disability in Western culture leads to the assignment of marginal status to those with visible deviances.

Childhood influences. Child-rearing practices and early influences (verbal and behavioral) are often stressed as having a major influence on a growing child's belief and value system. Actions, tone of voice, gestures, and the like are transmitted directly or indirectly to the child, and have a crucial impact on the formation of attitudes toward disability. Rearing practices that emphasize the importance of health, normalcy, and an aversion to sickness, illness, and long-term disability are not helpful. It can become difficult for disabled persons to reject the "suffering" role, because any attempt to do so is met with negative reactions. An association of a nondisabled person with a disabled person may be interpreted by others as implying some psychological maladjustment on behalf of the nondisabled person. In addition, a fear of ostracism discourages nondisabled persons from forming associations with disabled persons.

Aesthetic aversion. Repulsion and discomfort concerning amputations, body deformities, cerebral palsy, skin disorders, and so forth are, according to Livneh, important factors in the formation of negative attitudes.

Threats to body image integrity. An individual's own body image may be threatened by the presence of a disabled person. Many people experience a profound anxiety about becoming disabled, and therefore avoid and attempt to segregate and isolate disabled people (a view supported by Dunn and Herman, 1982). A fear of contamination or inheritance may lead to avoidance in both superficial (social intercourse) and in-depth (e.g., marriage) relationships.

Rejection of the strange/unusual. People tend to reject the strange because it does not fit into the structure of previous experience. Negative atypicalities of appearance cause distress because there is a general lack of experiential contact and exposure to visibly different people with disabilities. Richardson (1963) believed that negative stereotyping of disabled persons may occur because the prevalence of handicap in the general population is low. The novelty of encountering a handicapped person provides uncertainty for others as to how to behave. Siller (1976) measured nonhandicapped people's attitudes toward a wide range of disablements, and found, like Richardson, an uneasiness in his nondisabled subjects due to an uncertainty about how to behave coupled with emotional distress. Siller used personal construct theory to explain that people build up a construct system to predict events. Anxiety is experienced if a person becomes aware that his or her constructs are inadequate to deal with the task in hand—thus inadequacy and uneasiness are felt on confrontation with a disfigured person because so little experience has been gained with them.

Minority group comparability. This view upholds disabled persons as a marginal group subject to the same stereotypical reactions experienced by those occupying other devalued and inferior positions in society (e.g., certain ethnic, racial, and religious groups). The attitudes resulting from this allocation of marginal status are discriminatory and prejudiced, with many advocating isolation and segregation of disabled persons. This relates to the notion put forward by I. Katz (1981) of a fundamental tendency to see things of like quality as belonging together and being causally related. Thus negative states (sickness and deformity) are perceived as having negative causes (for example, wrongdoing by the sufferer or someone else). The person is seen as inferior across a broad range of nonvisible characteristics simply on the basis of a visible or known deformity.

Other Factors Involved in Negative Attitudes

Livneh's classification summarizes possible sources of negative attitudes toward visibly disadvantaged persons. Additional information in the form of the demographic characteristics of the holders of these attitudes is also a useful source of material for those who seek to modify attitudes toward those disadvantaged by their physical appearance.

Are there, for example, any sex differences in the attitudes held toward facially disadvantaged people? Shakespeare's (1975) review of research relating to attitudes toward handicapped persons suggests that either there are no differences, or females are more accepting than males. She pointed out that these findings are consistent with the normally found female characteristic of being more caring and protective toward others. Livneh's (1982) own review of the literature also concludes that females display more favorable attitudes toward physically disabled persons.

Livneh further believed that attitudes toward physically disabled persons are more positive in late childhood and adulthood and less favorable in early childhood, adolescence, and old age. Shakespeare (1975), on the other hand, reported that children have little reaction to disability at a preschool level, and cited some evidence to the effect that negative attitudes toward disability increase with the age of the child and are more common in secondary level schoolchildren (11 years and over) than in primary level schoolchildren (4 to 11 years) (see Chapter 6 for a review of children's reactions to facial appearance). On the whole, the age of adults seems to have little effect except that there is a slight tendency for younger adults to be more accepting than are older adults.

There are few clear findings concerning attitudes toward disabled persons and the education and socioeconomic status of the attitude holders. Livneh (1982) reported a trend for higher income groups to have more favorable attitudes toward emotionally and mentally disabled persons than lower income groups, but in the context of those with visible deformities, no consistent differences have been found. Livneh also reported most studies to have found a positive correlation between higher educational level and more favorable attitudes toward those with physical deformities. Shakespeare (1975) concluded that it is likely that prejudice toward handicap is spread fairly generally among different classes, occupation groups, and people of different educational levels, but offers little evidence to support this assertion.

Some researchers have examined personality characteristics as a factor in attitudes toward facially disadvantaged persons. The most common factors found in those people who are most accepting include higher self-concepts, lower levels of anxiety, a higher need for social approval, and a greater ability to tolerate ambiguity (Shakespeare, 1975). Similarly, Livneh (1982) reported that high levels of self-insight, body and self-satisfaction, and ambiguity tolerance, and a positive self-concept are associated with more accepting attitudes toward disabled persons. On the other hand, high levels of authoritarianism, aggression, and anxiety, a need for social approval, and ethnocentrism are related to a lack of acceptance of disabled persons.

In addition to the demographic characteristics of attitude holders, other factors that have been shown to play a part in the extent to which attitudes toward disfigured persons are negative include the type of disability or disfigurement, and the contextual variables against which the disfigurement or disability appear. As reported in Chapter 7, Rumsey (1983) has found that reactions to congenital facial disfigurements are more negative than reactions to facial injuries caused by trauma. People's reactions also vary if the same facial disfigurement is presented in different locations on the face, with disfigurements involving the communication equipment of the face (primarily the eyes and mouth) being less acceptable than those at more peripheral locations (such as the forehead, cheek, or chin). Livneh (1982) believed that those disabilities with the least functional implications (e.g., alcoholism) are reacted to least negatively. In an occupational setting, for example, employers were found to prefer physically disabled individuals to more functionally impaired ones (e.g., mentally retarded/emotionally disabled persons). Other writers have highlighted the effect that the severity of a deviation from normal appearance can have on the reactions of others. In the case of facially disfigured persons, Macgregor (1982) has noted that reactions to people with mild or severe disfigurements are less extreme than reactions to people with moderate disfiguration. Additional factors that have been shown to affect negatively people's attitudes toward disabled persons include the possibility that the disability might be contagious, and any lack of predictability of the prognosis for recovery from the disability.

In terms of the contextual aspect of attitudes toward disabled persons, S. Katz and Shurka (1977) have pointed out that disability per se is not the only variable that influences the degree of negativism toward disabled persons. They found that the framework within which the disability was presented appeared to have a stronger effect on the evaluation of disabled persons than any other individual factor. Katz and Shurka used three types of disability (amputation, facial disfigurement, and blindness), and provided contexts related to combat (war), a car accident, and a work accident. The subjects were 226 11th-grade schoolchildren from two high schools. The experimenters prepared five videotape segments. These comprised simulated life history interviews with (a) an amputee, (b) a man with a facial disfigurement, (c) a blind person, (d) a nondisabled man, and (e) a nondisabled soldier in uniform. Although few details of the content of the videotape are reported, the authors do mention that the contents of the interview, the background setting, and other aspects of the interview were kept as identical as possible. Subjects rated the stimulus person on thirty-six 5-point semantic differential scales dealing with intelligence, appearance, and vocational, social, moral, and personality factors. Subsequent analyses revealed significant main effects of the disability context and type (and a significant interaction between the two factors). Disabled veterans were evaluated more favorably than those disabled in car and work accidents (there was no difference between these latter two accident groups). The war-disabled blind person was rated more favorably than the war-disabled facially disfigured person and the amputee, although in general the "disability type had little influence on the evaluation of the disabled by the nondisabled." The military versus civilian contextual dimension seemed to have the strongest effect. The authors pointed out that the age of the subjects (one year prior to conscription) was likely to predispose the subjects to more favorable attitudes toward the soldiers. Richardson (1971) offered support for Katz and Shurka's finding in his report that facially disfigured veterans receive more positive evaluations than people with facial disfigurements caused by accidents or those with congenital facial disfigurements.

Knowledge of the factors involved in attitudes, and of demographic details relating to the holders of the attitudes, does not, of course, provide psychologists with a prediction of how well people's overt behavior will be related to the attitudes they hold. However, it can be hoped that as knowledge relating to attitudes increases, psychologists can use the information to suggest ways in which attitudes may be changed in order to make life more tolerable for those with atypical facial appearance.

What of the behavior and attitudes of facially disadvantaged persons themselves? Do such people share the negative attitudes held by others? Do they in some way contribute to the formation and maintenance of such attitudes toward themselves?

The Behavior and Attitudes of Facially Disadvantaged Persons

Some of the features of attitudes reported above may often be shared by facially disadvantaged persons themselves. For example, the perceived cause (context) of the disability or disfigurement seems to be an important factor for disabled people as well as for the other parties. S. Katz, Shurka, and Florian (1978) reported that those disabled in work or traffic accidents, or as a result of polio, had lower self-concepts than those injured while in the course of armed service (veterans). Similar findings have been quoted in the United Kingdom concerning those injured in the World Wars.

Morgan, Hohmann, and Davis (1974) presented evidence that many patients disabled by spinal cord injuries had a negative view of their future capabilities and expectations for social life. Morgan et al. interviewed 214 patients in all. Fifteen percent reported that in the future they expected either to be in worse health or dead; 18% expected to be in an institution, 13% expected no social life, and 19% expected no, or very little recreational pleasure.

Wright (1960) talked of disabled people holding expectations of being treated in deprecating ways and of "setting themselves up" in situations where they will be devalued. Livneh (1982) also discussed prejudice-inviting behaviors on behalf of disabled persons quoting examples of disabled people projecting an image of dependence, of seeking secondary gains, of behaving fearfully, and of appearing insecure of inferior. Livneh further maintained that behaviors such as these serve to create and strengthen prejudicial beliefs in the observer. He also talked of "prejudice by silence"—a lack of interest in social intercourse on the part of disabled persons and a lack of "public relations" attempts by disabled persons to emphasize positive aspects of themselves.

Several authors have suggested that these negative expectations and the internalization of negative attitudes toward the self may contribute to the development of a poor self-image by facially disadvantaged persons (see Dixon, 1977). Zimbardo (1981), among others, agreed that the way we feel about ourselves has a profound effect on all aspects of our lives. People with a sense of positive self-worth typically display poise and radiate confidence as outward signs of inner satisfaction. Such people are not highly dependent on the praise and social reinforcement of others because they have learned how to be their own best friends and biggest boosters. They do not crumble under criticism, or feel devasted by rejection. People with low self-esteem, on the other hand, are said to be more passive, more persuasible, and less popular. They tend to be overly sensitive to negative criticism, thinking that this confirms their inadequacy. They have more difficulty in accepting compliments and tend to be more neurotic. Kurtzberg et al. (1967) reported that New York jail inmates with abnormal physical traits (e.g., hump nose, protruding ears, jailhouse tattoos, conspicuous facial scars, or needle tracks) lacked a sense of self-worth, and believed that their physical appearance stereotyped them as boisterous, mean, aggressive, immature, low in intelligence, and addicted to violence. They reported that a large majority of these inmates expressed a conscious or unconscious desire to disassociate themselves from these stereotypes. (See Chapter 4 for a discussion of the effects of surgery on inmates' rates of recidivism.)

Techniques of Attitude Change

One other body of research relevant to attitudes toward facially disadvantaged persons needs to be considered here, and this is the research carried out on attitude change. A few researchers have specifically tackled the thorny problem of how to influence attitudes toward disabled or disfigured persons, and although much work remains to be carried out, there are a few trains of thought that seem to be worth pursuing.

Child-rearing practices that emphasise the importance of health and normalcy (very much in vogue in contemporary Western society) can lead to an aversion on behalf of children to sickness, handicap, or other visible deviations from the norm. Livneh (1982) indicated that the verbal and behavioral style adopted by parents in relation to disabled people can provide a major influence on a child's belief and value system. Actions, tone of voice, gestures, and the like are transmitted directly or indirectly to the child and have a crucial impact on the formation of attitudes toward disability. Bull (1985) has stated that "if we lead by our example, our children to behave less negatively towards those who are facially disfigured, then the associated psychological problems may be considerably reduced."

Attitude Change in an Educational Context

Children's attitudes and behavior toward facially disfigured persons are discussed in Chapter 7. Some studies have been carried out to examine the effectiveness of various educational strategies for changing children's attitudes toward disabled persons. T. Jones, Sorrell, Jones, and Butler (1981) divided seventy-four 7- to 9-year-olds into two groups. The children were then given a 5-hour program of activities planned to enable subjects to perceive and experience the needs of handicapped persons and to synthesize their perceptions. The activities included simulation of interactions with handicapped people and discussions. Jones et al. reported significant changes in a positive direction in subjects' perceptions. Perkins and Karniski (1978) gave 20 subjects (in the sixth grade) instruction concerning physical disablement. They found significant differences in the personal space employed by subjects on subsequently encountering disabled persons. Subjects approached disabled interactants to a significantly closer distance than did subjects in the control group, who had not received any instruction.

However, not all studies of educational strategies for attitude change have reported positive results. For example, M. Miller, Armstrong, and Hagan (1981), arranged for 71 nonhandicapped third- and fifth-grade students to be taught about five handicapping conditions over a 6-week period. The attitudes of these students were then compared to controls. Miller et al. found no significant differences in attitudes (despite the existence of trends in a positive direction). Other educational strategies concerned with attitude change that involve the use of the media are discussed below.

Attitude Change in Adults

Thoreson and Kerr (1978) examined several aspects of attitudes toward disabled persons, and suggested strategies for change. (They noted that attitudes are still predominantly negative despite current legislation to improve the status of disabled persons in our communities.) They recommended that people be educated to treat disabled persons more as humans than as people who are "sick" and that the problems facing disabled people should be illustrated as problems not unlike those all people experience. They also maintained that the idea of "acceptance" of disabled persons is intrinsically derogating, and that emphasis on "acceptance" as being desirable should be avoided.

Carver, Glass, Snyder, and Katz (1977) suggested that the "personalization" of a stigmatized person (e.g., by presenting personal information) tends to evoke sympathy in others. (Although this sympathy effect has been found in quite a few studies, it should be noted that it is highly susceptible to desirability artifacts). Carver et al. thought people may feel ambivalent about stigmatized persons. They may feel guilty about any negative attitudes to stigmatized people, yet will usually be reluctant to express these attitudes in the presence of the stigmatized people themselves. They may try to compensate for the guilt they experience by denying the negative feelings and evaluating the person more favorably. As the personalization increases, so should the favorableness of the evaluation. Gibbons, Stephan, Stephenson, and Petty (1980) (using crutches as the handicap) also looked at ambivalence theory by examining the effect that contact with handicapped people has on the evaluations of those people. They concluded that if the behavioral context involves a personalization of the handicapped person, then sympathy responses are likely, because it is relatively easy to deny any negative feelings. In these cases, the positive response to the handicapped person is likely to be greater than that to a nonhandicapped person. However, if the situation increases the salience of ambivalent feelings, especially the negative aspects (e.g., if the handicapped person is seen as the cause of the ambivalent feelings), then denial is less likely, and response amplification will occur, with the negative reaction to the handicapped person being stronger than it would be to a nonhandicapped person.

Attitude Change Among Facially Disadvantaged Persons

From the discussion in the preceding section it is evident that it is not only the attitudes of the general public that may to be changed, but also the attitudes of some facially disadvantaged people toward themselves. Little research on improving the self-attitudes of disabled and disfigured people exists. Attitudes toward the self, like attitudes toward other things, may differ between individuals in content, duration, intensity, importance, salience, consistency, stability, and clarity. There is a need to learn what each individual sees when looking at himself or herself (e.g., social status, roles, physical characteristics, skills, traits, and other facets of content), whether a disabled individual has a fair or unfair opinion of himself or herself, and whether he or she spends a great deal of time thinking about what effect his or her appearance has on other people.

The importance of self-esteem as a component of self-attitudes has been highlighted (Rosenberg, 1975). People with low self-esteem are more likely to be sensitive to criticism, and to be deeply disturbed when laughed at, scolded, blamed, criticized, and so on. They are more likely to be bothered if others have a poor opinion of them, are more likely to be disturbed if they become aware of some fault or inadequacy in themselves, and are more prone to lowering their self-esteem if they feel they are being misunderstood by others. The benefits of developing methods of boosting the self-esteem of facially disadvantaged people would be manifold, in terms of improving both self-attitudes and the quality of social interaction for all parties involved (see below for a discussion of social interaction involving disabled or disfigured persons).

The Media—Enemies or Allies?

Two additional ways in which psychologists can offer help to ease the problems facing those who are facially disadvantaged are first to identify ways in which values that work to the detriment of visually disadvantaged people are transmitted, and second to offer suggestions and practical advice as to how the influence of these values can be reduced or changed. From the ensuing discussion it will become evident that the media play a vital part in both these areas.

Currently our society relies heavily on the mass media for information both in print and nonprint form. Since its inception, the mass media have been influential and pervasive mirrors for societal standards. However, the type of information transmitted by the media has gradually changed over the years. Until the 1930s the work of newspaper reporters, for example, was structured—they were expected to hold a mirror up to an event. However, over the years, "in depth reporting" has become more fashionable, and reporters now go beyond the bare facts to proffer explanations as to why events occur, and to provide interpretations of the factual details. Developments such as these have fueled the debate concerning to what extent the media are acting more as shaping forces in our society than as mirrors of what already exists. To what extent are the media influencing our beliefs, attitudes, and behavior? This debate will doubtless continue for many years to come. Meanwhile, although many acknowledge that the media seldom bring about major attitude change, many also recognize that communicators can influence people's attitudes to some extent, and that such people certainly provide influential models of behavior for us all.

In what ways do the media work to the disadvantage of those toward the negative end of the physical attractiveness continuum? Berscheid and Gangestad (1982) speculated as to whether the media have been influential in skewing our perceptions of attractiveness. They questioned whether the media lead us to believe that attractiveness either is normally distributed in the population, with most deemed average and a few attractive or unattractive, or is skewed (as research into media depictions suggests), with most of us regarded as being below the "neutral" point. Berscheid and Gangestad believed that this skewed distribution promoted by the media may account for the increasing demand for plastic surgery (see below). Certainly there is no doubt that the high value placed on personal appearance in our society (and promoted by the media) exerts pressure on those who deviate in some way to strive to regain a "normal" appearance.

Television

It seems that the phenomenon of a skewed representation of physically attractive people also extends to the representations in the media of those with physical handicap. Donaldson (1981) analyzed a random sample of prime-time TV (85 hours) to determine the visibility and image of characters portrayed as handicapped. The results showed that handicapped persons were not highly visible, and were as likely to appear in negative roles as in positive ones. Donaldson concluded that prime time TV serves to maintain societal devaluation of the handicapped more than fostering positive attitudes and interactions.

Leonard (1978) (reported in T. Elliott & Byrd, 1982) studied the depictions of disabled characters on prime-time TV. She created demographic, dramatic, and personal profiles from an examination of the characters. Her conclusion was that TV does stigmatize people with disabilities. Of the disabled characters portrayed, 40% were depicted as children, and none were over the age of 65. They came from predominately lower classes of society and were usually unemployed. If they did have employment, it was in a low-status occupation. Most were excluded from important family roles, and the majority were depicted single. Almost one half of the portrayals were recipients of some type of abuse, both verbal and physical. Hero status was rare, but villain roles were also minimal. However, the story endings were more positive than those with nondisabled characters, in that most disabled characters experienced a miracle cure at the end of the program. Two-thirds were depicted as being succoured, and three-quarters as submissive. Personality traits included being dull, impotent, selfish, defensive, and uncultured. The disabled people were regarded as being objects of pity and care. Overall, Leonard concluded that the disabled characters were considered not quite human, and virtually immobile in society.

Donaldson (1981) examined televisions's depiction of disability and concluded that the percentage of TV characterizations of disabled individuals in 3-week period was conspicuously lower (0.4%) than the estimated 15% to 20% of the general population who are disabled. Portrayals of people with disabilities were reserved to major roles; they were absent from minor roles or background groups and crowds. Most of the roles were negatively characterized and implied that the disability was the central focus of the person's life. Many of the roles were associated with evil and evil intention. Rumsey (1983) found that the media seem to play a large part in the perpetuation of stereotyping, and pointed out that casting directors go to great lengths to select actors who "look right" to play particular parts. The gangster, for example, is often portrayed with a fearsome physical aspect, scarred as the result of previous violence and wrongdoings.

T. Elliott and Byrd (1982) have pointed out that the contemporary "average" American child spends 50% more time viewing television than going to school. Television is easier to absorb than most media because of its convenience and its auditory and visual impact. Marks-Greenfield (1984) believed that minority-status children and children of low socioeconomic status are typically the most vulnerable to having their concepts of reality shaped by TV. From the television they assess what different kinds of people are like, and how they should act toward each other—thus the TV influences their conception of social reality. Marks-Greenfield believed that very young children equate all of TV, except cartoons, with reality. Initially they believe that anything that happens on TV could happen in the real world; later on they believe that what they see on TV represents something that probably happens in the real world. The realistic style of entertainment programming leads to the continuing belief that entertainment does in fact represent social reality. For example, as early as the age of 3 years, "heavy" TV viewers in the United States have more stereotyped views of sex roles than "light" viewers (Marks-Greenfield, 1984). TV seems to be especially influential in forming attitudes and providing knowledge on topics in which the child lacks experience, such as disfigured and disabled people, perhaps. Children who have first-hand knowledge of a topic may be able to make a clearer separation between the real world and the TV world.

Advertisements

As a result of his own membership in the disabled population, Sheed (1980; reported in T. Elliott & Byrd, 1982) discussed the futility and degradation of dehumanizing advertisements and information that denies respect to people with disabling conditions, offering recognition in a purely superficial manner. Manstead and McCulloch (1981) considered the images that TV advertisements contain to be drawn from society at large, and that these can therefore be seen as in some degree reflecting prevailing cultural values. In addition, TV advertisements seem to play an important role in the influence of TV as an agent of socialization (Murray, Rubenstein, & Comstock, 1972). Media advertising of beauty aids, for example, may accelerate the processes that both create and emphasize visual distinctions, since they endorse the idea that attractive people have better prospects for happy professional and social lives. The fetish of beauty encouraged by advertising may persuade the public as to the desirability of possessing a face with perfect contours and fresh skin, with rows of shining teeth. Beauty is presented as the promise of complete satisfaction—by purchasing the products in question, the public can identify with the attractive, "contented" people in the advertisements (Kemp, 1982).

As the cosmetic industry expands, advertisements on TV, radio, billboards, and magazines become more and more sophisticated, emphasizing the need to be aware of and to control appearance. The boom in the cosmetic industry, plastic surgery, diet foods, and the fashion business are all indicators of the major economic investment made in appearance. The idea of "beauty one can buy" continues to spread. In the United Kingdom in 1977, 250 million pounds (about $400 million) was spent on beauty aids—presumably largely by those succumbing to the bias toward the physically perfect projected by the media, and in attempts to match up to the glossy images promoted by magazines. In the same year, 300,000 people were injured in the United Kingdom on the roads, 300,000 received plastic surgery for burns, 5,000 facial tumors were operated on, and there was an increase in terrorist attacks, muggings, and industrial accidents leading to visible injuries.

In the United States, television viewers are subjected to the same message again and again—beautiful people possess material goods, are loved, usually find success and happiness, and are worshipped from afar. Thus television advertisements can act as the "hidden persuader," filling our screens with beautiful people. Commercials use sophisticated techniques in attempts to manipulate viewers into wanting certain products. Tan (1979) reported an experiment in which a group of high school girls were shown 15 commercials emphasizing the importance of physical beauty; there was a control group who did not see the commercials. Those who did watch the commercials were more likely than the control groups to agree with statements such as "beauty is personally desirable for me," and "beauty is important to be popular with men."

Other Media

Women's magazines continue to offer advice on how to correct "faults" in appearance, encouraging readers to strive to match up to the glossy images projected by glamourous models. Most of us have a desire to conform to the standards that we believe are the norm for our society. A failure to do so sets us apart both in our own estimation, and in the estimation of others. Magazines project images of women with flawless inviting bodies, with young, firm, symmetrical breasts—thus exposing readers to a stereotyped ideal. The idea of "corrective" surgery is introduced, implying that there is a norm from which we have deviated, and that we should strive to correct. The implication is made that beauty (and therefore, happiness) will be gained by a painful, often expensive operation.

Weinberg and Santana (1978) in a survey of comic books reported that 57% of those characters depicted as having some form of disability were villians and another 43% were heroes. None of these characters had neutral status. Weinberg and Santana pointed out that many of the evil characters were described as having distorted eyes and highly arched eyebrows.

T. Elliott and Byrd (1982) believe that the stereotypic depictions of disability in the mass media are substantially modeled after presentations of disability found in the influential realms of classical and modern literature, for example, Melville's Captain Ahab scarred and with a missing leg—obsessed in his pursuit of Moby Dick. D.H. Lawrence described the plight of Lady Chatterley, who was unable to touch or to be touched by her paraplegic husband, a man she thought of as having no soul. In mythology, Vulcan, the god of fire, is depicted as having shriveled legs and being ridiculed when serving the gods on Mount Olympus at a banquet. Oedipus was blinded for sinning against his family. (However, the hunchbacked Quasimodo, the facially disfigured Cyrano de Bergerac, and the "Elephant Man" are notable because they are deformed and good.) Similarly in children's literature the wicked Captain

Hook is portrayed as having a prosthetic device, Pinocchio has an ever-growing nose, and the ugly Rumpelstiltskin is prone to kidnapping children.

Adams (1985) pointed out that as early as the age of 4 to 5 years, children begin regularly to hear stories that pair ugliness with badness, while beauty is continually paired with goodness, kindness, innocence, and tenderness (e.g., Snow White, Cinderella, Alice in Wonderland). Similarly, in pantomimes children are taught to hiss and boo at the ugly "bad guy," and they learn that the hero of the piece can only marry the beautiful princess and live "happily ever after" once he has been transformed into a handsome prince. Adams commented that adults have been subjected to similar messages for years, in more refined forms. He offers the example of the movies, where the hero is usually handsome but the villain sleazy and unattractive.

J. Taylor (1981) reviewed media content research relating to the disabled. To use a person's physique to discover his or her inner nature has a long history in literature. Disabled people have had a negative literary press. Taylor believed that care should be taken from very early in life to shape positive attitudes toward atypicality, because the children of today will be the playwriters, producers, and media executives of the future. Heese (1975) also discussed the portrayal of handicapped persons in literature, and noted that from the Bible to the Koran to Thomas Mann, handicapped people are portrayed as different, and that distance from and rejection by the environment is stressed. Heese also commented on literature produced by handicapped people, noting that such literature is often produced to deal with their individual and social problems, and mainly consists of serious accusations made by them against society, with the authors rarely transcending this to become objective.

Harris and Harris (1977) analyzed written fund-raising appeals for disabled persons over a 4-year period in three popular magazines. They found that 77% contained an element of succumbing (i.e., depicting disabled persons as suffering and dependent). They commented that appeals to pity and fear may generate large sums of money, but that they also have unwanted consequences, including the perpetuation of negative stereotyping and the incubation of unfavorable self-evaluations among disabled persons. T. Elliott and Byrd (1982) have noted that television telethons have been a source of well-intentioned but degrading presentations of people with disabilities. Appeals for help for those living "hopeless" lives do not give accurate information, and although they may raise funds, they tend to reinforce stereotypes. Advertisers and fund raisers could adopt more "coping" themes, stressing the adjustive, positive, and active/independent dimensions of disability (Shakespeare, 1975).

This message, it seems, needs to be brought home even to government officials. The Department of the Environment in the United Kingdom provided an example of an unhelpful depiction of a disfigured person when carrying out an adveristing campaign in 1978–1979 designed to persuade drivers of the desirability of wearing seat belts. They created a character called "Billy Blunders" who might be lurking round the next corner ready to cause an accident. It was interesting to note (Rumsey, 1983) that the photographic representation of Billy Blunders depicted a young man with a badly repaired cleft lip/palate.

From the above, it is evident that the media (in particular, television) promote a level of attractiveness and an image of disability that are detrimental to those with a less than perfect physical appearance. However, rather than merely criticize the media, perhaps it would be more productive to accept that the media are an integral part our society and that they are here to stay. We believe that efforts should be made to offer constructive criticism as to what sort of changes could be made, and how the media could be used to the benefit of those who are facially disadvantaged.

How the Media Can Help

Rumsey's (1983) research with 7-year-olds, which highlighted the influence of the media in stereotypic judgments of facially disfigured persons (see below), suggests that in the search for ways to improve attitudes toward facially disadvantaged persons the daunting task of enlightening the general public as to the falsehoods in myths and legends passed from generation to generation may not be as important (for children at least) as the task of tackling the pervasive representations of characters currently freely available to the general public via the media. The biggest problem for facially disadvantaged people seems to be the biases the media have toward depicting (positively) attractive and physically perfect characters. Altering this biased view of the world may seem to be an almost impossible task, yet in the past few years legislation concerning racial equality has had far-reaching effects on television, radio, and comic content, and perhaps (although to a lesser extent) on advertising. Although realistically the likelihood of legislation concerning facial prejudice is remote, the possibility of change does exist provided sufficient pressure can be applied.

There has been some evidence put forward (Kemp, 1982) that there are signs of change in the world of advertising. Consumer research and public opinion are playing a progressively larger part in the formation of advertising policy. The feeling among the advertising agencies, it seems, is that many would like to get away from images such as the "glamourous housewife" often used in the advertising of domestic products, since the majority of the general public recognize this image as unrealistic, and thus lacking sophistication. However, although it could be that public opinion concerning advertisements may swing in favor of those with mundane levels of attractiveness, it seems unlikely that those with physical abnormalities will be included in advertising campaigns. Perhaps not even the media could successfully project the desirability of a distorted face.

Thomas and Wolfensberger (1982) discussed the portrayals of disabled persons in advertising, stressing that conveying a positive ideology in relation to people with disabling conditions is much more important than technical expertise in the promotion of positive images of handicapped persons. Wright (1974) offered some examples of "good" advertising, using the situation of a blind person crossing the street, and suggesting an approach such as the blind person saying "I'm an ordinary person, just blind. Don't shout or address me as if I were a child. Don't ask my wife does he take cream in his coffee. Ask me."

Positive Uses of Television

Some researchers have attempted to harness the power of the media in attempts to influence attitudes toward the disabled in an positive direction. Haefner (1976) used 10 color TV spot announcements aired during prime time on the three major United States networks in three specific urban areas. The announcements were based on themes of the importance of hiring and retraining disadvantaged individuals and considered these people as those who might be discriminated against. Potential employers had been contacted prior to exposure to the advertisement, and had been required to complete a questionnaire concerning their attitudes toward disabled people. A further test was administered following the showing of the advertisements. The results suggested that the intensive campaign had a significant effect on the employers' behavioral intentions to hire or train disabled people in the experimental cities. (However, no data are available as to whether any employers actually took on any disabled employees.)

The value of the media as educational tools has long been recognized. Despite the seeming enormity of the task of changing society's values and moving public opinion in favor of facially disadvantaged persons, efforts could be well invested in using the media to improve public education and in trying to increase the public's awareness of the causes and effects of various visible abnormalities. Hoyt (1978) reported an approach that employed a television series designed to capitalize on the curiosity children have about disability. The programs were made to show to nondisabled children the similarities they have with disabled children. Hoyt reported that his young viewers began to show a degree of attitude change, liking disabled children because they were interesting, and because they wanted to know them personally.

Potter (1978) has also discussed the ability television has to generate questions concerning types of disability. He pointed out that these questions can be incorporated into a classroom strategy for attitude change by teachers, and can also be responded to by parents. He suggested that adults could guide children's viewing and that they could teach them to watch television critically and to learn from what they watch. T. Elliott and Byrd (1982) emphasized that fantasy should be distinguished from reality, and discussion should be encouraged in order to counteract one-sided viewpoints. Wherever possible, children should be given first-hand experience as well as the third-hand encounters they have through television. For example, ethnic stereotypes could be countered by exposing children to people from different ethnic groups.

Television could also easily be used to capitalize on adults' curiosity concerning disability. Many opportunities have been missed, particularly in the United Kingdom, to use documentaries to educate the public as to the problems faced by facially disadvantaged persons. In the United Kingdom the recent Falkland Islands crisis is a good case in point. Many of the survivors of the fighting were badly disfigured, and will remain so for life. It seems that these survivors have been kept out of the public eye (as witnessed by their absence from the victory celebrations following the return of the forces to the United Kingdom). However, volunteers from among the victims could undoubtedly be found who would be willing to undergo media exposure for a "good cause." The nature of their injuries could be explained, with parallels drawn with more everyday occurrences of disfigurement. The reactions that such people are likely to encounter from others could also be discussed, in the hope that this would provoke concern and thought from people as to how conditions for disfigured persons might be improved. It may be that this concern could then be passed on to younger generations, who seem, in the light of the results of Rumsey's (1983) research, to be the most prone to react negatively to abnormalities of appearance.

A documentary was screened on British TV that included footage of patients in a military hospital, injured as a result of the Falklands war, the London bandstand bomb blast, and the conflict in Northern Ireland. The ordeal of the fight for fitness, the problems for those who did not achieve the necessary fitness standard to stay in the Forces, and the dedication of the staff were discussed. However, although the film included some close-up footage of injuries, the predominant focus was on functional impairments, and facial injuries were notably absent from close scrutiny—as was a detailed consideration of the social problems that were likely to ensue following discharge from hospital. A subsequent follow-up program did address some of the social problems encountered by one particular soldier who had been badly burned in the Falklands conflict. The favorable public response to the program indicated that this medium is much underused in the search for ways in which public education about disfigurement might be increased.

In the United States several TV documentaries have been screened that have dealt with the experiences of various facially disfigured people. Although the documentaries employed very different techniques to convey the experiences of subjects, each one seemed poignant and effective in the message put across to viewers. All were reportedly well received on their initial screening in America. In addition to illustrations of possible formats for documentary program, models for educational advertisements can also be found on the Public Broadcasting System in several regions of America. Short film sequences explaining problems associated with epilepsy, kidney disease, and other conditions are regularly inserted in TV advertising breaks. Many adopt the maxim "See the person first, not the disability" (T. Elliott & Byrd, 1982). Although there is a notable lack of film sequences dealing with problems associated with disfigurement, the experience already gained of this type of public education could be used for purpose in other countries.

Media Other than Television

How can other forms of the media be used to facilitate an improvement in the stereotyping of disfigured persons? Some researchers have used purposely made films designed to break down stereotypes by providing accurate information about disabled persons. Thredkeld and DeJong (1982), for example, have evaluated the usefulness of viewing a movie "First Encounters" concerning the interaction strain between disabled and nondisabled persons. Using 84 nonhandicapped students as subjects, they found that the showing of the film was effective in increasing the willingness of subjects to engage in relatively less intimate, one-off encounters with disabled persons, but this effect did not apply to more extended and intimate interactions.

Can literature be used to change children's behavior toward disabled persons? Dobo (1982) argued that children's literature can help nonhandicapped children overcome their fear and come to accept disabled peers. He suggested exploring literature in the classroom by reading to children, and following up the reading with provocative discussion. This can help the teacher discover what the students know, feel, or believe regarding disabilities and disabled people.

Various educational strategies involving media other than television have been used to try to improve attitudes toward disfigured and disabled persons. Shortridge (1982) examined the perceptions of 424 nondisabled elementary level schoolchildren after exposure to a structured learning experience dealing with what it would be like to be handicapped. Shortridge found significant positive shifts in subjects' perceptions of a handicapped peer's play capabilities, intelligence, and self-concept. Ibrahim and Herr (1982) tried two educational modes. One group role-played a disability (to do with speech pathology and a hearing problem) for 3 hours. The other group saw "informational" films and a slide show concerning handicap, and then had a discussion. Both groups acquired a more positive orientation toward disability even when measured 6 weeks after the experience.

Zakariya (1978; reported in T. Elliott & Byrd, 1982) discussed the effectiveness of a curriculum developed with the purpose of preparing a class for the mainstreaming of students with disabilities into the classroom. The units of the curriculum included simulation activities, class discussion with guest speakers, movies, slides, and videotapes of disabled children. Zakariya reported that the students responded with questions to guest speakers and teachers that were indicative of an empathic interest in the disabled. Donaldson and Martinson (1977) reported a study in which 96 students enrolled in a psychology course were assigned to four groups. A panel discussion involving six individuals with visible physical disabilities was viewed live by one experimental group, while another viewed the discussion via closed circuit TV, and a third listened to the discussion via audiotape recording. Donaldson and Martinson reported positive trends in attitudes for the live and videotape groups, whereas the audio presentation group did not differ from the control group.

Handlers and Austin (1980) combined five activities in an attempt to alter the existing attitudes of high school students. The activities included simulation exercises, first-hand contact with severely disabled persons, and the viewing of a selected film. An examination of the pre- and posttest scores indicated a positive shift in the attitudes of the young students toward disabled people. Sadlick and Penta (1975) presented TV programs of a well-rehabilitated quadriplegic to senior nursing students. The subjects answered a pretest, viewed the film presentation, and took an immediate posttest and a second posttest 10 weeks later. Significant changes in attitudes in a positive direction were found, with the change still evident (although slightly diminished) after the 10-week time span. However, the nurses, as members of the helping professions, could have been likely to be positive toward those with disabilities even before viewing the film. Whether other types of people would also show a positive shift was investigated by Staffieri and Klappersack (1960), who used a film designed to promote positive impressions toward individuals with cerebral palsy. The subjects (from a sophomore psychology course) did not show any significant attitude change following the showing of the film (the authors believed this was due to the lack of emotional appeal in the film).

Hafer and Narcus (1979) reported a study in which subjects viewed a film designed to inform about and encourage positive attitudes toward cerebral palsy. They reported that these subjects scored significantly lower on the attitude questionnaire than did subjects in the control group who had not seen the film. A second posttest 6 weeks later revealed no significant differences in attitude scores between the two groups. Westervelt and McKinney (1980) found no significant changes in fourth-grade children's attitudes following the showing of a film about disabled children in wheelchairs. They concluded that a film presentation alone is not sufficient to change attitudes concerning disability. Similarly, Monson and Shurtleff (1979) pointed out that filmstrips were only effective in influencing children's attitudes if, in addition, teachers exemplified positive attitudes toward disabled persons themselves, and provided a good role model of behavior for the children to copy.

From the evidence presented above, it would seem that in many cases it is possible to influence attitudes toward disabled or disfigured persons in a positive direction through the use of the media. However, regardless of the positive results of some of the studies reported above, it is acknowledged that attitude change is a complicated business. It is all too easy to overstimate the ability of the media to change attitudes, and in most cases modification is more likely than any degree of radical change. Any new communication transmitted by the media enters a situation where norms and standards are already firmly established, and where already the mind is typically made up. Liebert (1975; reported in T. Elliott & Byrd, 1982) has pointed out that for effective attitude change, both the cognitive and affective components of attitudes must be addressed by a blend of rational and emotional appeals relevant to the needs of the viewer. Arguments that will not alienate or threaten the audience must be employed, since the greater the anxiety the more likely the attitudes will be negative toward the stimuli eliciting the anxiety. Given that currently the majority of portrayals of disability primarily occur in the context of dramas and other program utilizing suspense, it is no wonder that negative attitudes are perpetuated. There is little doubt that television with its vast audiences has played, and will continue to play, a decisive function in maintaining and reinforcing attitudes toward facially disadvantaged persons. Let us hope that audiences will soon tire of the empty glamour and beauty so pervasive on our screens. The time to initiate accurate and nonstereotypical portrayals of people at all points on the physical attractiveness continuum seems long overdue.

The Provision of Health Services for Facially Disadvantaged Persons

There are several aspects of health care provision for those seeking facial plastic surgery to which psychologists can usefully contribute. One way is by promoting an accurate knowledge of the advantages and disadvantages of surgical intervention to improve appearance. All too often, television programs and magazine and newspaper articles comment on the miracles of modern surgical methods, describing new procedures designed to perfect appearance and provide the promise of complete satisfaction. The underlying message seems to be "If there is an aspect of your appearance you don't like, never fear, plastic surgeons are here to correct it." Rarely in the media, it seems, is there an informed discussion of the problems and disadvantages that can be associated with plastic surgery. What is badly needed is an awareness of the personal and interpersonal consequences of surgery, not only for those with fairly marked deviations from the norm, but also for those with minor blemishes, considered well within the normal range of appearance.

Issues that need careful consideration include first, at what stage of development should surgical intervention be employed? For facially disadvantaged children and adolescents, the balance between waiting for physical growth to be completed and the psychological problems associated with waiting is a precarious one. E. Clifford (1974), when discussing craniofacial malformation, suggested that the longer the person has had to accommodate to a malformation the greater the dependence on that malformation, and the greater the problems on its removal. Fantasies may develop, and surgery may become the great solve-all. The prospective patients may dream that, following surgery, no one will recognize them, and imagine that many aspects of their behavior will change. Pertschuk and Whitaker (1982) stated that craniofacial surgery patients aged 6 to 13 years presurgically fare better than those of 14 and over. The latter, they argued, are more prone to social isolation and problems relating to their self-concepts and mood state. Postoperatively most patients improved, with significant correlations between changes in appearance and changes on several measures including self-concept and trait anxiety being found. J. Weiss and Eiser (1977) recommended that removable appliance treatment (e.g., orthodontic braces) should be completed by the onset of puberty, because it is likely that teasing may become a particular problem then.

Children are not the only ones who are likely to be at a disadvantage while waiting for surgery. Waiting lists in the United Kingdom for National Health Service facial revision operations are particularly long (in some cases up to 10 years). Rumsey (1983) has indicated the problems that this can cause. In many hospitals, facially disfigured patients with no functional impairment receive low priority in a section of the health care system that is seriously underresourced. People who are facially disfigured in some way should warrant particularly speedy attention, whether it be in the form of surgery or some other kind of support. Munro (1981) maintained that an anomaly of the face should take precedence over any physical defect, and quotes the World Health Organization, which stated that "an anomaly should be regarded as requiring treatment if the disfigurement or functional effect is, or is likely to be an obstacle to the patient's physical and emotional well being."

It seems that in general behavioral scientists are in favor of early intervention. However, there are sometimes good physiological and technical reasons why surgery should be delayed until growth has finished. For such cases, Busch-Rossnagel (1981) recommended intervention strategies to reduce existing/potential developmental handicap resulting from atypical physique. Techniques suggested include the use of cosmetic prostheses, learning to control abnormal postures/expressions (for further discussion of social skills techniques, see below), and the alteration of the patient's social environment so the deviation is accepted by significant others (this latter suggestion represents quite a tall order!).

When surgical intervention is decided upon, additional considerations such as the amount of hospitalization that will be necessary, and how the patient will cope between operations (when the extent of unsightly disfigurement due to the surgery is likely to be considerable), need to be carefully thought through. In addition, the issue of how the patients will adapt to the change in their appearance remains. Help may be required by patients who will have to learn new behavior patterns to cope with different reactions to their new appearance from others.

Does Facial Surgery Always Improve Appearance?

Prospective facial surgery patients and their families frequently believe that surgery can provide a magical cure-all, which will either remove the blemish and/or create the appearance they desire. To what extent is this a valid belief? Well-controlled studies of the effects of aesthetic surgery are few. The early psychodynamic approach to plastic surgery took the line that patients requesting surgery were frequently emotionally disturbed, and that surgery would merely cause them to channel their underlying psychopathology to some new symptom (see W. Baker and Smith, 1939; Hay, 1970). More recent data suggest that severe psychological problems occur only in a minority of patients (Cash, 1985; Reich, 1975).

Kalick (1977) is one of the few contemporary researchers who has attempted to examine the effects of plastic surgery. Subjects rated photographs of patients before and after surgery on a number of personality dimensions (none of the patients were grossly deformed prior to surgery). Kalick found that surgery did increase the physical attractiveness ratings. In addition, the people were perceived very differently in terms of their personality and other characteristics. In particular, the perceived social desirability of women appeared to be significantly increased. They were perceived as kinder, more sensitive, more sexually warm and responsive, more competent as marriage partners, and more likely to marry the person of their choice. There was also a significant change in patients' perceived social and professional happiness. Cash and Horton (1983) tested the hypothesis that rhinoplasty precedures improve physical attractiveness and foster more favorable attributions of personality characteristics by others. They also used photographs of patients before and after surgery (however, unlike Kalick, Cash and Horton attempted to control for possible effects of patients' hairstyle, hair color, cosmetics, etc.). Psychology undergraduates rated the photographs for self-assertiveness, interpersonal attractiveness, intelligence, life success, personal likeability, and physical attractiveness. Cash and Horton reported that 45.3% of the data reflected significantly more favorable perceptions as a result of the rhinoplasty, with 44.2% of ratings showing no difference. (Ten and one-half percent of ratings showed less favorable attributions, but Cash and Horton thought that the physical attractiveness of these particular stimulus individuals was unaffected, or only weakly affected, by the rhinoplasty procedure.)

Arndt, Lefebvre, Travis, and Munro (1986) investigated whether the appearance of 24 children with Down's syndrome was rated more positively after facial surgery to make their features more socially acceptable. Arndt et al. found that lay raters judged the postoperative appearance of the children as slightly less attractive than the preoperative appearance, although the childrens' parents rated them as significantly more attractive postoperatively, in addition to reporting happier personal, family, and social lives. Arndt et al.

suggested that the positive psychosocial consequences associated with surgery may be more circumscribed than originally expected, and largely the result of parental satisfaction and hope for the future integration of their children into the "normal" world. Similarly, Lefebvre, Travis, Arndt, and Munro (1986) reported the results of a study of 25 children with Apert's syndrome. Parents' ratings of the children's appearance improved significantly 1 year after facial surgery. In addition, the self-esteem of the children was also significantly higher 1 year postoperatively than it had been preoperatively. (It should, however, be noted that the children's self-esteem level had dropped again 4 years postoperatively.) Lefebvre et al. concluded that the children did "most certainly" benefit from surgery (although this conclusion appears to be based on the rather tenuous self-esteem data), and that the parents saw the surgery as a major therapeutic intervention in their children's lives.

Macgregor (1981) has offered three categories of reasons (unsubstantiated by data) as to why in some instances "successful" cosmetic surgery may be followed by dissatisfaction from the patient. First, there are reasons that are attributable to the patient (the patient has had surgery to please someone else; the patient has serious preexisting psychological problems; the patient expects surgery to solve his or her life problems; the patient's expectations of the likely aesthetic result of surgery are unrealistic; the patient is dependent on others for his or her level of self-esteem). Second, dissatisfaction may be attributable to the surgeon. Macgregor pointed out that, like architects who build buildings that have no relationship to the people who will live in them, some surgeons, in their zeal to achieve anatomic perfection, build noses and faces that bear no relationship to the people who must live with them. She offers the example of a woman who was referred to a surgeon on account of her breathing difficulties. On the morning of the operation, the surgeon suggested removing a small hump in her nose. Anxious that the operation should go well, the patient agreed. However, after her operation she found that the surgeon had also changed the tip of her nose (and that he had presented her with a bill for the additional cosmetic surgery). Previously, she had felt proud of her nose, and confident of her physical appeal; however, postoperatively this was lost—she felt that she had acquired a hard and stern countenance, and that she was no longer attractive. She felt she had lost her identity. Macgregor also felt that some surgeons may fail to prepare their patients adequately concerning what is involved in the facial surgery procedure. Alternatively, they may make a hasty evaluation of the patient, or may fail to describe adequately what the patient's appearance will be like postoperatively. A third source of dissatisfaction may be attributable to the interaction between the patient and the surgeon—for example, personality conflicts or poor communication.

In addition to Macgregor's attributions of postoperative dissatisfaction, the reactions of significant others to postoperative changes in the patient's appearance seem to be particularly important. R. Devine (personal communication, 1982) noted that following cosmetic surgery many patients discover that their friends do not, in fact, notice that a particular feature has been altered, but instead make general comments on their appearance, for example, "your holiday must have done you good." Sometimes, however, reactions are more negative, and postoperative dissatisfaction is often attributed to the reactions of friends or family (Reich, 1975). Cash and Horton (1983) put forward the idea that some significant others react negatively to the increased "marketability" of a loved one, and respond in a nonsupportive manner in order to restore the equity they felt previously existed. Problems of a different nature can also be caused by significant others. Many patients experience more attention from others postoperatively than they had when their appearance had been less attractive. Some patients revel in this attention, but others find it galling that the increased attention must be due to their increased level of physical attractiveness rather than to internal qualities and behaviors. Macgregor (1981) offered the example of Jack, who had a rhinoplasty procedure at the age of 14 because of breathing difficulties. Subsequently he was pursued by females who had previously paid him little attention. He found this distressing because internally he did not feel he had changed at all—he did not feel that his more attractive external image was a reflection of his real self.

Munro (1981) assessed the effects of orbital hypertelorism on 12 patients prior to surgery, and concluded that none of the subjects were living "normal" lives. He found that very positive psychological changes occurred after surgery at all ages. Patients and parents quickly forgot the severity of the preoperation situation and it was necessary sometimes to remind them with the use of photographs. Other researchers also quote high rates of satisfaction among postoperative patients. Cash (1985), for example, quotes figures of 76% to 87% rhinoplasty customers being satisfied. However, Jensen (1978) mentioned the diversity of techniques, approaches, theoretical orientations, and so forth that exist, and stated that patients' actual social behavior and experiences with others may not always improve postoperatively. From an experimental point of view, it is, of course, very difficult to establish accurately the relationship between surgery and improvements or decrements in the quality of patients' lives. The very circular effects, both pre- and postoperatively, of person's self-esteem, his or her social behavior, and the behavior of other people make the researcher's task very difficult. Predictions of whether surgical intervention is likely to benefit a particular patient are difficult to make, whether or not a dramatic improvement in appearance is likely.

Additional Factors Affecting Postoperative Satisfaction

Residual disfigurement can pose a particular problem. This can take the form of scarring or a reduced level of the original deformity. Macgregor (1981) stated that some patients consider residual scarring to be even worse than the original defect. Despite words like "incision" and "skin grafts," the notion still exists in some patients that surgical scars will be invisible. Patients frequently fail to hear what doctors tell them, and ambiguous phrases such as "there may be some residual scarring" make no impression before surgery. Kapp-Simon (1980) stated that those who remain deformed after surgery can find themselves in an unenviable situation. Before surgery, there was no doubt in the eyes of onlookers that the patient had a gross defect, and thus questions as to the nature of the disfigurement were not necessary. After surgery, however, although the defect had been improved, problems can be caused by the deformity that still remains. The status of the disfigurement has become unclear. Kapp-Simon reported that some patients regretted surgery, and one in particular recounted the dilemma caused by those people who on the one hand had told him that appearances aren't important, but on the other hand had also urged him to have surgery, implying beauty was important after all. Such potential confusion following surgery should be borne in mind, because it could lead to fractured self-concepts and problems concerning people's personal identity, especially because residual deformity following surgery is much more common than is popularly believed (Rumsey, 1983).

The type of disfigurement plays a part in the likelihood of whether cosmetic surgery will improve appearance or not. First, the site of a disfiguring feature is important. The importance of the face in social interaction and impression formation has been discussed elsewhere, as has the case for early intervention to provide surgical and/or psychological support for facially disfigured people. However, individuals can experience equal distress from disfigurements to other parts of the body (hands, breasts, legs, etc.).

The etiology of a disfigurement is also an important factor. Munro (1981), for example, believed facial deformities due to trauma to be more easily accepted and understood by others than are congenital deformities, which may produce the greatest adverse psychosocial reaction. Rumsey et al.'s (1982) work has provided support for this idea. They found that the general public react more negatively to a facial port wine stain (a congenital disfigurement) than to trauma scarring consistent with injuries sustained in a road traffic accident. This suggests that improvements to congenital disfigurements (even if only to the extent that the disfigurement was changed to look more like a traumatic injury) would be better received by the general public.

Posttreatment satisfaction of those with congenital deformity may be higher than those with traumatic injury. The latter have had an experience of what it is to have a "normal" appearance, and many entertain the ideal that they would like to be returned to their former unblemished selves. Congenitally disfigured people, on the other hand, have never experienced life without a visible abnormality, and may perhaps be more modest in their aspirations. Graber (1980), for example, has pointed out that in the case of dental abnormalities, those with congenital disfigurements have greater posttreatment satisfaction than those with traumatic injuries. This, Graber suggested, is because the latter want to be returned to a "normal" state—and this is often unrealistic.

Here, then, are some of the factors that need to be borne in mind when the potential advantages and disadvantages of surgery are being assessed. There is still much to learn about the psychological outcomes associated with facial surgery (longitudinal research is especially needed). However, whatever the likely outcome of such research, Jensen (1978) believes that surgeons would do well to remember that the patient is more than a living organism upon which techniques may be practiced. Perhaps psychologists can help by proffering reminders of these issues and by encouraging an assessment of each individual case on its own merits. There is, however, one modus operandum that psychologists can suggest to surgeons and staff. Kalick, Goldwyn, and Noe (reported in Kalick, 1982) looked at the satisfaction of patients with port wine stain and found that patient satisfaction is accounted for to a surprisingly large degree by what the surgeon and staff do—how considerately they treat the patient in addition to the physical results they produce.

The Motivation of Patients to Seek Surgery

An additional way in which psychologists could help disfigured people, and those involved in their care, is to make health care professionals more aware of the complex phenomenon of people's motivation to improve their appearance. In the United Kingdom patients may have difficulty obtaining the necessary referral from their general practitioner to a plastic surgeon, encountering attitudes such as "We're in the business of treating sick people, and patients who want referral to plastic surgeons aren't really sick" (R. Devine, personal communication, 1982). Similarly, in British National Health Service hospitals, social and/or psychological reasons for seeking surgery are considered second best, and patients citing such reasons for wanting surgery may receive lower waiting list priority than prospective patients who cite physical problems (e.g., difficulty in breathing, problems with speech, etc.). Many patients are well aware of this situation, and feel discouraged from revealing the full extent of the social and psychological problems they are experiencing. Despite the higher priority given to those experiencing physical problems, Rumsey (1983) found that when patients are questioned by someone other than medical personnel, the most frequently mentioned motives for seeking surgery are social ones—embarrassment, self-consciousness, increased sensitivity, feeling uncomfortable meeting others, a wish to improve social life, and the like. Similarly, Reich (1982) reported a survey of 3,000 patients in which questions were asked in an attempt to discover the predominant reasons for requesting surgical improvement in appearance. He stated that 60% of his sample reported self-consciousness in interpersonal relationships, 25% reported social isolation, 10% stated that an employment situation was involved, and 5% reported other adverse situations.

The finding that social and psychological problems are the predominant drive behind the desire for cosmetic surgery is hardly surprising. Colligan et al. (1980) believe that the largest part of the increase in demand for reconstructive facial surgery could be attributed to the increased value placed on appearance by contemporary society. Additional social factors include the ways in which people cope with adverse life situations. Bereavement and divorce, for example, can exacerbate concern over appearance (Colligan et al., 1980).

Reich (1982) pointed out that, in addition to the physiological implications of plastic surgery, plastic surgeons also need to be aware of the psychological and social ramifications of the patient's desire for surgery. They need, for example, to be aware of both internal and external motivations for surgery (Edgerton & Knorr, 1971). External motivations include a desire to please others, a response to peer pressure (nicknames, teasing, harassment, exclusion from groups), and socio-cultural factors. Parental pressure can be a particularly potent source of motivation. Graber (1980) quoted work by Baldwin and Barnes (1966), who surveyed 375 orthodontic patients and their parents using a detailed questionnaire. Information was sought concerning socioeconomic background, ethnic identity, motivation, dental health, the personality characteristics of the child, and so forth. The authors reported that the mother was usually the motivating individual and that many mothers had themselves undergone orthodontic treatment when they had been young. Some mothers reported feeling guilty about their child having inherited their dental faults. Others who had not received treatment in their youth did not want their children to suffer any of the negative consequences of less than perfect dental appearance that they themselves felt they had experienced. Many parents believed that treatment would lead to improved social and work possibilities for their children in later life. Warford (1973) reported that youngsters seeking orthodontic treatment expected that straighter teeth would increase their popularity, improve their speech, improve their looks, lead to less teasing about their appearance, and lead them to having more friends. However, Warford also commented that the degree of parental influence, not the degree of malocclusion, was the key factor in seeking treatment. Several researchers have commented that middle- and upper-class patients predominate in the field of orthodontics. For these people, straight teeth (and hence an enhanced physical attractiveness), are seen as a means of social advancement. (Chapter 9 briefly mentions other studies involving dental appearance.)

Reich (1982) pointed out that the explosion of outdoor activity and the popularity of exposing the "body beautiful" may be unhelpful. Some may feel their appearance causes others to be derisive toward them, and that treatment may make their social environment less threatening. Some may experience a sense of personal inadequacy as a result of a failure to reach an acceptable standard of appearance. Perhaps they may feel that their disfigurement is an obstruction to career prospects or to social ambitions, and that an improvement in appearance might aid prospects in these areas (see Linn, 1966).

Approaches to Patient Care

Once the decision has been made to seek cosmetic surgery, how can psychologists contribute to the quality of patient care? Strauss (1980) pointed out that the medical response to disfigurement is the result of a rational and scientific framework. Similarly, Rumsey (1983) noted that although training curricula for many health service professionals in the United Kingdom now encompass more psychology and sociology, the current emphasis on the medical model in British National Health Service hospitals allows little time for social and psychological rehabilitative concerns. Instead, the emphasis is shifting more and more toward the "efficient" use of staff time, hospital facilities, and available beds for inpatients. Many nurses and rehabilitation staff are led to believe that the medical model (i.e., concern for the physiological needs of the patients) is the most efficient and professional approach to patient care. Issues such as the motivation of patients to seek surgery and their expectations of treatment are all too often ignored, and less and less time is left for the more humanistic focus needed by those who often have to cope with problems of psychological/social rather than physiological functioning, even though addressing these issues may turn out to be *more* cost-effective in the long run. Kligman (1985), for example, reported that physicians typically underestimate the psychological pain experienced by patients with skin discoloration (such as vitiligo, albinism, and port wine stains). Porter, Beuf, Nordlund, and Lerner (1978) reported that many vitiligo patients are embarrassed by the disease, and often stated that they were socially or sexually impaired. Yet they received little sympathy from physicians. Similarly, N. Bernstein (1976) pointed out, concerning burns patients, that improved surgical treatment in burn care means that more people survive with incredible disfigurements. These, however, often lead to devastating psychological and practical problems for patients, families, and staff of intensive care units, and are issues that cannot be ignored if effective rehabilitation of burn patients is to be achieved.

The participation of behavioral scientists in the evaluation, planning, and treatment of patients should be recommended. The social and psychological problems likely to be caused by disfigurement due to traumatic injury are apt to be considerable. In addition, for those seeking elective facial surgery, the main motivation is likely to be psychological/social. A team approach to patient care should be adopted, with health care professionals of many disciplines (e.g., occupational health, social work, psychiatry, and psychology, as well as surgeons, nurses, etc.) all working together. Some successful examples of this approach are operating in the United States. The United Kingdom, however, still has some way to go. Many hospitals have yet to implement a comprehensive team approach to facial surgery and burn patient care. Although some successful examples exist, all too often the membership of the health care teams is limited, with behavioral scientists frequently excluded. This exclusion can to some extent be explained by the chronic underresourcing of psychologists in the British Health Service. However, it is also incumbent on our profession to demonstrate the useful and important role that psychologists can play.

The benefits of including behavioral scientists in the care of disfigured patients are potentially manifold. Possible activities include groups for present and past patients. These provide the opportunity for discussion of problems such as interaction with peers, how to deal with curiosity and stares, and coping with feelings of guilt and blame. Groups can also be offered to nursing staff—many experience bouts of fatigue and depression, and conflicts between wanting to make every effort to heal the patient, but at the same time worrying about the likely quality of life for people who are so badly disfigured. In addition, the activities of psychologists and social work staff can usefully include regular psychosocial ward rounds. These can be used to discuss behavioral management issues, the psychological assessment of personality problems, and how to help patients and families gradually deal with the realities of their situation and to encourage the development of realistic expectations concerning burn surgery—that is, what improvements can actually be made. In addition, some basic social skills training could be possible (see below).

Cahners (reported in N. Bernstein, 1976) made comments on the care of burn patients that are applicable to the majority of disfigured patients. She has stressed the need for the provision of social services. Patients are likely to experience much anxiety about leaving the sheltered environment of the hospital. Staff need to contact schools, businesses, and other places to warn them of particular problems such as the inability to wear uniform, for example. "On the spot" education concerning the nature of patients' injuries has also been shown to be useful. Fellow students or co-workers can be taught what has happened to their colleague's body, the sorts of treatment they have undergone, how their self-esteem may have been lowered, and so on. Follow-up work such as this is sometimes necessary for months after discharge.

There is an urgent need to redirect the attention of those responsible for the allocation of funds within health services toward the discharge planning and rehabilitation of facially disfigured patients. Although the widespread provision of a comprehensive rehabilitation service seems in most cases a long way off, there are many activities that would be relatively easy to incorporate into the care of disfigured people. Contact needs to be made and maintained with patients' families in order to provide advice and support. Volunteers could be used to provide extra services (e.g., camouflage makeup) on a regular basis. Regular groups could be provided for patients, families, and staff. These have been shown to have great potential, both in terms of establishing mutual respect and encouragement and for improving the quality of communication between health professionals, patients, and families (Rumsey, 1983).

The training of medical staff should be extended to include not only medical aspects of care, but also interviewing techniques, rudimentary counseling skills, and an appreciation of the value of assessing patients' attitudes and psychological and social needs. The approach to training should be electric and pragmatic, with the aim that staff should be capable of offering well-reasoned and adequately informed psychosocial support and evaluation to the patient.

There is undoubtedly an urgent need to facilitate sympathetic communication between patients and staff. A greater awareness, instilled at the training stage, of patients' psychological and social needs can only be beneficial to this cause. L. Bailey and Edwards (1975) lend weight to this point of view with their recommendation that attention should be paid to the establishment of rapport based on mutual respect, honesty, and confidence, stressing that an understanding of patient dynamics is helpful in establishing clear communication.

Ways of Offering Help Directly to Facially Disadvantaged People

There is little doubt that many of the suggestions presented so far for helping facially disadvantaged people have to be viewed in the long term. Changing the ingrained values of a society, changing attitudes, even changing the health care system are undoubtedly complex affairs. Although attention should not be directed away from these areas on account of the daunting nature of the task, something more immediate is needed. Facially disadvantaged people need direct, practical help, and they need it quickly.

The questions psychologists need to consider are pragmatic ones. For example, what type of help is going to be most effective? For some, counseling could provide the answer.

Counseling

The availability of a sympathetic, supportive ear could work wonders for many facially disadvantaged people. Any improvements in their self-concepts, any increased understanding of the perspective of others, and any lessening in the preoccupation with the self that could be facilitated by a counselor could be of great benefit. Regular or even occasional chats with someone able to empathize with the problems associated with facial handicap could even in some cases obviate the need to contemplate surgical intervention. More research is needed into the types of counseling that would be the most helpful.

The appearance of the counselor.   Facial appearance and counseling has been a topic of some research; however, the emphasis has been on counselor appearance rather than on counseling those disadvantaged by their facial appearance. Strong (1968) asserted that a client's perception of counselor attractiveness is based on perceived similarity to, compatability with, and liking for the counselor, and that if these factors existed, self-disclosure would be facilitated. These thoughts have led some researchers to examine the effects of the physical attractiveness of the counselor on the client's perceptions. Cash, Begley, McCown, and Weise (1975), for example, asked subjects to assess a brief videotaped self-introduction of a 30-year-old male professional counselor in either a physically attractive or an unattractive condition. For both male and female subjects, the physically attractive counselor was perceived more favorably than in the unattractive condition, in terms of both interpersonal attraction and credibility.

Lewis and Walsh (1978) also used a videotaped presentation. They reported that female subjects rated an attractive female counselor as more competent, professional, assertive, and interesting than the counselor in an unattractive condition. Although the results of these two studies were taken as evidence of the positive effects of counselor physical attractiveness on clients' perceptions of counselors, Corrigan, Dell, Lewis, and Schmidt (1980) have interpreted the results of these studies (and also results reported in a study by Cash and Kehr [1978]) as reflecting the debilitative influence on clients' perceptions of counselor *unattractiveness*, rather than the facilitative nature of counselor physical attractiveness. The point is also made that the results of the above three studies were produced from video or audiotaped presentations of the counselor, with client impressions based on a single, initial contact with the counselor—a situation hardly representative of the usual counseling process. Whether this debilitating effect of unattractiveness would generalize to facially disadvantaged clients has yet to be examined. It may instead be that unattractiveness in the counselor may enhance the perceived similarity between the facially disadvantaged client and the counselor, thus increasing the interpersonal attraction between the two, and facilitating the counseling process. The only evidence currently available that may be relevant to this issue is from a study by Strohmer and Biggs (1983). They examined the potential benefits of having disabled counselors for disabled clients and they concluded that this tactic is not necessarily effective, reporting that client perceptions of the counselor expertness or attractiveness were not affected by the presence or absence of a disability.

Zlotlow and Allen (1981) pointed out that counselor physical attractiveness is a complex composite of attributes, and that it is mediated by a substantial number of additional characteristics. The influence of physical attractiveness is greatest during the earliest stages of impression formation, whereas its impact over more extensive interactions may be substantially modified by the behavior of the person being evaluated. A physically attractive person may have a head start in developing rapport, but attractiveness is still not an adequate substitute for technical skill or social competency.

The appearance of the client.   What of the appearance of the client? Are the disadvantages that are associated with unattractiveness in social interaction also involved in the therapeutic process? It seems that for some counseling situations, they may be. Schofield (1964), among others, has emphasized the major extent to which counselors and therapists prefer to work with young, attractive, verbal, intelligent, successful ("YAVIS") clients. In addition, several investigators have indicated that physical attractiveness ratings ascribed by counselors to clients are significantly related to more favorable impressions formed by counselors of physically attractive than of unattractive clients.

Hobfoil and Penner (1978), for example, conducted a study using graduate students of clinical psychology as subjects. These trainee psychotherapists evaluated the self-concepts of attractive and unattractive "clients" who were presented through a video and audiotaped presentation. Subjects judged the attractive clients to have better self-concepts than the unattractive clients. Hobfoil and Penner pointed out that this form of stereotyping may produce differences in the clients' self-concepts where none previously existed. Nordholm (1980) showed 289 health professional black-and-white head and shoulder photographs of physically attractive or unattractive "patients." The attractive stimuli were judged to have more socially desirable personality traits; to be more intelligent, more friendly, less complaining, less aggressive, and more responsible; and to have a better motivation and a greater likelihood of improvement than physically unattractive patients.

Barocas and Vance (1974) used professional student counseling staff as subjects. They reported that counselors' attractiveness ratings of male and female undergraduates were significantly related to client prognosis (but were unrelated to other measures of interview performance, initial clinical status, and final clinical status). Other correlational evidence from this study suggests that physical attractiveness may be a more salient cue for inferring clinical status in female rather than male clients. The authors also suggested that male counselors may be more consistently influenced by the physical attractiveness of clients than female counselors. Cash, Kehr, Polyson, and Freeman (1977), using photographs and audiotaped interviews as stimulus materials, reported that physically attractive people are perceived by college students as likely to need less therapeutic intervention for psychological problems than unattractive people. They noted that the unattractive stimuli who were presented as being quite extensively disturbed were particularly likely to be recommended by subjects to seek professional assistance. Jones, Hansson, and Phillips (1978), who also used photographs as their stimulus material, reported that physically attractive individuals are less likely to be selected by college students as showing symptoms of psychopathology.

Schwartz and Abramowitz (1978) carried out an investigation of the clinical judgments of male psychotherapy trainees. They concluded that many of the psychodiagnostic and self-judgments made by their sample seemed to be relatively well insulated from the impact of variations in client physical appearance. Subjects did, however, expect unattractive "clients" to terminate therapy sooner than attractive "clients." Schwartz and Abramowitz suggested that this might be a consequence of the belief of the trainee therapists that the clients might fail to provide sufficient social incentive for the therapists to promote a successful therapeutic engagement. Consequently they warned supervisors to be alert to subtle manifestations of covert prejudice against physically unattractive clients in their trainees.

Sandler (1975) carried out a study notable because of its subject sample of 123 practicing therapists from different parts of the country. By using photographs of people who were judged low, moderate, or high in physical attractiveness, attached to a "problem oriented record," Sandler investigated the effects of client physical attractiveness on various judgments of the therapists. Therapists were asked to assess the clients' likely level of intellectual functioning; the motivation for treatment; the prognosis, level of pathology, probable duration of treatment, and type of therapeutic intervention recommended; and the therapists' interest in treating such a client. Overall, Sandler found only one significant correlation—a relationship between client attractiveness and therapists' judgments of intellectual functioning. Sandler noted, however, that "single male therapists" and "analytically oriented male therapists" produced significant positive correlations across the majority of dependent measures.

Here, then, are suggestions that a client's level of physical attractiveness may affect the therapeutic process in some way. Once more, however, the studies quoted above are prone to methodological weaknesses. Frequently undergraduate students or trainee counselors were used as subjects, and "clients" were briefly presented by means of photographs and audiotapes, or by means of videotaped presentations—hardly representative of a true counseling situation. However, the evidence is consistent enough to ask the question whether in fact the counselor perceptions reported above may have some basis in fact. Is there a link between physical appearance and mental health? Are physically unattractive people more liable to experience mental health problems than physically attractive people?

Physical appearance and mental health.   Unfortunately, little research examining this issue is at present in existence. Cash (1985) has stated that depressed college students and psychiatric outpatients and inpatients are more likely to be dissatisfied with their bodies and to view their physical appearance as ugly. He found that the personality characteristics of physically attractive people reflected a pattern of somewhat greater self-acceptance, sociability, internal locus of control, cognitive inquisitiveness, psychological androgyny, and independence, whereas the pattern for unattractive individuals was somewhat more asocial, external in locus of control, cognitively constrained, self-protective, and lower in self-esteem. Cash quoted an unpublished doctoral dissertation by Noles (1983), who found that depressed and nondepressed undergraduates did not differ in their objective level of physical attractiveness. However, the depressed subjects were significantly more dissatisfied with their body parts and their appearance than the nondepressed subjects. Noles reported that depressed students tended to negatively distort their attractiveness, believing that they were less attractive than their peers had actually rated them. (Noles noted that the ratings by nondepressed students were distorted in the opposite direction, i.e., they had a tendency to inflate the attractiveness ratings assigned to them by peers.)

Some other researchers have examined possible links between physical attractiveness and mental health. Archer and Cash (1985) found a modest, but significant relationship that schizophrenic psychiatric patients were less physically attractive than nonschizophrenic patients. Pertschuk (1985) has suggested that the unkempt, unattractive appearance of mentally disturbed patients serves to perpetuate their condition because it means that other people are likely to keep the patient at a distance, thus further confirming a sense of unworthiness in the patient.

Farina et al. (1977) studied three groups of females, one consisting of hospitalized psychiatric patients, one of university employees, and the third of shoppers. Using photographs and face-to-face ratings, the hospitalized psychiatric patients were found to be less physically attractive than the normal controls. In a second study with hospitalized psychiatric female patients as subjects, Farina et al. reported that the more unattractive the subject the more likely she was to receive a diagnosis of schizophrenia, and the more inadequate were ratings of her contemporary interpersonal behavior. Napoleon, Chassin, and Young (1980) published a partial replication of Farina et al.'s study. In general the results stood up to the replication. In addition Napoleon et al. reported, using high school yearbook photographs, that psychiatric patients were premorbidly less attractive than their classmate controls, and also that they declined further in attractiveness before their hospitalization. They concluded that being physically unattractive may predispose an individual to a number of negative social outcomes, one of which is mental illness.

Despite some indicators from the research findings quoted above, much more research is needed before a firm link between physical appearance and mental health can be established. In particular, research is needed concerning why some objectively unattractive individuals manage to cope while others cannot, and require help to function adequately.

Self-Help Groups

Self-help groups hold promise as a means of helping facially disadvantaged people. They have been well proven in other areas such as those dealing with alcohol problems, groups providing support for those suffering from particular disease, and those catering for the problems encountered by minority groups of various sorts. The efficacy of self-help groups for facially disadvantaged persons has been the subject of some debate. Although some workers in the field have thought that they hold promise (e.g., Rumsey, 1983), others (e.g., Piff, 1985) have maintained that facially disfigured people in particular do not want to meet others similarly afflicted, because in some way they would feel they were having to parade their own disfigurement when in fact they would prefer to hide it. However, subsequent experience in the field has led Piff (personal communication, 1986) to believe that group meetings and self-help groups can in fact have a valuable function for facially disadvantaged persons. They provide the opportunity for discussions, for exchanges of views and experiences, and for mutual support. In addition, they lend a kind of legitimacy to the problems faced by facially disadvantaged people with the recognition that social and psychological problems are the norm rather than the exception among facially disfigured or ugly people

Another technique that holds much promise for offering direct help to visibly disadvantaged persons is that of social skills training.

Social Skills Training

In the last decade there have been many developments in the area of non-verbal communication and an increasing awareness of its importance in social interaction. Technological advances, especially those relating to film and video equipment, have enabled researchers to examine increasingly detailed aspects of the components of nonverbal behavior. As research escalates, realization of the importance of behavior transmitted through the nonverbal channel and of the reciprocal nature of social interaction has grown. These technological and research advances have facilitated the development of social skills training (SST). The approach recognizes the importance of the use of skillful social behavior in interaction. SST techniques are designed to examine, and if necessary, separate out the verbal and nonverbal components of social behavior, and to teach (usually through a mixture of instruction, modeling, behavioral rehearsal, reinforcement, and homework assignments) a new and more socially acceptable repertoire of skills to enable patients/clients to communicate and influence their environment more effectively.

SST has developed as a method of teaching, in a systematic way, the skills of social interaction. It is primarily concerned with changing overt social be-havior. However, although the approach makes no direct attempt to change other aspects of the person's experience, as the person becomes more socially skilled, changes in other, more 'internal' dimensions may occur. The person may become less anxious and depressed and feel less inadequate and more confident as a result of becoming more effective in social communication.

Does the approach work? There is little doubt that a person's behavioral style in social interaction has a considerable effect on the impressions other people form of him or her. Research by Kendon (1967), for example, re-vealed that subjects whose interviewer did not look at them for part of the interview thought the interviewer had lost interest in them. Washburn and Hakel (1973) examined pairs of subjects, one of whom was assigned to be an "interviewer" and the other a "job applicant." The "interviewer" was in-structed to be either enthusiastic or unenthusiastic, and to emit high or low levels of gestures, eye contact, and smiling. Observer subjects rated the inter-viewer. The enthusiastic interviewer was perceived as being younger, as liking the job better, and as being more easily approachable, interested, consider-ate, and intelligent. Interestingly, the "applicants" in this condition were also rated more favorably by the observers, even though the former were given no instructions. The authors postulated that this was probably a direct result of the behavior of the interviewer. This view lends weight to the notion that the level of social skill employed by facially disadvantaged people during social interaction could have important effects on the reactions of others.

But what about the potential of SST techniques for those disadvantaged by their appearance? Snyder et al. (1977) have illustrated that the way others treat us is in large measure the result of our treatment and expectations of them. Thus it follows that much is to be gained from studying the effects of the facially disadvantaged person's behavior and expectations in social interaction. Perhaps the negative feelings that many ugly or disfigured people report concerning their experiences and expectations of interaction may be sufficient to create the kind of self-fulfilling prophecy mooted by Snyder et al.

Intuitively, SST is likely to be useful for those disadvantaged by their appearance. Kalick (1982) reported cosmetic surgery clinic sessions where staff have said they wished a particular patient was more outgoing and expressive, and that the physical defect would be less noticeable if this were the case. Rumsey et al. (1986) reported, in a preliminary study to examine the potential of SST for facially disfigured people, that the use of a high level of social skill by a confederate resulted in favorable impressions and behavior from subjects, whether the confederate appeared to be facially disfigured or nondisfigured.

Kapp-Simon (1980) provided a note of caution concerning the carrying out of plastic surgery without attendant attention to social skill. She reported the case of an 18-year-old who was changed from an ugly outcast into an attractive and socially desirable woman. She did not, however, possess the social skills to enable her to cope with her new status. She felt uncomfortable with (although flattered by) male attention. She married someone she had only dated a few times—unfortunately her husband turned out to be a transvestite. Kapp-Simon cautions that patients who have lived for many years with their deformity may need help following surgery in adjusting to their changed status in society. With such help, a positively modified self-perception can result in a more assertive and more adaptive self-presentation. This in turn leads to experimentation with new social skills, and a more confident self-projection. Thus the social responses received from the environment may be reordered, and adaptive social development may be reinforced. Underlying the assumption that SST has potential for those disadvantaged by their appearance is the notion that there is a link between physical appearance and social skill.

Is There a Link Between Facial Appearance and Social Skill?

Several researchers have recently addressed this issue. Although the evidence is limited that facially disadvantaged people are to some extent lacking in social skill (see below), more researchers have tackled the other side of the coin—the question of whether there is a link between facial attractiveness and social skill. The findings of these researchers are difficult to draw together coherently, because the multifaceted nature of social skill has meant that different researchers have concentrated on different aspects of behavior, and have used different units of analysis. In some cases, considerations of experimental control have led to the usage of highly contrived interaction situations, many of which have limited generalizability to the wider setting of everyday social interaction. However, despite the methodological problems, the literature is still worth reviewing, because a greater understanding of the effects of physical appearance and social skill in interaction can only be beneficial to those whose facial appearance handicaps them in social encounters.

A major component of the physical attractiveness stereotype of "What is beautiful is good" (Dion et al., 1972) is the belief that attractive people are, in fact, more socially skilled. Adams (1977b), for example, proposed that attractive people receive more favorable expectations from others in interaction. It therefore follows that they may enjoy better social exchanges, develop more favorable self-images, and come to manifest more confident interpersonal behavior patterns in subsequent interaction.

Reis, Nezlek, and Wheeler (1980) examined the link between physical appearance and social skill by asking undergraduates to complete a social interaction diary. They found that attractive males interacted more often and for longer periods of time with a greater number of different females than did unattractive males. (Attractive males also interacted less often with fewer male friends.) Attractive males felt a greater percentage of their interactions with females were mutually initiated, rather than self- or other-initiated (Reis et al. took this to imply greater self-confidence). For female subjects attractiveness did not relate to the quantitative aspects of social participation. In terms of quality, however, attractiveness correlated positively with both reported intimacy and satisfaction for both sexes. In addition, this correlation increased in strength over time.

Reis et al. (1982) tried to eliminate the artifacts that had occurred in Reis et al.'s (1980) study in an examination of how attractiveness relates to social participation. They asked the question, "Do beauties have more social interaction than other people because they are aesthetically pleasing, or is it because they are more socially skilled?" They reported that physical attractiveness influenced the social experience of both sexes in their sample of college students. Physical attractiveness appeared to be related positively to the amount of intimacy and self-disclosure in interactions. In addition, physically attractive males were more assertive and lower in fear of rejection by females than were unattractive males. Attractive females, on the other hand, were less assertive and lower in trust of the opposite sex than their unattractive counterparts. In fact, the authors found a certain skills deficit in attractive women. However, they argue that despite this deficit, other people expect them to be more socially adept, creating a generally enjoyable experience for them both. They noted that Berscheid (1980) found less satisfaction among college beauties in later life, and speculated that maybe after having learned to enjoy a kind of socializing that has been enhanced in a large part by the reactions of others to one's appearance rather than to one's social competence, a deficiency in social skill endures that becomes consequential once beauty fades, and other people no longer provide the spark to social interaction.

Edgemon and Clopton (1978) looked at the relationship between physical attractiveness, physical effectiveness, and self-concept. They found that for males, ratings of physical attractiveness and physical effectiveness were minimally related to each other, and that these two dimensions were not related to subjects' self-concepts. For females, however, the correlations between the measures were very high, indicating strong relationships between the three factors.

Larrance and Zuckerman (1981) examined the relationship between attractiveness and one component of social skills, the ability to accurately send facial expressions of emotion, which they judged from male and female undergraduates' expertise at sending nonverbal facial cues of emotion. Judges rated facial and vocal qualities from videotape and audiotape recordings. They found that facial attractiveness and vocal likeability were related to an increased accuracy in the sending of facial and vocal cues of pleasant (but not unpleasant) emotions. They speculated that attractive people may find their faces to be the focus of attention and may consequently make a special effort to use them more effectively in communication. They acknowledged that the elucidation of the origin of the association between attractiveness and sending ability is still required, and noted that attractiveness may serve as both cause and effect, with attractive people learning to use their physical appeal, and such usage in turn further enhancing their attractiveness. There is evidence that physically attractive people may be more aware of the way they appear to others than unattractive people. Lipson, Przybyla, and Byrne (1983) measured the amount of time students spent looking at themselves as they walked beside a long wall of reflecting glass that acted like a mirror. They found (as did McDonald and Eilenfield, 1980) a significant positive correlation between the time subjects spent looking at themselves and their physical attractiveness.

Kupke, Hobbs, and Cheney (1979), using psychology undergraduates as subjects, found that physical attractiveness and the amount of personal attention paid by males to females significantly predicted female attraction for males (using psychology undergraduates as subjects). The results of this study, and of a subsequent study by Kupke, Calhoun, and Hobbs (1979) suggested that males may directly influence their heterosexual desirability in initial interactions by engaging in this type of conversational behavior.

Fugita, Agle, Newman, and Walfish (1977) used a technique whereby a confederate pushed a concealed button each time she was engaged in direct eye contact by male subjects. The results indicated that subjects looked more at attractive confederates than at unattractive ones and also that high-self-concept males looked more than low-self-concept males (at both the attractive and unattractive female confederates). It would seem that males with high self-concepts are more adept at using powerful eye contact cues than are low-self-concept males. However, it should be noted that one methodological problem associated with this study is the difficulty of assessing the level of eye contact associated with a high level of social skill. (Perhaps, for example, some of the high-self-concept males were gazing too much—thus making the cointeractant feel uncomfortable).

Chaiken (1979) reported a study in which psychology undergraduates were trained to deliver a persuasive message. They were then videotaped, and rated for physical attractiveness, vocal confidence, direct gaze, speech rate, and smiling. It was found that physically attractive communicators elicited greater agreement from targets than did unattractive communicators (although there was no difference in the number of people agreeing to be interviewed). The attractive communicators were perceived as somewhat friendlier than the unattractive communicators. The former were also significantly more fluent speakers, and had marginally faster rates of speech, although there was no difference in ratings of vocal confidence, gaze, or smiling behaviors. Attractive communicators also described themselves more favorably on several dimensions than unattractive communicators (e.g., persuasiveness, attractiveness, interestingness, and optimism about getting a good job).

Dion and Stein (1978) used 10- to 12-year-old children subjects. They were designated attractive or unattractive by peer consensus (although these ratings may have been contaminated by the influence of the children's preexisting levels of social skills). Two independent judges then rated the children on perceived forcefulness, persistence, and skill in devising peruasive arguments while engaged in conversation in opposite-sex dyads. They found that attractive and unattractive children employed markedly different interaction styles, in that the attractive children were more successful in influencing a peer's behavior, than were unattractive children.

Kleinke et al. (1975) manipulated attractiveness and gaze. Females previously rated as being high in attractiveness received more consistently favorable ratings (on six bipoplar adjective rating scales) from male undergraduate subjects than females rated as low in attractiveness. If highly attractive females gazed at a low level (10% instead of 90%), it did not make a significant difference to the ratings. If low-attractiveness females gazed at a low level, ratings of them were disproportionately unfavorable.

Steffen and Redden (1977) also used male college students as subjects. The authors used three questionnaires to measure the social competence of subjects. (The Social Avoidance and Distress Scale was used to measure the reported distress experienced by people in a variety of social situation, the Social Behavior Reporting Form (SBRF) measured the frequency of an individual's social behavior in various social setting, and the Peer Rating Inventory, which is similar to the SBRF except that it is completed by a friend, was used to give a peer rating of a subject's behavior in various social situations.)

On the strength of their scores on these three measures, subjects were divided into high-competence and low-competence groups. The men who were designated as high in competence were judged by two independent female raters as being more physically attractive and more socially skilled than low-competence men. Steffen and Redden found that highly competent subjects' response latencies were not as disrupted by negative feedback in a 5-minute opposite-sex dyadic interaction than were the response latencies of low-competence subjects. In addition, high-competence men used a wider range of responses than low-competence men in response to negative feedback. Steffen and Redden made the important methodological point that the unit of analysis when measuring social competence is all too often the response of the subject. The true unit of analysis should be the interaction itself. Feedback is important, and competent subjects are able to receive behavior and to modify their own behavior in response.

Adams and Read (1983) found that high levels of facial attractiveness in undergraduates were associated with more frequent interaction attempts than were medium or low levels of facial attractiveness, and that attractive people were more likely to internalize the view that they are highly socially skilled. However, they reported that more attractive female undergraduates viewed themselves as being less effective at integrating and understanding a broad range of social stimuli, and as having poorer control of interpersonal situations than women of medium or low facial attractiveness. Adams and Read also reported that unattractive female undergraduates were less likely to engage in frequent interaction attempts. In addition, they were likely to use less desirable interaction styles than attractive people, including elements such as demanding, interrupting, and being opinionated, submissive, or antagonistic. They pointed out that many published studies have suggested that positive interaction styles are associated with physical attractiveness, but have failed to document (even if many have implied) that there are correspondingly undesirable interaction characteristics associated with physical unattractiveness.

Young (1979) has illustrated that physically attractive people can in some cases elicit more self-disclosure from other parties in social interaction. The ability to elicit self-disclosure is considered by some researchers as being a positive element of social skill, because self-disclosure (especially of the mutual variety) can lead to an improvement in the quality of social interaction for both parties (see Pelligrini, Hicks, Meyers-Winton, & Antal, 1978). In Young's study, subjects were shown photographs of physicians (a somewhat unrealistic procedure) and were asked to report their willingness to disclose their symptoms and fears concerning (a) private parts of their body (those concerned with elimination or sex), (b) mental illness, and (c) nonprivate parts of the body. Young reported that subjects were more willing to disclose symptoms in all categories to physically attractive than unattractive physicians. Young also noted that subjects had a same-sex preference for the physicians, especially in the disclosure of personal and mental symptoms.

Arkowitz, Lichtenstein, McGovern, and Hines (1975) compared high-frequency-dating males with low-frequency-dating males on a number of behavioral measures of social skill in live interactions with a female confederate. Only one behavioral measure—the number of conversational silences— adequately discriminated between the two groups. They believed, however, that social skill deficits were present, but that the particular behavioral measures employed were not sensitive to the differences. Glasgow and Arkowitz (1975) used a rather artificial "get to know situation" in which opposite-sex dyads engaged in 10 minutes of unstructured conversation that was videotaped. They found female social science students who had a low frequency of dating to be characterized by a social skill deficit. In male students, however, low frequency of dating was related to negative self-evaluations but not to a social skills deficit. The authors postulated that low-frequency-dating men may be reasonably socially skilled, but overly critical of their own performance. Such overly critical self-evaluation might be an important factor in mediating social anxiety and inhibition in men.

Mitchell and Orr (1976) examined the relationship between self-judged physical attractiveness and opposite-sex behavior as part of a large survey of the interaction patterns of 963 college students. The findings suggested that a self-rated negative physical image was related to significantly high levels of heterosexual difficulties. The authors measured (using self-report techniques) subjects' anxiety, avoidance tendencies, and self-perceived and other-perceived social interaction competencies. They found no relationship between subjects' self-judged physical attractiveness and self-perceived social competence in opposite sex interactions. However, subjects who rated themselves as unattractive believed others would rate them as less socially skilled than individuals who perceived themselves as attractive. The self-rated unattractive also reported a significantly higher tendency to avoid opposite-sex situations.

Shea, Crossman, and Adams (1978) pointed out that data that have been provided by self-evaluative measures have lent support to the existence of a relationship between the personality style of attractive individuals, and the impressions formed of them by others. However, using objective measures of 294 undergraduate subjects, they found that attractive and unattractive subjects did not actually differ in their personality styles. They used Maddi's (1968) distinction of the core (enduring, structural) characteristics of personality, and peripheral (self-evaluative more superficial) traits, and suggested that any "attractive = good" stereotype that may exist affects only the peripheral aspects of personality.

Thus it can be seen that the majority of evidence favors the view that physically attractive people exhibit a greater level of social skill in interaction than do physically unattractive people. Much less research has been carried out on whether social skills deficits are common in facially disadvantaged people.

Social skill deficits in facially disadvantaged persons.   Priestley, McGuire, Flegg, Hemsley, and Welham (1978) define social skill as the ability to manage the exchanges and problems of everyday life effectively. Using this definition, many visibly disfigured people may be deficient to some extent in their use of social skills. In the field of mental health, Condon (1966, reported in N. Bernstein, 1976), found the body motion and facial patterns of individuals who are emotionally disturbed to lack the variability and rhythmic mobility observed in "normal" people. Condon also noted a parallel lack of variability in the speech stream of disturbed subjects, giving a sense of monotony and flatness to the total behavioral presentation.

Rutter and Stephenson (1972) examined the visual interaction of 20 schizophrenic and 20 depressive patients. It was found that both groups spent proportionately less time in looking at the interviewer, and used shorter glances than did subjects in the psychiatrically normal control group. They put forward the idea that the reduced level of looking may be interpreted by others as an inability or unwillingness to interact, and thus may act as a discouragement to others to initiate interaction. Libet and Lewinsohn (1973) compared the social skill level of depressed and nondepressed undergraduates. They found that the group of depressed subjects were less socially skilled than the nondepressed individuals, in that they emitted behavior at a lower rate than subjects in the control group, interacted with fewer "safe" people, and allowed a greater time to elapse between the occurrence of a behavior from another person and taking action themselves. Libet and Lewinsohn concluded that a deficiency in social skills is an important antecedent for depressive behavior.

Argyle, Trower, and Bryant (1974) studied seven patients with personality disorders and neuroses. Having stated that inadequate social behavior has long been regarded by some psychologists and psychiatrists as an important factor in psychiatric disorders, they reported common difficulties in social behavior among their sample. These difficulties included the initiation of conversation; taking an interest in others; the appropriate use of nonverbal signs such as appearance, expression, looking, and gestures; and suitable use of the voice. In a later report (Trower, Bryant, & Argyle, 1978) they noted that behavioral deficits in their sample of socially inadequate patients resulted in them being rated as significantly more cold, nonassertive, socially anxious, sad, unrewarding, and uncontrolling than the socially skilled patients. On sociometric tests, these patients were found to be significantly less dominant, less sociable, and less self-accepting.

Studies in a nonclinical setting.   Studies in the nonclinical field are relatively few and far between. However, there are areas of research that appear to have a direct bearing on the issue of social skill deficits in facially disadvantaged persons. Some researchers have highlighted a link between unattractiveness and social skill deficits. Krebs and Adinolfi (1975), for example, commented that physically unattractive college students tend to be more asocial and socially isolated. D. Jackson and Huston (1975) noted that physically unattractive college students tend to be less interpersonally assertive, Goldman and Lewis (1977) (but not Bull and Stevens, 1981) that they tend to be less socially skillful in initial peer encounters, and Cash and Soloway (1975) that they are less self-disclosing.

Observations reported in Rumsey (1983) suggest that facially disfigured people in various settings appear to others to be withdrawn and depressed. Many disfigured people tend to exhibit lower levels of eye contact, use a more monotonous tone of voice, and initiate conversation less often than do non-disfigured people, leading to social behavior that seems to reflect shyness, defensiveness, and depression. Rumsey (1983) noted that for facially disfigured people, the level of social skill a person possesses may often be more predictive of success in social situations than the presence or absence of a facial disfigurement.

Kleck and Strenta (1980) carried out a laboratory study that supports the observations reported in Rumsey (1983). They led subjects to believe they were to interact while "wearing" a facial scar—(these were applied through the use of makeup). Kleck and Strenta reported that those subjects who thought they had a facial scar (whether or not in fact they did have one) were more likely to focus on the gaze behavior of other nondisfigured interactants, and to believe that this gaze behavior reflected their physical "defect." (For more detail of this experiment see above.) This preoccupation with appearance was also noted in the confederates used in Rumsey's studies. Her confederates reported experiencing a wide range of emotions while "disfigured," including shyness and a preoccupation with the effect that their appearance was having on others. Many reported that they felt they would prefer to avoid interaction whenever possible, because they were wary of possible negative reactions to their appearance from others.

Social skill deficits in shy and lonely people. The problems disfigured and handicapped people encounter in social interaction can be considered to be somewhat akin to those encountered by shy people. Zimbardo (1981) believes that shyness is not often caused simply by a lack of self-confidence, or unfounded fears about social situations, but that it may be more a matter of not having or not practicing certain social skills. (This is thought to be particulary applicable to those in the middle range of shyness—they do not have the social skills essential for keeping the machinery of human relationships functioning smoothly.) To be shy is to be "difficult to approach, owing to timidity, caution or distrust." Zimbardo stated that many shy people become caught up in the web of egocentric preoccupations, and stop tuning in to what other people are saying and feeling. They rarely notice the tears and hurts of others, because their own psychological survival becomes an all-consuming obsession. Zimbardo believed that developing specific and successful social skills is an important part of helping people to overcome shyness. Building a positive self-esteem is also important. The way we think about ourselves has profound effects on all aspects of our lives. People with a sense of positive self-worth typically display poise and radiate confidence as outward signs of inner satisfaction.

Some researchers have pointed out that social skills deficits are common in loneliness. Peplau and Perlman (1979), for example, defined lonelines as a social deficiency. Loneliness exists to the extent that a person's network of social relationships is smaller or less satisfying than a person desires (i.e., there is a discrepancy between the desired and achieved levels of social interaction). Thus it can be seen that loneliness may be a state applicable to many unattractive, disfigured, and handicapped people. Characteristics that reduce a person's desirability (such as a visible stigma or unpleasing appearance) may limit the person's opportunities for social relationships.

R. Weiss (1973) and others have suggested that a lack of social skills may be associated with loneliness. However, there are conflicting results here. Indices of social skills are not comprehensive enough since they do not tap the quality of relationships (also shown to be an important factor in loneliness). W. Jones, Hobbs, and Hockenbury (1982) found that lonely people tend to give less attention to their partner. They found that an increased use of partner attention during dyadic interactions resulted in significantly greater desirable changes in scores of loneliness and related variables. Statements in the literature concerning loneliness have recently begun to emphasize the role of deficiencies in social skill, for example, passivity (Brennan, 1982); lack of assertiveness; greater shyness and self-consciousness (Jones et al. 1982); problems of inhibited sociability, for example, difficulty in making friends naturally and with ease (Horowitz & French, 1979); and less self-disclosure (Chelune, Sultan, & Williams, 1980). Many of these studies, however, have been carried out using self-report techniques. This begs the question of whether the reports of social skill problems of lonely people derive from genuinely self-recognized behavior difficulties, or from the general tendency of lonely individuals to rate themselves negatively on various dimensions. (Most of the research is also correlational, not causal.)

Peplau and Perlman (1979) found that in dyadic interactions people scoring high on loneliness scales tend to interact with less awareness of or concern for others, with less responsiveness, and in a more self-focused or self-absorbed manner (this was observed in actual behavior, not through self-report). It was found that they made fewer partner references, continued the topic discussed by partner less, asked fewer questions of the partner, and emitted fewer partner attention statements. In a second study, Peplau and Perlman reported that those scoring high on loneliness scales were given instruction in conversation skills. It was found that increasing the frequency of partner attention statements resulted in significant reductions in self-reported loneliness and related self-perceptions, thus suggesting that loneliness involves behavioral manifestations of deficient social skill, and that such deficits are causally linked to feelings of loneliness. Peplau and Perlman speculated on the mechanism of interactions involving lonely people. They suggested that if a partner receives less attention, then the interaction will be considered less socially rewarding, leading to rejection and disinterest. On the other hand, it may be that lonely people recognize their social skill deficits, and therefore expect to be rejected by others. In a circular manner, less interest and acceptance are shown, and loneliness is experienced as a result. In either case, the probability of friendship formation is reduced—especially friendships of an intimate and lasting nature.

Here, then, is the evidence relating to possible social skills deficits in facially disadvantaged persons. Previous research has also been indicative of several potentially helpful approaches of the social skills approach for those disadvantaged by their appearance.

Potential Applications of SST for Facially Disadvantaged Persons

Gresham (1981) reviewed the use of social skills training (SST) techniques with handicapped children, and concluded that SST represents a potentially effective approach to the successful mainstreaming of handicapped children into a nonhandicapped population. More specifically, Morgan and Leung (1980) examined the effects of assertion training on 14 physically disabled undergraduates' acceptance of disability. Following training sessions they found significant improvements on measures of acceptance of disability, self-concept, and social interaction skills in comparison with subjects in a control group. They concluded that assertion training may be an effective way to increase people's acceptance of disability.

Rusalem (1973) made the point that a general deficiency in social skills can result from the social isolation that often accompanies disability, especially in those with handicaps that limit mobility. Few of the more difficult situations they encounter have been experienced before disability; consequently many do not have the experience or repertoire of behaviors needed to cope adequately with such situations, or with the "stigma" of physical disability. For some, this may lead to a reduction in social participation and an avoidance of the general public. Rusalem believed a multifaceted treatment package to be required, including methods of improving communication with physicians (especially in connection with reducing anxiety from misunderstood comments concerning disorders, medicines, or treatment). Rusalem pointed out that such programs generally have good face validity and often encourage staff acceptance. In addition, social skills programs might be a useful way to establish broader based behavioral intervention programs, especially in areas where psychological input in the rehabilitation of disabled persons has previously been avoided (see above).

Heimberg, Montgomery, Madsen, and Heimberg (1977), A. Rich and Schroeder (1976), and Lange and Jakubowski (1976) have all concluded that treatment procedures that combine behavioral rehearsal (role play), modeling, and coaching (live feedback and instructions) are effective treatments for social skills deficits. However, they also pointed out that these are techniques that are not widely used with handicapped persons, despite evidence that many handicapped people are lacking in social skills.

Dunn, van Horn, and Herman (1981) have examined the use of SST with spinal cord–injured patients. They pointed out that life with a visible handicap requires management of the social consequences of asking for help, refusing help, patronization, the discomfort of acquaintances, the handling of embarrassing situations, and so forth. Their spinal cord–injured patients were given both paper-and-pencil and videotaped measures of performance, and demographic information was noted. Subjects were then divided into four groups. Group one was given social skills training only. Group two was given SST together with a modeling film. The third group was given the film only, and the fourth group was used as a control. All groups were retested 4 weeks after the original completion of the paper-and-pencil tests and the videotaped measures of performance. Dunn et al. found no differences between the subjects on the subjective measures. Subjects in groups one and two, however, showed greater before/after differences on the behavioral measures than groups three and four. Subjects who were exposed to video feedback, modeling, and instructions also made significant gains in their performance in the sorts of situations that severely handicapped individuals must face on reentry to society. Dunn et al. concluded that SST is a relevant procedure for male spinal cord–injured subjects (but noted that no long-term follow-up was carried out).

SST and the treatment of shyness and loneliness.   Some successes have also been reported with the use of SST in the treatment of shyness (an affliction that may affect many facially disadvantaged people). Zimbardo (1981), for example, incorporated SST techniques into his suggestions for helping shy people. He commented that "caught up in a web of egocentric preoccupations, they stop tuning in to what other people are saying and feeling. They rarely notice the fears and hurts of others because their own psychological survival is an all-consuming obsession." Zimbardo believed that four basic changes are called for: first, in the way shy people think about themselves and about shyness (they need to understand themselves and their shyness better, and they need to build their self-esteem); second, in the way shy people behave (they need to develop specific and successful social skills); third, in relevant aspects of the way in which other people think and act (they need to help people who are shy); and fourth, in certain social values that promote shyness (we need to learn ways to alter our shyness-generating society).

Pilkonis, Heape, and Klein (1980) also thought SST techniques to be useful in treating shyness. They believed SST can be effectively used on both an individual and a group basis—group therapy can provide a good opportunity for interpersonal learning and feedback from a variety of other persons. Techniques such as discussion, role-playing with interpersonal and video feedback, monitoring of activities outside the group, and the setting of tasks between sessions were suggested. Topics such as the development of conversational skills, strategies for establishing new relationships, difficulties in interacting with authority figures, problems in intimate relationships, and the management of loss or rejection are mentioned. They recommended a "problem solving" approach to interpersonal difficulties where participants are encouraged to define difficulties as specifically as possible, to generate a range of possible solutions, to anticipate the consequences of each alternative, and to decide on the best approach to overcoming the problem. Pilkonis, Lewis, Calpin, Senatore, and Hersen (1980) believe that by using SST techniques it is possible to influence quite complex social behaviors, providing the patients are not grossly deficient in social skills. (It should be noted, however, that these recommendations resulted from the reporting of a one-patient sample.)

Peplau and Perlman (1979) have reported findings concerning one aspect of social skill as a modulator of loneliness—the perceived level of control over the amount of social contact in which a person engages. They quoted Schulz (1976), who had groups of undergraduates visit elderly people over a 2-month period. It was found that patients who could choose and predict the times of visits reported less loneliness than those whose visitors just dropped in, even though the amount of time involved was the same. Peplau and Perlman suggested the fostering of three coping mechanisms for loneliness: first, the use of strategies to alter the desired level of social contact; second, strategies to alter the achieved level of social contact; and third, ways of altering the perceived gap between the desired and achieved levels of social contact.

SST and facially disfigured persons.   Rumsey's results (Rumsey, 1983; Rumsey et al., 1986), which are discussed in more detail above, indicated that SST techniques may be a promising application to facially disfigured people who are experiencing problems in social interaction. She pointed out, however, that SST techniques need to be used with great care, because many individual differences exist both in the types of deficits in skill, and in the types of problems encountered by disfigured persons. In addition, many disfigured people are highly sensitive to anything involving their appearance. Nevertheless, many might wish to learn how to behave in a more natural manner, to avoid being apologetic and to cease hiding from others. Any investment in video equipment that can be made by those assisting in rehabilitation or training efforts would seem worthwhile. Video enables disfigured people directly to observe their behavior from the perspective of other people. Thus they can be helped to examine the effect their behavior has on other people, and with increased understanding can perhaps reduce the resentment felt as a result of their negative interpretation of the reactions of others. Video recordings of SST techniques also have useful applications. Dunn (1982) has compiled a video recording of the application of social skills techniques to the sorts of social problems commonly encountered by spinal cord–injury patients. Similar videos could be compiled for use by groups or individuals in both in- and outpatient settings, and at worst could provide some initiative for discussion and practice of social skills techniques relevant to improving the quality of social interaction for those disadvantaged by their appearance.

Although public education regarding problems encountered by disfigured persons is desirable, it is unlikely to provide any answers for them in the short term. It would therefore be beneficial for many facially disfigured people if they could be helped toward an acceptance of their appearance, and if they could be helped to learn strategies to cope with it.

A note of caution about SST. SST would seem to provide considerable potential as a technique for alleviating problems experienced by facially disadvantaged persons in social interaction, and as a means of offering direct practical help to such people. However, there are a few cautionary points to be borne in mind when considering the use of the approach. Wilkinson and Canter (1982) noted that SST has developed very rapidly in the past few years, and its progress has been somewhat marred by overenthusiasm. It has becomes a fashionable term used loosely by some to encompass most of human activity. Therefore, a critical approach is needed in the assessment of material purporting to promote the merits of SST.

Rumsey (1983) made the point that people vary widely in their deficits and talents in social behavior. There are wide individual differences among facially disfigured persons in the ability to both encode and decode social information. Individual programs tailor-made to requirements are desirable for the majority of those desiring help with social interaction problems. Yardley (1979) also noted that the skill of the individual therapists is all-important in SST, and that trainers should be carefully chosen. There is perhaps a danger that because SST handbooks are proliferating, many would-be helpers may try their hand at SST, with insufficient knowledge of the workings of social behavior at their disposal.

Marzillier (1978) noted that it is only recently that social skills training methods for treating social problems have developed to any degree. To date, many of the studies that have examined the effectiveness of SST have been carried out in the sphere of mental health. In addition, many studies have been beset by design difficulties and methodological problems—for example, lack of control groups, the relative skills of individual therapists, placebo effects, the length of treatment time, and a lack of adequate follow-up. Dunn et al. (1981) pointed out that as yet there is no single measure of social skillfulness; thus multiple measures must be used, complicating the issue still further.

Future research will also have to tackle the mammoth task of unraveling the relative importance of the various components of nonverbal behavior. As Reece and Whitman (1962) pointed out, many components are involved in an individual being perceived as a "warm" person (shifts in posture toward the other interactant, smiling, verbal reinforcers, direct eye contact, etc.) or a "cold" person (inappropriate eye contact, slumped posture, lack of smiling, fidgeting, etc.). It will be difficult to fully examine the effectiveness of social skills training until a substantial body of research has been carried out. Marzillier (1978) stressed the desirability of carrying out further research into SST, and has suggested two ways in which the efficacy of treatment can be investigated systematically. First, there are the effects of SST on a single person. The advantage of such an approach is that the programs are individually tailored to tackle specific deficits. Although in an experimental setting it might be shown that certain behaviors are more likely to achieve a certain goal, a competent response is something that is appropriate for an individual in a particular situation. SST misapplied (or too generally applied) could have the effect of coercing the individual into adopting unsuitable rigid, stereotyped behavior patterns. Working on an individual basis, it should be possible to increase a person's behavioral repertoire so that the person is free to choose from a variety of behaviors. However, the results of unsuccessful case studies are rarely reported, and in any case conclusions drawn from case studies using one person have limited generalizability. Rumsey (1983) elaborated this point in her comments concerning the potential benefits of individual SST programs for disfigured people (see above). However, although individual programs are desire for the majority of such people, they are less beneficial in terms of assessing the general effectiveness of SST techniques.

Second, Marzillier noted that it is possible to examine the effectiveness of SST techniques using experimental and control groups. The advantages here are that generalizations are more valid, and that a consideration of the effects of particular SST techniques on several people would reduce potential contamination from placebo effects. On the other hand, group approaches to SST are insensitive to individual needs, and the averaging of results across the group might camouflage the fact that some patients did not improve, and may even have become worse.

Despite the relative lack of outcome research, however, the approach has gained popularity in the last few years, and is being used in such diverse areas as in schools and hospitals, in community work, with student populations, in counseling, and in management training. Reports of this preliminary work are encouraging (see Priestley et al., 1978), and it seems that there may be great potential in the application of SST techniques to those who suffer problems in social interaction as a result of their physical appearance. Dunn (1982) stated that not only is SST an effective approach to social rehabilitation for handicapped patients, but it would also be beneficial for those who are interacting *with* handicapped persons. He made the important point that the social environment of a physically abnormal person is likely to be complex because of the conflicting attitudes and emotions about people with disabilities held by nondisfigured people (see Chapter 7). The ambivalence felt by members of the public can create social discomfort and may lead to a lack of honest feedback for people with disabilities.

This point concerning the role of the social environment, and the beliefs and attitudes of interactants, highlights one of the major drawbacks of the

SST approach. There are some pyschologists who think that SST pays too little attention to the cognitive aspects of social behavior problems. Morrison and Bellack (1981), for example, have highlighted the importance of social perception skill. They believe that in addition to the ability to interpret interpersonal behavioral cues, interactants must also be able to take account of the beliefs and expectations of others in interaction. Participants must learn to read the social environment, and to develop social sensitivity in order to know when particular skills will be effective. Morrison and Bellack thus believe that any behavioral analysis of social interaction that fails to take account of social perception skills is incomplete. Another question that the SST approach leaves unanswered is the extent to which important aspects of the person's behavior are due to deep-seated underlying personality traits that would produce similar behavior regardless of the person's current appearance. Alternatively, are the behavioral deficits directly attributable to the person's physical flaw and the resulting self-perceptions and responses by others (Kalick, 1982)? N. Bernstein (1976) has pointed out that it would be grandiose to assume that simply by giving people instructions as to how to use appropriate eye contact, how to gesture effectively, and the like, one could alter the whole social framework or personality pattern of a disfigured person. On a similar theme, Yardley (1979) advocated a combination of treatment using both verbal insight and more SST-oriented behavioral techniques.

It is to be hoped that the relationship between cognitive elements, personality, and social skills will be illuminated and understood more thoroughly in time. Meanwhile it seems that efforts to increase the self-awareness and self-confidence of those with abnormalities of facial appearance would be well spent.

Conclusion

This chapter presents suggestions as to how psychologists might go beyond description and explanation to provide a relevant and informed contribution to the easing of the problems encountered by facially disadvantaged people. These suggestions include ways of tackling negative attitudes held by the general public and techniques for improving public education concerning facial disfigurement. In addition, methods of offering help directly to facially disadvantaged persons are discussed—for example, through the provision of more effective health care and rehabilitation for those undergoing surgical intervention, through counseling, self-help groups, and/or the use of social skills training techniques. It is hoped that these suggestions may provide an impetus toward the practical help much needed by facially disadvantaged persons.

Chapter 9

Some Final Remarks

In this final chapter we will briefly mention some studies of facial appearance that do not readily fit in with the organization of the previous chapters. We then discuss what is meant (so far as is known) by facial attractiveness. The possible influences of individual perceiver differences and context effects on reactions to faces are mentioned. An overview is then presented of the theoretical explanations that have been put forward to account for some of the findings mentioned in this book. This chapter ends with some further suggestions for future research.

Other Studies Concerning the Social Psychological Aspects of Beauty

In 1978 Adams and Crossman made the point that, "From a scientific perspective little is known about the psychological importance of beauty." We trust that having read this book readers will be aware of research conducted since 1978 (and earlier) that could be deemed to involve scientific study of the social psychology of facial appearance. Indeed, one of the criteria that we adopted to decide which studies to describe and which to ignore or merely cite was their scientific rigor. This led to certain social psychological aspects of facial appearance research being omitted from the main chapters. Many of the omitted studies examined the effects of isolated facial features in rather basic ways.

Studies have examined, often in ecologically invalid circumstances, the effects of eye color, pupil size, glasses, beards, hair, and dental appearance. A brief overview of these studies is presented below. Better research is needed on these topics because they, along with the use of makeup, may be relevant to attempts to help improve the facial appearance of disfigured and unattractive people.

Dental Appearance

W. Shaw (1981a) examined the effect on perceivers' ratings of varying children's dental appearance (by using a photographic superimposition procedure). He pointed out that, "A review of the literature regarding the social implications of dentofacial anomalies reveals a paucity of systematic research." Shaw found, as did Sergl and Stodt (1970), that the variations in dentofacial appearance (i.e., normal, or prominent, or crowded, or missing incisors, or hare lip) had significant effects. However, Shaw also wisely varied background facial attractiveness, and he found this to have a stronger effect on ratings (as did W. Shaw and Humphreys [1982], and also W. Shaw, Rees, Dawe, and Charles [1985], who noted that their attractive female stimuli were rated as *less* friendly, kind, and honest). W. Shaw (1981a) made the valid point concerning research on dental appearance that, "It is, of course, imperative that investigations based on photographs be complemented by naturalistic studies." Unfortunately, extremely few such studies have been conducted (Bull and Stevens' [1980] study, described in Chapter 7, was a rather basic attempt at such a study). Shaw concluded that, "While awaiting the outcome of further research in real life settings where true interaction has taken place, it seems reasonable to anticipate that dentofacial anomalies of sufficient severity to mar a child's facial attractiveness may represent an important social disadvantage. Although the magnitude of this handicap is difficult to define in precise terms, the available evidence indicates that parental concern and desire to have such anomalies corrected in their children is well placed."

Ten years earlier M. Burns (1972) similarly held the view that normalization of dental appearance can be justified on psychological grounds, even though he also noted that there was a "relatively sparse amount of research on the subject found in the literature." He argued that, "Malocclusion, being an easily recognized physical defect, constitutes a major cause of abuse and may lead to humiliation in the overly sensitive individual. . . . As a result the target of the abuse may withdraw from his peers. Frequently, he may smile with his mouth covered by his hand, smile with his lips together, or not smile at all." Unfortunately, no evidence was cited to support the last sentence. Burns also stated that the primary psychological impact of malocclusion does not result from the response of others but from the individual's own reaction. Although, again, the evidence for this is far from strong, if it is a significant aspect then the rapid psychological benefit that Burns argued results from orthodontic improvement in appearance could occur.

However, such rapid changes in self-image (as well as any changes brought about by now being treated differently by society) must depend on the extent to which individuals feel a need for their dental appearance to be improved. Research has shown not only that many children and adolescents with "good occlusions" report dissatisfaction with their dental appearance, and vice versa (Lewit & Virolainen, 1968; W. Shaw, 1981b), but also that parents rather than children desire improvements in youngsters' dental appearance (Baldwin & Barnes, 1966), and that adults and orthodontists by no means share views about which aspects of dental appearance merit improvement (W. Shaw, Lewis, & Robertson, 1975).

These problems notwithstanding, Jenny (1975) suggested that, "If children's teeth do not naturally meet the norm for aesthetic dental appearance, the response of families to sociocultural expectations and pressures produces a culturally valid need for orthodontic intervention." She argued that treatment of severe malocclusion "can produce psychological rehabilitation of an individual whose dentofacial handicap might otherwise lead to a life of antisocial behaviour." However, no real evidence was supplied by Jenny to support this contention, and the research described in previous chapters in this book is not strong in suggesting that facial appearance has a definite, more powerful effect for antisocial behavior than other ecologically valid factors.

In fact, even though studies (e.g., Linn, 1966) have found people to rate dental appearance as likely to be very important in many real-life situations, only a few have examined whether this is indeed the case. Rutzen (1973) interviewed 252 people 5 years after their orthodontic treatment had been completed, and their data were compared with that of an untreated malocclusion control group. Small and "barely statistically significant" differences (most $p < .05$, one-tail) were found in occupational rank but not in educational level, in whether married/engaged but not in whether "going steady" or dating, in self-assessment of personal appearance but not in questionnaire self-esteem, and in anxiety but not in neuroticism or extraversion. He concluded that "the low level of differences may be due to the infrequent use of malocclusion as a basis for social discrimination," and/or that the untreated group somehow, via "compensation," came not to differ greatly from the treated group. Similarly, Helm, Kreiborg, and Solow (1985) found in adults who all had malocclusions at age 15 years that those who subsequently received orthodontic treatment did not have higher occupational status at age 30. The treated group did express greater satisfaction with their dental appearance, and they recalled experiencing significantly less teasing from schoolmates (presumably posttreatment, although this is by no means clear from Helm et al.'s paper).

In 1981 Korabik stated that although many health professionals had noted improvements in dental appearance to have positive psychological implications, "this evidence is anecdotal, and controlled research is needed to confirm the premises." She asked undergraduates to rate for "intelligence, morality, adjustment and personal feelings" photographs of adolescent girls' faces (with mouths closed) taken before and after orthodontic treatment. The ratings were summed per photograph to form an "interpersonal attraction" index, and it was found that the post-orthodontic treatment summated scores differed from the pretreatment scores and from those for the control group. Korabik claimed that "the results of this study verify the claim that orthodontic treatment can have psychological as well as physical benefits for those who receive it." However, we consider this claim to be going beyond Korabik's evidence. She showed merely that orthodontic treatment affected ratings in an ecologically weak situation. As previous chapters in this book attest, it by no means follows that such ratings would affect behavior in real-life settings. Also, Korabik varied no other factors against which the power of the orthodontic treatment could be pitted. Variations in other aspects of facial appearance could have stronger effects than orthodontic manipulation. Secord and Backman (1959) also found orthodontic appearance to influence personality ratings, but they noted this to be a far less memorable aspect of facial appearance than most other aspects, especially the eyes.

Before we move on to studies that have examined effects of variations in the appearance of the eyes we should note that knowledge concerning the social psychology of dental appearance has increased little since 1970 when Stricker stated that

> The literature concerning psychological aspects of dental malocclusion is replete with theoretical speculation much of it psychoanalytic in origin and much of it unsubstantiated by research data, whatever its inherent merits may be. Case studies are present in profusion, almost always demonstrating striking changes in self-concept, emotional health, and level of social adjustment of the patient following orthodontic correction of a malocclusion. Needless to say, these are carefully selected cases and yield little information about the extent to which the phenomena being described are widespread and generalizable. Solid research data, based on sound experimental design, are rare, and programmatic research, in which one investigator addresses himself to a particular research area over a number of years and allows the results of early studies to shape the design of later ones, is almost unknown.

Ocular Appearance

Pupil size.   More research has been published on the social psychology or ocular appearance than of dental appearance. In response to Striker's final sentence (above) it can be said that one researcher (i.e., Hicks) has regularly published research concerning the appearance of the eyes. However, this research has rarely, if ever, had high ecological validity.

Hicks has shown to subjects "retouched" photographs of faces with various pupil sizes, as did Hess (1975), who found that subjects who saw the face of a woman with apparently large pupils rated her as having more positive attributes than did those who saw the same woman with small pupils. Hicks has repeatedly noted results that do not fit in with Hess' notion (and the belief of users of belladonna) that increased pupil size should occasion more positive ratings. He has observed an inverted U-shape relationship between pupil size and positive ratings for opposite-sex faces (Tomlinson, Hicks, & Pellegrini, 1978), and an inverse relationship between pupil size and positive ratings for same-sex judgments (Hicks, Reaney, & Hill, 1967), which Hess (1975) noted. Furthermore, Hicks has found data to support the notion that the effect of pupil size depends upon the "background" attractiveness of the face

(Hicks, Pelligrini, & Tomlinson, 1978). (Note Shaw's finding on dental appearance and "background" facial attractiveness mentioned previously.) Thus when other aspects of facial appearance are varied, pupil size may not be among the most powerful factors. Kirkland and Smith (1978) varied not only apparent pupil size but also pupil highlighting ("the small patches of reflected light") in one infant's facial photographs. They found female shoppers, when asked which photograph of the infant "makes the baby look more attractive," not to select the one with dilated pupils but to choose the one with highlighted pupils (whether they were large or small in size).

Some support for Hess' notion about the effects of pupil size was, however, found by Bull and Shead (1979), whose only facial variable was pupil size. They noted Stass and Willis' (1967) finding that enlargement of pupils of a person of the opposite sex increases that person's attractiveness. (That is, subjects were introduced to two people of the opposite sex, one of whom had, via drug manipulation, enlarged pupils. These subjects were asked to select one of the two persons to be their partner in an experiment. Both adult male and female subjects more frequently chose the person with the larger pupils and none mentioned pupil size as a reason for their choice.) Bull and Shead found males over 16 years of age to rate as more "good-looking" photographs of females with apparently large pupils. They found that 10-year-old boys rated as more good looking the female faces with small pupils, as did the 16- and 20-year-old women. The finding for the 10-year-old boys fits in with McLean's (1974) finding that children under 14 years of age did not assume larger pupils to indicate greater happiness, whereas those over 14 years did so. Bull and Shead found no effects of males' pupil size. They concluded that, "Many *post hoc* explanations might be offered for the reactions of men to females' pupil dilation. It seems that children have larger absolute pupil sizes than do adults. If this is so, then men might perceive women with larger pupils as younger. Also, of course, a man might be chauvinistic enough to take pupil dilation in a woman to be indicative that she has some interest in him. Why women seem to react as they do to other women's pupil enlargement remains to be explained, though Simms (1967) found male homosexuals to have preference for women when they had smaller pupils."

Hess (1975) also reported, as did Hicks, Williams, and Ferrante (1979a), that when asked to "draw in the size of pupils" in a smiling or scowling face, college students drew larger pupils on the smiling face. However, children below age 15 years did not do so. Tarrahian and Hicks (1979) also found American children aged below 11 years not to draw larger pupils on a happy face. However, "children reared in the Persian culture . . . that can be described as 'pupil-intensive'" did so from age 8 years. (Chapter 6 examined other research on the developmental aspects of reactions to facial appearance.)

Although the present book has purposely not focused on the effects of facial expression, it should be stated here that any effects of increased pupil size may well also depend on the overall facial expression. P. Bull (1983) suggests that Hess was wrong in believing that pupil dilation indicates positive affect, and that such dilation could be better understood merely as an index of arousal (see also Hicks, Evans, Martin, and Moore, 1978), the concomitant facial expression indicating positive or negative affect.

Hess (1975) reported that when men saw a picture of a woman with large pupils their own pupils dilated, as did those of women in response to men. He did note, however, that such dilation to faces with large pupils did not happen in same-sex pairings. Q. Jones and Moyel (1971) found apparent pupil size not to influence how friendly males thought photographed people would be. However, they did find iris color to have an effect, and it is to studies of this factor that we now turn.

Iris color. Jones and Moyel's subjects indicated that they considered more friendly the faces that had light rather than dark irises (as shown in black-and-white photographs). A possible explanation of this finding could be Worthy's (1974) hypothesis that there is a relationship between people's iris color and their sociability. However, this hypothesis is in the opposite direction to Jones and Moyel's finding. Other research that has examined Worthy's hypothesis has been conducted by McLean (cited in Hess 1975), T. Robinson (1981), Markle, Rinn, and Bell (1984), Hicks, McNicholas, and Armogida (1981), Hicks, Williams, and Ferrante (1979b), and Williams and Hicks (1980), and strong support for the hypothesis has not been found.

Feinman and Gill (1978) found females to prefer men with dark-colored eyes and males to prefer women with light-colored eyes. Even so, at present there is little research upon which to base recent media debate that via the use of colored contact lenses one could enhance one's appearance. However, there has been a little more research on the social effects of another form of vision correction, that of spectacles.

Spectacles. Terry and Zimmerman (1970) argued that, "It is generally assumed that social rejection is anxiety inducing, and, thus, a spectacle image, itself, which connotes social rejections, should be anxiety inducing. We reasoned that wearing spectacles leads to the formation of a negative, spectacle image, which is anxiety inducing, and that contact lenses contribute to a reduction of anxiety." They found that contact lens wearers felt anxious when asked to wear spectacles (without lenses) in an interview role play. Even though their study has its limitations, Terry and Zimmerman were wise enough to realize that, "The present investigation does not shed light on the dynamics of the underlying assumption" that the wearing of glasses "leads to a negative self concept." (Terry and Brady [1976] found females who usually wore glasses to rate themselves as less physically attractive, particularly their eyes.) Terry and Zimmerman wondered whether self-knowledge of the glasses was sufficient to cause this assumed effect, or whether there must "be a perception that other persons are also aware." What does research tell us about the social psychology of spectacles?

Terry himself sought to answer this question. He and Kroger (1976) found subjects to rate people as less attractive when they wore glasses. However, they did not cite the work of G. Thornton (1943, 1944), who found positive social effects of glasses in that people photographed wearing glasses were rated as higher in honesty, dependability, industriousness, and intelligence than when the same persons were photographed without glasses, nor that of Manz and Lueck (1968), who found similar effects in Germany.

From his overview of work on this topic Terry (1982) concluded that "the presence of eyeglasses is associated with positive evaluations of task-relevant characteristics and negative evaluations of social characteristics." We believe, however, that better quality research is necessary concerning the social psychology of spectacles before such a conclusion can be made.

Argyle and McHenry (1971) showed that the initial effects of glasses (which in their study were positive) on the reactions of others can be readily eliminated as other information about the wearer becomes available. Although we have repeatedly made a similar point concerning the effects of facial appearance, we should not ignore (especially in the light of our chapter on facial disfigurement) Terry's (1982) suggestion that the wearing of spectacles may to some extent prevent others from troubling to realize what, in fact, lies behind them. Kellerman and Laird (1982) made the related point that any effects of glasses may be dependent upon individual differences. Certainly the literature on ocular appearance does suggest that other factors interact with this variable. Therefore, any advice concerning the social psychological effects of ocular appearance would seem premature. But what of other aspects of facial appearance that individuals to some degree are able to vary? Most men can choose whether or not to have a beard, and in many societies women's use of makeup is common. Both sexes can exert choice concerning hair length and color. We will now examine what research there is on these topics.

Beards

Little social psychological research has been conducted on this topic, and what there is seems rather basic. In 1969 Freedman reported that female students rated a bearded male face as more masculine, mature, independent, and sophisticated than a nonbearded face. Similarly, both Roll and Verinis (1971) and Kenny and Fletcher (1973) found students to rate a bearded face as more masculine, strong, and sincere, but also more dirty (versus clean). Pancer and Meindl (1978) found beardedness to lead to more positive ratings. However, Feinman and Gill (1977) found their female students to like least a man with a beard. They put this finding down to the possibility that their Wyoming students were more conservative than the Chicago, Midwestern, Memphis, and Canadian students of the above four studies. Whether this be true or not, it again points to the need for studies of the social psychology of facial appearance to vary factors in addition to single aspects of the face. A similar conclusion applies to studies of hair color and length.

Hair Color and Length

The previous study of beardedness by Roll and Verinis (1971) also examined effects of hair color. They found male and female Midwestern students to rate male blond hair as "valued," black hair as potent, and red hair
as least valued, potent, and active. Lawson (1971), however, found male and
female New York students to rate more positively dark hair than blond hair,
although again it was red hair that was least positively evaluated. Lawson also
examined the effects on their ratings of the raters' own hair color and he
found this to have an interactive effect in that subjects rated more positively
hair of their own color. Thus, Lawson's main effects were largely the result of
their being more dark-haired subjects in his sample than blonds or redheads.
    Feinman and Gill (1978) claimed to have found a "tremendous aversion to
redheads." However, since they failed, unlike Lawson, to take into account
the subjects' own hair color, no gross generalization of this finding can be
made, save to nonredheads, perhaps. Feinman and Gill did, however, note
the effect of sex of subject and they found that whereas females indicated that
they liked males with dark hair, males showed (just) a preference for females
with blond hair. In their study of male hair length K. Peterson and Curran
(1976) did bother to take into account female students' own hair style.
Overall, short-haired males were evaluated more favorably and "as resem-
bling more the male stereotype" than were long-haired males, especially by
females who described themselves as more conservative. The females whose
personality, sexual experience, and background suggested that they were
more liberal showed some preference for long-haired males. Peterson and
Curran concluded that, "Preference for another individual is a function not
only of the characteristics of the person being observed but also to some
extent a function of the characteristics of the observer."
    Pancer and Meindl (1978) failed to note any aspects of their subjects other
than their sex. They found female and male Canadian subjects to rate drawings of long-haired males as less educated, intelligent, and happy, but more
open-minded and younger than short-haired males.
    Whether these finding concerning hair length and color would still hold
today is impossible to say since a variety of factors (e.g., the media—see
Chapter 8) are likely to have an effect. The picture may be rather clearer
concerning the effects of makeup since in Chapters 2, 3, and 4 the reported
effects of facial attractiveness were often achieved for female stimuli by the
use of cosmetics. Studies employing makeup that were not presented in those
chapters are now briefly described.

Makeup Cosmetics

One of the first studies of the effects of lipstick was conducted by McKeachie
in 1952. This study found that male interviewers (students) rated female interviewees when these were wearing lipstick (of which no details were given) as

more talkative, anxious, frivolous, and interested in the opposite sex, and less conscientious. Graham and Jouhar (1980) presented a review of the role of cosmetics as a physical attractiveness variable. They noted that the use of makeup usually occasions ratings of greater facial attractiveness (as they did in 1981; see also Graham 1985), and that this has some of the consequences we have already described in earlier chapters. Graham and Jouhar did not, however, focus on the possible nonpositive effects of facial attractiveness or on the unskilled or inappropriate application of makeup.

Their (1981) finding that with professionally applied facial makeup females were rated as more sociable, interesting, confident, and secure was taken by them to suggest that "make-up enhances evaluation of the more outgoing aspects of personality." This may well be the case, but whether a woman wishes to be rated in this way may affect her makeup usage. L. Miller and Cox (1982) found that whereas women's degree of "public self-consciousness" was related to the extent of their makeup usage (see also Buss, 1985) their "private self-consciousness" was not. Those high in public self-consciousness were more apt to believe that by wearing makeup they could improve their social interactions. Miller and Cox suggested that degree of makeup usage may act as a cue to "a woman's values, sexual desires, availability," and Graham and Jouhar (1981) thought that there may exist a "positive cosmetic stereotype which carries its own concept 'what has been cared for is good.'" Cash and Cash (1982) pointed out that "few systematic studies have examined individual differences in women's use of facial makeup or the possible psychosocial effects of such use." They also found makeup usage to relate somewhat to public self-consciousness, to less social anxiety, and to a more flawed and personally unacceptable body image. When asked to imagine (!) themselves being in a variety of situations in which cosmetics usage would be a possibility, women who said that they would use makeup rated themselves as likely to be more self-confident in that situation, and less likely to avoid such a situation.

Cash, Rissi, and Chapman (1985) also examined correlates of makeup usage. They found high-quantity users to be more feminine and more liberal on sex role questionnaires. Cosmetic usage was not related to self-esteem nor to locus of control for affiliative outcomes, although it was to achievement outcomes, with high users being less external in their causal explanations for achievement success. Cash et al. concluded that, "To date, the psychology of physical appearance has largely reflected a 'passive stimulus perspective', as studies often focus on static attractiveness as a fixed, immutable characteristic of a person. A shift in this paradigm is called for in the direction of a dynamic, transactional perspective." With this we would wholeheartedly agree, particularly in the light of Chapters 7 and 8. We can conclude this section on dental and ocular appearance, face and scalp hair, and makeup, by stating that little quality research is available to assist those who wish to change their facial appearance in these ways. This is particularly so since research has also tended to ignore the question of what actually constitutes facial attractiveness.

What Is Facial Attractiveness?

In the previous section of this chapter we briefly mentioned studies concerning the social psychological effects of varying facial appearance by using makeup, and we stated that most of the studies employing this variable as a facial attractiveness factor had been described in previous chapters. Now we will consider what is known concerning the question of what actually constitutes facial attractiveness, whether this be an interfacial or intrafacial variable. This is a particularly important question in the light of the fact that the vast majority of research on the social psychology of facial appearance has used attractiveness as the main independent variable. However, as Patzer (1985) pointed out, "physical attractiveness is essentially not a quantitative trait;" it cannot (as yet, if ever) be measured with any instrument, but is merely assessed by the rankings or ratings people allot to various faces.

Interjudge Agreement

Early studies by Iliffe (1960) in the United Kingdom and by R. Udry (1965) in the United States found that there existed strong interjudge agreement when ranking female faces for how pretty they were. The sex and locality of the several thousand readers who responded to Iliffe's and Udry's requests printed (along with the faces) in national newspapers had minimal effects on the rankings. In the United States respondents' social class had no effect, although in Britain the interjudge agreement was smaller, but still very high, for "lower" class judges than for judges of a "higher" class. Respondent age differences had little effect unless the respondents were aged over 55 years, when they ranked as less pretty than did younger respondents "a very young" woman's face, and ranked as more pretty "a very mature face." Minimal overall differences between the United States and the United Kingdom rankings were found. One can conclude from these studies, and from the many studies of attractiveness mentioned earlier in this book that typically report significant and high interjudge agreement concerning rankings/ratings, that people usually agree on the question of how attractive certain faces are. Patzer (1985) went so far as to state that "people's perception of another person's physical attractiveness can be accurately predicted." He pointed out that, "Even though no objective or absolute answer exists to the question of who is physically attractive, or what determines physical attractiveness, people do agree."

What Determines Facial Attractiveness?

Even though Patzer (1985) stated that "no objective answer exists to the question . . . what determines physical attractiveness," he argued that one criticism that could be directed toward research on attractiveness is its lack of attempts to examine what might constitute facial attractiveness.

Terry and Davis (1976) asked male and female students to rate for attractiveness the faces of five males and five females, in full-face form and in the form of isolated features. Correlations between the rating given to a full face and the ratings given to its isolated parts revealed that mouth, then eyes, then hair, and then nose correlated strongest with full-face attractiveness. This order reflected that found by Terry and Brady (1976) for self-ratings. Terry (1977) found similar relationships when the separate features were rated within the context of the full face. McAfee, Fox, and Hicks (1982) also found mouths to more strongly affect ratings than did eyes.

Lucker and Graber (1980) attempted to determine which aspects of facial appearance contribute most to subjective judgments of normality/abnormality. They pointed out that "while much psychological research has documented the plight of the unattractive, investigators have not been successful in identifying the physiognomic components of attractiveness or even in delineating, a range of 'acceptable' and 'unacceptable' appearances based on facial dimensions. . . . In no case have actual measurements of facial form been related to evaluations of the pictured individuals." Lucker (1981) noted that Cox and van der Linden (1971) (who employed silhouette facial profiles) found faces judged to be unattractive to be "more convex" and to have "greater soft tissue thickness in the lower third of the face," and that Hildebrandt and Fitzgerald (1979) found, using frontal photographs, that infants rated as "cuter" had "short narrow features, large eyes and pupils, and larger foreheads."

Lucker and Graber (1980) commented that in the practices of facial surgery and orthodontics it is common to focus on both frontal and profile representations of the face, whereas almost all psychological research has employed only frontal views. They (as did Lucker, 1981) argued that given recent advances in the techniques of facial surgery, and in the light of research findings concerning the social effects of facial appearance, "it seems imperative to identify those clusters of facial lineaments that people find to be unaesthetic and potentially stigmatizing for the individuals possessing them." In their study children aged between 10 and 13 years were asked to decide whether there was "something wrong/nothing wrong" with the photographed (in black and white) faces of children of a similar age. Both a frontal and a profile view of each face were provided simultaneously. X-rays of the faces taken from both perspectives were available to provide a large number of facial measurements. Correlations between each of these measurements and the observers' judgments were calculated, and it was found that 19 of these were significant for the male faces and 37 for the female faces. These measurements were combined into "general categories dealing with specific regions of the face." For both the male and female faces "one cluster dealt with protrusion of the mandible (lower jaw) and lower teeth relative to the rest of the skull, another with the protrusion of the maxilla (upper jaw) and upper teeth relative to the rest of the skull, and the third with the relative position of the mandible and maxilla and their respective dental structures." An additional two categories were found for the female faces and these were the "size of the upper face, and the width of the face from a front-on-view." Via the use of principal components analysis these variables accounted for 62% of the variance in observers' judgments of the male faces and 75% of that of the female faces. Lucker and Graber concluded that their "results support the contention that . . . society has a clear standard for facial appearance." However, they pointed out that the facial measurements that they found most strongly related to subjective evaluations dealt with "anter-posterior lateral variability," thus "traditional physical attractiveness research has introduced some serious artefacts because of its reliance on frontal photographs." In real life people's faces are mostly seen in three dimensions and we would agree with Lucker and Graber that future psychological research on the social effects of facial appearance should bear this in mind, as should research on facial recognition.

However, Pittenger, Johnson, and Mark (1983) found frontal and profile views of the same photographs of faces to lead to moderately similar ratings of attractiveness. They stated that "while there are plausible reasons to suppose *a priori* that different representations might not be equivalent, no empirical tests appear to have been reported." They asked undergraduates to rate for physical attractiveness the separately presented frontal and profile photographs of a number of children. The correlation between the mean ratings of the front and profile views across stimulus persons was found to be $+.48$ ($p <$ .01). Nevertheless, Pittenger et al. noted that "for many individuals the different representations are far from equivalent." They concluded that "neither front or profile photographs . . . can serve as the basis for a physical metric that fully captures attractiveness. Whether or not use of multiple two-dimensional representations will suffice to solve the problem is unknown. It may be necessary to use three-dimensional, perhaps even dynamic, representations to develop a general, clinically applicable set of measures linking the physical structure of the face with its perceived attractiveness."

Berry and McArthur (1985) attempted to relate subjective judgments of faces to physical measurements of these faces. Yearbook photographs of male students were rated by other students for their attractiveness, for a number of personality traits, and for a number of other factors such as mature face/babyface and close-set eyes/wide-set eyes. Aspects of each face were measured by "projecting each of the faces onto a flat wall surface and measuring 11 characteristics of the face using a ruler." High interrater agreement was found for the trait ratings, for attractiveness, and for "babyfacedness." Babyfacedness was found to correlate significantly with perceptions of warmth, honesty, naivete, and kindness, these correlations being rather stronger than the largely significant correlations of these trait ratings with rated physical attractiveness. Although rated attractiveness and babyfacedness were found to be moderately correlated ($r = .38$, $p < .05$), multiple regression analysis revealed that attractiveness had a rather weaker (and independent) impact on the trait ratings than did babyfacedness. In terms of measurements of the faces, babyfacedness was positively related to having large eyes, round eyes, a narrow chin, and high eyebrows. (Berry and McArthur made no mention of relationships between rated attractiveness and facial measurements.) They concluded that, "The impact of a babyface was independent of the well documented impact of physical attractiveness," and we would urge future research to note this finding.

Berry and McArthur correctly pointed out that most research on the social psychological effects of facial appearance has tended to be atheoretical in nature. (A later section of this chapter will focus on this point.) Their own explanation of the effects they found for babyfacedness concerned the notions that, "The appearance characteristics that seem to elicit protective behaviors and inhibit aggressive ones involve a quality referred to in the literature as 'babyishness,'" and that there may be "overgeneralizations of such impressions to adults who exhibit some of the characteristics of a babyish appearance."

In the same vein, M. Cunningham (1986) found, using micrometer measurements, "the neonate features of large eyes, small nose, and small chin" to correlate positively with the attractiveness ratings that male undergraduates gave to full-face photographs of females (who were Caucasian, or Negro, or Oriental). The attractiveness ratings were also positively correlated with "prominent cheekbones and narrow cheeks," "high eyebrows, large pupils, and large smile." He suggested that one reason for the paucity of research on this topic could be that, "The pseudosciences of phrenology and physiognomy may have made measuring the face seem disreputable to some scientists." In the second part of his study Cunningham found that females whose faces had "neonate, mature and expressive features were seen as being more bright, sociable and assertive . . . but with more vanity and a greater likelihood of having an extramarital affair." (See Chapter 2 for more research on this last point.)

Thus Berry and McArthur (1985) found the babyishness of adult male faces to influence positive reactions to them, and M. Cunningham (1986) found similar effects for adult female faces, although the assumption his subjects made of a relationship between female attractiveness and the likelihood of having an extramarital affair may not necessarily be deemed "positive." (See Gillen [1981] and Tanke [1982] for more on the notion that female facial attractiveness may be related not merely to general goodness—as suggested by Dion et al. [1972]—but also to sexuality.)

Cunningham concluded that his results "demonstrated that beauty is not an inexplicable quality which lies only in the eye of the beholder." However, he did concede that "such results do not preclude some variability in judgments of attractiveness" across subjects. It is to this topic of individual differences between perceivers in their reactions to facial appearance that we shall turn once we have noted Stritch and Secord's (1956) important finding for future research that, "Alteration of a physiognomic attribute in otherwise identical prints of a face will induce perceptions of change in other facial characteristics."

Individual Differences Between Perceivers

In his 1986 paper (mentioned previously) Cunningham also made the point that in their judgments of attractiveness "Females may use slightly different standards than males." Most of the studies cited in this book did not find or report significant sex of subject effects. Morse, Gruzen, and Reis (1976) found "no differences in the way males and females evaluated the attractiveness of stimulus persons." However, they did find that when rating opposite-sex people along a number of personality and "sex appeal" dimensions men stated that they placed more emphasis on facial appearance than did women, who said that they were more affected by men's personal qualities. Lakoff and Scherr (1984) discussed the same point while arguing, as have several studies cited in our previous chapters, that the ways in which female stimuli are evaluated in terms of their facial appearance may differ somewhat from how males are judged. Morse et al. (1976) found few differences in their findings between American and South African subjects, but as Lakoff and Scherr (1984) suggested, cultural factors have rarely been examined in studies of the social psychological effects of facial appearance. Huston and Levinger (1978) correctly made the point that, "Research investigating individual differences in the traits attributed to others based on physical appearance and the value persons place on such traits remains to be done." Fairly recently Rand and Hall (1983) found that females had more accurate self-perceptions than did males of their own level of physical attractiveness, but that this difference was not due to the ratings by others of the males' attractiveness being less consensual than those for the males stimuli. Secord and Muthard (1955) found no overall difference between male and female subjects' reactions to females' photographs, although there were some sex of subject differences for certain photographs. Secord and Muthard found effects of the age of their adult male subjects and they suggested, as do we, that investigation of the effects of perceiver personality characteristics on reactions to faces warrants further study. Indeed, this may be a major weakness in the literature.

Very early on in the history of psychological research on the social effects of facial appearance Fensterheim and Tresselt (1953) suggested that the judgment of people "from their physical appearance would seem to be an area in which the observer makes a great contribution to the percept." However, few studies have found evidence for this and therefore, as argued by Warr and Knapper (1968), person perception may to some degree be a process similar to object perception. Nevertheless, Fensterheim and Tresselt did find some evidence that observers "most liked" the head and shoulders photographs of which "were attributed values that most closely resembled those of the S." This notion that our evaluations of individuals based on their facial appearance may be influenced by the extent to which we find the individuals to be similar to ourselves is deserving of more research.

Lucker (1976) found the attractiveness ratings given to photographs of males and females to be influenced by the subjects' self-ratings of attractiveness. He found that unattractive subjects gave significantly higher target attractiveness ratings than did attractive subjects. Tennis and Dabbs (1975), however, found that unattractive males gave lower attractiveness ratings to targets than did attractive men. Langlois and Downs (1979) noted that children behaved more prosocially when interacting with peers of similar attractiveness to themselves. Paschall (1974) found, even though there was high interrater agreement concerning target attractiveness ($r = .82$), that the higher subjects rated themselves for physical attractiveness the lower the ratings they gave to attractive persons. Interestingly, "raters who were considered by other raters to be of medium attractiveness rated targets higher than did raters who were themselves either high or low in physical attractiveness." (See Patzer [1985] for a wider discussion of the possible effects of research also employing medium, as well as merely high or low, levels of attractiveness.) Thus, effects of stimulus facial attractiveness may be qualified by other attractiveness factors such as the attractiveness of the perceiver.

Another possibly important attractiveness factor ignored by most research on the social psychology of facial appearance is that of context effects. Let us now examine research on this topic.

Context Effects in Reactions to Faces

Other Faces

In Chapter 2 we presented details of research that has found people to evaluate a stimulus person more favorably when this person appears to be married to a facially attractive spouse. In these studies the control condition of an unassociated male and female found no effects on the reactions to one person of the presence of the other. Melamed and Moss (1975) in their unassociated condition found, however, that ratings of female targets' photographs were affected by the female photograph presented alongside. When the accompanying, unassociated female was attractive the targets were rated as less attractive (and vice versa). This contrast effect was also found in their second study, in which some subjects were told that the target female was not associated with the two women whose photographs were presented alongside hers. Other subjects were told that the three women in each photograph were friends. Their ratings of the target women showed not a contrast effect, but an assimilation effect. That is, when targets were associated with attractive females they were rated higher (and vice versa).

Kenrick and Gutierres (1980) noted that contrast effects are a consistently reported finding in studies of perceptual judgments. In their second study they found a contrast effect similar to that observed by Melamed and Moss in their unassociated condition. Presenting a photograph of an attractive female to males just before they rated a female of average attractiveness led to lower ratings than did no such presentation. Kenrick and Gutierres found a similar effect when asking males to rate a photographed target female while they were watching a television program that contained beautiful women, or during a program that did not. In their third study Kenrick and Gutierres again found a contrast effect, and this time a sequential rather than a simultaneous context manipulation was employed. They pointed out, however, that they "have not elucidated the cognitive mediators underlying our obtained effect. . . . it would be of some theoretical interest to investigate the cognitive processes responsible."

Geiselman et al. (1984) did not find an association between the target and the context faces to be important in determining whether a contrast or an assimilation effect was found. Contary to the findings of Melamed and Moss (1975), of Kenrick and Gutierres (1980), and of Kernis and Wheeler (1981), they found assimilation effects in their unassociated condition. Only for successive rather than simultaneous presentation of context was there a hint of a contrast effect. However, Melamed and Moss found contrast effects with both forms of presentation. Thus a clear answer to the question of whether reactions to a face are affected positively or negatively by the context of other (unassociated) faces awaits future research.

Reactions to faces may also be affected by other context effects such as the arousal level of the subjects.

Subject's Arousal

Stephan, Berscheid, and Walster (1971) asked male subjects to read some paragraphs before rating a female based partly on her photograph. Those males who read "an article depicting a romantic seduction scene between two young people" rated the female as more attractive than did those who read "an article depicting the sex life of herring gulls." No effect, however, was found on personality evaluations of her. Stephan et al. suggested that reading the seduction article was sexually arousing and that this arousal caused the heightened attractiveness ratings.

A similar explanation involving arousal was offered by Dutton and Aron (1974), who found that females were rated more positively by subjects who were on a narrow rope bridge over a deep gorge. Carducci, Cozby, and Ward (1978) found some evidence that males' ratings of a female were more positive after reading an article or viewing slides concerning romantic seduction than concerning sticklebacks. However, this effect was modified by whether the target was attractive or unattractive (as deemed by prior determination). Similarly, a study by Pelligrini, Hicks, and Meyers-Winton (1979) found that the attractiveness level of a female target influenced whether or not males' evaluations of her were affected by their success or failure on a task.

Several other studies have manipulated subject's arousal in a rather more direct way. In 1966 Valins led subjects to believe that their heart rate had increased as a result of the presentation of certain ("semi-nude females") slides but had not changed in response to other similar slides. The male students rated as more attractive the slides accompanied by this enhanced feedback. However, higher ratings were also given to slides accompanied by a (false) decrease in heart rate. Although Valins' study may have suffered from a number of methodological weaknesses, somewhat similar effects were found by Kerber and Coles (1978) and by Woll and McFall (1979). Kerber and Coles pointed out that a person's affective state must surely influence their reactions to other people. With this we would agree, and future research should examine the effects of individuals' affective state on their reactions to facial appearance, particularly in the light of Hatfield and Sprecher's (1986) suggestion that the prearousal attractiveness level of a stimulus may determine whether arousal will occasion an increase or decrease in aroused subjects' rating of the stimulus.

Somewhat similar effects to those of Valins (1966) were found by May and Hamilton (1980), who observed that listening to certain types of music increased the attractiveness ratings given to photographed individuals. Hartnett, Gottlieb, and Hayes (1976) found that the arousing presence of an attractive person influenced task performance, as did Donley and Allen (1977).

Although studies of the effects of context and arousal have not produced consistent findings, we believe the notion that context influences the social psychological effects of facial appearance to be one that should be incorporated into any attempt to develop a theory that tries to organize and accommodate the research findings presented in this book. It is to such theories that we now address ourselves.

Theoretical Explanations

While drawing together previous research and ideas about the social psychology of facial appearance, we looked for a theoretical framework (or frameworks) that would account for the research results. However, it soon became apparent that the diverse nature of the research topic makes it, in our view, a worthy illustration of the current controversy over the value of theories in social psychology. Some of those involved in this debate have criticized the labors of others who try to develop rules and predictions for highly complex areas of social behavior (Gergen, 1975). It is thought that a preoccupation with a particular theoretical viewpoint can result in too much effort being expended on experimental manipulations of relatively unimportant variables and too many research findings having only very limited generalizability. This may occur since in the pursuit of evidence for or against a particular viewpoint, it is all too easy to lose the link between the results obtained and their correspondence with everyday behavior outside of the laboratory.

Sorell and Nowak (1981) argued that "due to variations in the theoretical frameworks, research designs, and operational methods employed by physical appearance researchers, many findings lack empirical and interpretive comparability, clarity and continuity. To correct existing difficulties in physical appearance research, and to render future research useful as a basis for understanding the importance and function of appearance variables as developmental phenomena, an integrative conceptual framework is necessary."

Often theory-based research does little more than test the usefulness of a particular theoretical viewpoint. King (1986) recently argued that "the nature of theory in social psychology is such that the same behaviour may be subject to several different interpretations and predictions of future behaviour and may even depend upon the particular theoretical interpretation applied." It is the opinion of some (for example, Elms, 1975; Hebb, 1974; Triandis, 1975) that social psychology has not as yet provided anything like the level of understanding hoped for. Many argue that the roots of social psychology should remain firmly in the study of everyday behavior, and should concentrate on naturally occurring events, rather than becoming lost in the search for ever more sophisticated theories. Indeed, Gergen maintained that principles of social behavior cannot readily be developed, because the facts on which they are based do not remain constant or universal. Social psychologists would perhaps do better to concentrate more on the acquisition of knowledge related to specific issues, with the aim of applying the knowledge to problems of a more practical nature—if necessary, mixing concepts from "different" theoretical approaches.

Sorell and Nowak (1981) pointed out that most of the research literature concerning the social psychology of facial appearance comprises single-shot, isolated studies. They noted that

> Attempts have occasionally been made to interpret results within one or another theoretical framework. For example, Barocas and Karoly (1972) and Elder (1969) adopt an exchange theory perspective in looking respectively at social responsiveness and marriage mobility as related to appearance; Murstein and Christy (1976) interpret the association between appearance and marital adjustment in terms of equity theory; [N.] Cavior and Dokecki (1973) tested the relationship between physical appearance and self-concept from a symbolic interactionism perspective; and Langlois and Stephan (1981) have suggested a social learning [or reinforcement] model as appropriate for understanding the relationship between physical appearance and the development of peer relations in childhood. Nevertheless, the majority of studies are atheoretical. Because the assumptions guiding the conception and design of physical appearance investigations are often unstated, it is difficult to relate such studies to one another and to interpret findings in relation to the overall functioning of appearance variables.

Others, however, express faith in the more traditional approaches to research in social psychology. Schlenker (1974) maintained that theories are useful in providing a framework for the orderly accumulation of knowledge. Wrightsman (1977) noted that theories serve as ways of organizing information, and help us to see whether groups of facts and figures do, or do not, hang together—thus indicating gaps in knowledge, and highlighting implications and relationships that may not have been evident from the raw data alone. Undoubtedly, theories have the important function of stimulating research aimed at clarifying or redefining a particular issue.

It had originally been intended to include a "theoretical" chapter in this book. It was found, however, that although many major theories contained aspects that could account for some of the research findings under review, no one theoretical perspective deserved pride of place. Furthermore, the vast majority of the publications cited in this book made little or no mention of theoretical perspectives. Certainly there was no theory that could in any way provide a comprehensive explanation of the research findings concerned with the effects of facial appearance. Consequently, it was decided that there was little to be gained by presenting a comprehensive theoretical review, thus making the proposed "theoretical" chapter to a large extent redundant. A brief review of those theories considered to have some potential relevance for the research reviewed in the book is presented below.

Cognitive Explanations/Attribution Theory

A cognitive explanation of the research findings mentioned in this book concerns the notion that people do not react to a real or objective environment, but react in terms of their limited perceptions of (a) that environment, and (b) their own reactions based on their perceptions. Clifford and Bull (1978), and Berscheid, Graziano, Monson, and Dermer (1976), among others, have argued that the cognitive operations of the perceiver not only suffer from processing limitations, but they are also inextricably interwoven one with another and with what are sometimes naively taken to be separate social factors.

A. Miller (1982) pointed out that commonly "People are conceived as having limited capacities to process information about the social world. Stereotypes are functional in the sense of reducing the complexity of this world. The phenomena associated with stereotyping are thus attributable to processes that are fundamental to human thought—categorization, concept formation, and judgmental inference, among others." He noted that various definitions have been offered of stereotyping, but that all seem to agree that stereotyping, whether this be probabilistic or absolute in nature, is concerned with acts of social judgment that, whether valid or invalid, are based on some salient feature of an individual, for example, facial appearance.

Attribution theory focuses on the process by which people infer stable, internal characteristics from the overt actions or physical appearance of others. Miller noted that humans are prone to committing the "fundamental attribution error," that is, they perceive the causation of behavior to lie within other individuals, even when such behavior is under situational constraint. Furthermore, he suggested that cognitive research had shown that "we are all inclined to hold initial expressions or impressions with conviction, and to seek information that supports such images." However, "there is nothing evil, immoral, or inferior about stereotyping. Its central operating characteristics—

categorization, inference, anticipatory thinking, and planning—are obviously adaptive, functional." Nevertheless, since a stereotype may be used to justify conduct toward its object, "Not recognizing these matters would seem to fall short of acquiring a full appreciation of the issues involved," which is likely given that most people may frequently be unaware that they are stereotyping. Miller suggested that stereotyping can be used beneficially, such as in the phrase "Black is beautiful."

Attribution theory, Miller noted, emphasises that "to bring the social world into more manageable dimensions, the individual imposes structure, seeking constancies or invariances. . . . a central premise concerns our overwhelming tendency to view the actions of others as having causes or intentions," which exist within the individual. R. Jones (1982) made a similar point and added that what people have inferred about another person will influence not only what they believe (often erroneously) they can "remember" about that person, but also how they subsequently behave toward the person. Furthermore, Jones argued that people often behave in ways that almost force individuals to conform to these expectations and stereotypes of how they will behave. Thus the limitations and needs of cognitive processing can create self-fulfilling social behavior. R. Jones (1982) went on to point out that the implicit personality theories so formed "may play more of a role in our perception of others than the actual characteristics of others," and that they might be expected to play a large role in our impressions of others when working from memory. He claimed it to be "one of the ironies of modern social psychology that the overwhelming message of research on attribution processes is that in seeking to understand and predict behavior, we often, even usually, do not behave in the rational, analytic manner postulated by attribution theory." Space does not permit a fuller discussion of attribution theory in general. However, the reader can judge from the research cited in our previous chapters the extent to which Jones' claim is true regarding facial appearance, including the negative first impressions that may be the result of facial deformity/unattractiveness and their effect upon avoidance behavior.

Snyder (1981) made the point that, "It is a basic fact of social life that we form impressions of other individuals whom we encounter in our day-to-day lives. In our relationships with others, we seem to want to know not only what they do but why they do what they do. To the extent that we think we understand the global attributes that underlie the specific actions of other people, we may feel better able to understand their actions and to predict their future behavior."

Self-Fulfilling Prophecy Explanations

Snyder (1981) was particularly concerned with the notion that one person's stereotyped beliefs about another, which may well be erroneous, may exert an influence on subsequent interaction. In Chapter 3 we cited the study by Snyder et al. (1977) that found that males' beliefs about the facial attractiveness of a woman with whom they were having a telephone conversation influenced not only their own conversational style, but also that of the woman. (In Chapter 3, however, we noted that Reingen et al. [1980] did not find such a powerful dyadic effect.) Snyder (1981) asserted that, "An individual, having adopted stereotyped beliefs about a target, will: (1) remember and interpret past events in the target's life history in ways that bolster and support these current stereotyped beliefs; and (2) will act upon these current stereotyped beliefs in ways that cause the actual behavior of the target to confirm and validate the individual's stereotyped beliefs about the target." He presented a well-argued case to support these assertions. However, little research involving facial appearance has been so well designed as to be able to test these interesting suggestions.

We have just mentioned the studies by Snyder et al. (1977) and Reingen et al. (1980). Mathes (1974) argued that a "beauty-is-good stereotype" would lead people to reinforce "attractive people for engaging in desirable behaviors and unattractive people for engaging in undesirable behaviors." However, he found that his data did not support this argument. Mathes suggested that "a reinforcement approach in which physical attractiveness is seen as a positive reinforcer producing various effects such as being liked" might offer a better explanation of his data.

Reinforcement Theory

Reinforcement theory is based on the premise that we like those people who reward us. In addition, a principle of secondary reinforcement states that we like people who are associated with pleasant events, and dislike those who are connected with unpleasant events. Thus reinforcement theory has been used to explain that people generally like physically attractive others because they find them rewarding (perhaps they are aesthetically pleasing, or are considered a high-status commodity), and may dislike the physically unattractive or disfigured (perhaps they make us feel uncomfortable, or are threatening, or unaesthetic).

Byrne et al. (1968) were among the first to argue that a reinforcement notion could be used to explain findings concerning the interpersonal effects of facial appearance. They suggested that attraction toward a person would be a function of the positive reinforcements offered by, or expected from, that person, and that, "Given the proposed reward value attached to physical attractiveness, it is hypothesized that interpersonal attraction is greater toward an attractive than toward an unattractive stranger." They found that "cues to physical attractiveness . . . possess . . . acquired reward value."

In 1968 there existed little research on facial appearance that Byrne et al. could have used if pressed on the tautologous nature of their statements. If there is validity in the more up-to-date notion that "what is good is thought to be beautiful" this would cast doubt on the usefulness of a simple, causative reinforcement explanation based on the longer established research finding that "what is beautiful is thought to be good." However, even though a reinforcement explanation of the effects of facial appearance may seem little more than a tautology, some of the findings mentioned in this book (e.g., on dating and on selling) might be as well explained by reinforcement theory as by any other theory currently available. One statement by Byrne et al. (1968) is particularly interesting given the findings discussed in our chapter on facial disfigurement. They noted in their second study that "there is no evidence of a positive effect of attractiveness but rather a negative effect of unattractiveness." Byrne et al. could have discussed the implications of this finding for a reinforcement explanation that is based solely on the assumed rewarding or positive effects of facial attractiveness, rather than also on a notion of the negative or cost effects of unattractiveness.

The notion of rewards versus costs forms part of Piliavin's theory of helping (Piliavin, Piliavin, and Rodin, 1975), and this notion merits wider application to various social effects of facial appearance.

Equity Theory

Equity theory makes some attempt to focus on the balance between rewards and costs. It holds that people deserve their rewards or costs. One of the main premises of the theory is that it is particularly comforting to believe in a world that is predictable and equitable. We are incapacitated if we think that we do not have some degree of control over our fates—people cannot believe, for the sake of their own sanity, in a world that is governed by random reinforcements (M. Lerner, 1970). If we perceive inequity, we act to restore balance. One way of restoring equity, and therefore predictability, is to convince ourselves that a person who reaps rewards (e.g., is facially attractive) in some way deserves them, and/or that one who incurs costs (e.g., the unattractive victim of fate) somehow is at fault and deserves these. In the present context, this would mean that a person would be regarded as being ugly or disfigured through a fault of his or her own. Lerner believed that we have to tell ourselves that we are different from the "victim," or else that we would behave differently if we found ourselves in the same situation, in order to dispel fears that the misfortune could also happen to us. Equity could also be restored by reassuring ourselves that the victim deserved to suffer. Lerner argued that we have a need to believe in a "just world" where good things happen to good people and bad things only happen to bad people, and that we construct explanations in order to bolster such beliefs.

Although it could be argued from our research review that static aspects of facial appearance influence the explanations and expectations that people hold about others, it would not be true to say that there is strong evidence that facial appearance has been shown to exert powerful effects on people's lives. Adams (1977a; see Chapter 6), among others, has argued that such expectations should have important developmental consequences. A symbolic interaction perspective could be relevant here.

Symbolic Interaction Theory

Symbolic interaction developed from the ideas of theorists such as Cooley (1912), who introduced the notion of the "looking glass self," and the idea that a person's self-concept is significantly influenced by what he or she believes others think of him or her. The "self" idea is formed from (i) the imagination of what our appearance is like from another's viewpoint; (ii) the imagination of the other's judgment of that appearance; and (iii) the person's self-feelings (for example, of pride or shame). Mead (1934) postulated that the self-concept arises in social interaction as an outgrowth of the individual's concern about how others react to him or her. The individual learns to interpret and anticipate the reactions of others, and learns to interpret the social environment as others do. This incorporation of how the "generalized other" would respond provides the major source of internal regulation, and eventually comes to guide and maintain behavior, even if external forces are no longer present. The individual develops self-attitudes consistent with those expressed by others, and consequently comes to value or demean himself or herself in the same way that others accept or reject him or her.

The symbolic interactionist viewpoint states that through interaction, a person comes to hold an internal conception or interpretation of the opinions and attitudes of others. There exists a positive relationship between how a person perceives others respond to him or her and how a person feels about himself or herself:

actual   perceived
response $\longrightarrow$ response $\longrightarrow$ self-concept $\longrightarrow$ behavior
of others   of others

Symbolic interactionists emphasize the vital significance of interaction as the means of defining the self-concept. Thus the theory would seem to predict that if a facially disfigured person experiences some sort of faulty interaction, and perceives negative reactions from others, he or she will develop a negative self-concept. Since the self-concept is seen as being constantly redefined (Charon, 1979), the experience of consistently positive or negative responses in the course of social interaction may lead to an increase (for the physically attractive) or a decrement (for the ugly or disfigured) in the feelings the person has about himself or herself. These feelings are believed then to feed back into social interaction via the behavior of facially attractive or unattractive persons. Of relevance here is Kelley's (1971) notion of covariation. If an individual wishes to know to what extent others' treatment of him or her is due to an aspect of him or her such as clothing, he or she can purposely vary the attire and any differential treatment can be noted. However, although some aspects of facial appearance may be covaried in this way, others (e.g., deformity/disfigurement) may not. In essence symbolic interaction theory suggests that individuals play a role suggested to them by the social feedback they receive from others.

Role Theory

Role theory is a loosely linked network of hypotheses based on a theatrical perspective. It attempts to explain behavior solely in terms of roles, role expectations and demands, role skills, and the reference groups that operate on participants. Although lacking in precise predictive validity, comments made by researchers under the auspices of role theory may be of relevance to the material quoted in this book.

Goffman (1963) maintained that in encounters, we act out a "line"—a pattern of verbal and nonverbal acts that are used to express a view and an evaluation of the situation and its participants. "Face" is the social value a person claims for himself or herself. A person is described as being "in" or "maintaining" face when the line he or she takes presents self-image that is internally consistent, that is, the image is supported by judgments and evidence conveyed by other participants in the encounter. When "in face," a person typically feels confident and relaxed. To be in the "wrong face" means that information is brought forth about the person's self-worth that cannot be integrated into the "line" that he or she is taking. He or she is "out of face" when not taking the kind of line that people usually expect. He or she then feels ashamed or inferior, especially if that image has been relied upon in the past.

Secord and Backman (1964) stated that "role strain" occurs when group members do not hold expectations in common, or when they act contrary to expectations. If expectations are unclear or consensus is low, there may be strain and disagreement. Intuitively, it seems possible that role strain may result from interaction with ugly or disfigured people. A person with a facial disfigurement represents something out of the ordinary. Most members of the general public will not have had enough previous contact with disfigured people to have built up a clear set of expectations and norms either for the behavior of the facially disfigured or for themselves. They will not be sure of the role that the facially disfigured person will adopt. In a similar manner, the disfigured person will be unsure of possible reactions to the deformity. He or she may wish to take the role of someone with a normal appearance, since he or she may consider himself or herself to be a "normal" person who has the misfortune to have a physical defect. However, others may expect him or her to adopt the sort of role considered appropriate for someone who is handicapped or sick (Macgregor, 1974). Hence, the disfigured person may end up feeling trapped in a role enactment.

Summary

In summary, each of the theories outlined here could provide a form of theoretical framework for some of the research examined in this book, and might prove useful as guidelines for future research. However, none of the perspectives is by any means comprehensive, and at present there seems little to choose between them. Indeed, since the theories have been developed largely to accommodate the results of research that has often been of limited ecological validity, they may not be of much use to future and, it is hoped, more valid research. McArthur and Baron (1983) stated that their ecological theory of social perception's emphasis on dynamic stimulus displays provided a needed balance to the "laboratory-based," photographic tradition of research that constitutes the majority of published studies on the purported social effects of facial appearance. They argued that, "The emphasis on the dynamic relationship between perception and action directs attention to the rather neglected question of social perceptions within ongoing relationships, where perceptions are informed by actions and where people really do have the opportunity to perceive one another's invariant attributes. The emphasis on perceived affordances provides a vital alternative to the trait analysis of social perception." They subsequently added that, "However, it is acknowledged that the detection of some of these properties requires extensive perceptual learning and in the absence of such learning, may require inference."

Thus future theoretical development may well need to combine into one perspective the more appropriate aspects of extant theories. We believe strongly that future theoretical developments concerning the social psychology of facial appearance should take note of McArthur and Baron's more dynamic perspective. However, we might here usefully summarize the extant major relevant theoretical perspectives reviewed above. These seem to concern the following points:

1. A discrepancy between how a person sees himself or herself and how others see that person is distressing (equity and role theories).
2. The degree to which a person evaluates himself or herself positively or negatively can have implications for social behavior (symbolic interaction).
3. The reactions of others are important, because a person is reliant on the behavior and opinions of others for molding his or her own behavior (symbolic interaction, self-fulfilling prophecy, and reinforcement/social learning theories).
4. Interaction is important for the forming of internal conceptions, and as part of the interpretation of the opinions and attitudes of others (attribution and symbolic interaction theories).

The lack of relevant theoretical rationales was one of the major reasons why in 1974 Berscheid and Walster were of the view that "an interest in physical appearance variables relegated one to the dustbin of social science." We trust that having read the present book readers will not be of the same opinion regarding its authors.

As stated at the beginning of Chapter 2 Walster et al. (1966) found that the only predictor of individuals' liking for (and desire to date again) a "computer-dance" partner was partner physical attractiveness. Twenty years later Walster (now Hatfield) point out (see Hatfield & Sprecher, 1986) that,

"Against the advice of some senior colleagues, who believed the finding was 'theoretically uninteresting' and therefore unworthy of consideration by professional journals, she wrote up her 'serendipitous finding' as she called it then." Hatfield and Sprecher noted that

> It was not, of course, that we didn't suspect appearance played some role in how a person was regarded by others. But this was the early sixties—when appearance was almost universally regarded as a frivolous and superficial attribute. At this time people requesting plastic surgery to modify some aspect of their appearance were routinely subjected to tests to ascertain that they were free of psychopathology—a certification difficult for the candidate to achieve since a request for plastic surgery was itself considered a symptom of neuroticism. During this era the only reasonable justification for orthodontic surgery and treatment, or indeed routine dental treatment, was considered, by insurance companies, dentists, and clients alike, to be improvement of "function"—not aesthetic appearance.

They pointed out that nowadays "judges, juries, and lawyers representing clients whose appearance has been adversely altered through the negligence of others take into consideration more than just impaired physical function. The probability that a disfigurement also leaves the victim with impaired self-esteem and impaired social and economic opportunities is also considered."

However, we would contend that the current picture is far from clear concerning the actual real-like effects of facial appearance, including changes therein. Although Hatfield and Sprecher recently stated that from "the evidence indicating that good-looking men and women have an enormous advantage in life . . . a person might be tempted to conclude that everyone must be profoundly concerned about appearance, that wise individuals should do all they can to make themselves as appealing as possible, and that any other course is foolhardy," they immediately pointed out that life is much more complicated than this. Future research must address this fact, and it is to further comments on this topic that the final part of this concluding chapter is addressed.

Further Points for Future Research

Herman, Zanna, and Higgins (1986) recently argued that, "Physical appearance research has entered its adolescence: it is now asking subtler questions, and discovering subtler relationships between variables. But obviously, it is far from mature, either in terms of its empirical knowledge base or its conceptual organization." This claim may be just a little premature, but we trust that it turns out to be true.

Stimulus Choice

Future research should get away from showing facial photographs to undergraduates and measuring their reactions to these using rating scales or questionnaires. Due consideration must be given to how the facial stimuli are to be presented. Barnes and Rosenthal (1985) found in their study that "when actual people are used instead of photographs, the strong effect of physical attractiveness may become diluted by the amount of other information available." (Earlier in this chapter we mentioned Argyle and McHenry's [1971] finding that the initial effect of spectacles soon dissipated as the interaction progressed.) La Voie and Adams (1978), and Lyman, Hatlelid, and Macurdy (1981) have argued that in this field the traditional, rather basic research methodology employed by the majority of investigators is in need of considerable improvement. Lyman et al. suggested (i) that many investigatory procedures on this topic have been so constrained in presenting stimuli as to bias the results and to lead to erroneous conclusions, and (ii) that physical appearance is by no means always the first information that we receive about another person. Benassi (1982) found information about individuals' facial attractiveness only to influence his subjects' responses when it was made available to them prior to, rather than after, information about the individuals' performance.

Knapp (1985) made the point that future research should examine how generalizable are previous findings using photographs to understanding the behavior typical of daily interactions, particularly those that require a degree of psychological commitment and mutual influence from those involved. He observed that "the analysis of face-to-face message behavior combined with reports from participants as well as observers can be noted in several studies although I could not find any that combine all these elements." One of our own studies (Rumsey et al. 1986) may be among the few to do this. Knapp argued that research on facial appearance should "examine interactive situations, make multiple observations over time, treat appearance as a multi-meaning phenomenon, operationalize perception differently and account for the influence of a wider variety of contextual factors."

Studies Over Time

It is certainly the case that research on the social psychology of facial appearance has rarely taken the trouble to determine whether the noted "one-shot" effects have temporal persistence.

Future research could also become longitudinal by examining more extensively those individuals who, for one reason or another, undergo a pronounced change in their facial appearance such as via facial surgery procedures or via the natural changes that occur during childhood and adolescence (see Sussman, Mueser, Grau, & Yarnold, 1983). Another way in which a shift away from slavishly using undergraduates as subjects (and/or as stimuli) could be achieved is by assessing the importance of facial appearance across the life span (Adams, 1985; R. Jones & Adams, 1982; Maruyama & Miller, 1981) and for the elderly (Dushenko, Perry, Schilling, & Smolarski, 1978; D. Johnson, 1985).

More studies of the effects of facial appearance should be conducted involving various races (I. Bernstein, Lin, & McClellan, 1982; Moss, Miller, & Page, 1975), cultures (Himmelfarb & Fishbein, 1971), and nationalities (Bull & David, 1986; Secord & Bevan, 1956).

Choice of Dependent Variables

Greater effort should also be put into employing more worthwhile and ecologically valid dependent variables. Sigall and Page (1972) chided social psychologists for not paying sufficient attention to their choice of dependent measures. They argued that, "The measures employed to assess subjects' responses frequently are haphazardly thrown together questionnaires, rating scales and the like." They also pointed out that many of the dependent measures used in research in this area are clearly open to bias. They suggested that demand characteristics and norms about people not disclosing their "true" feelings about others would be reduced by use of the "bogus pipeline" technique in which subjects are led to believe that their psychophysiological responses to the presented interpersonal stimuli are also being monitored. Although the interpretation of actual psychophysiological data may be as problematic as is that for "paper-and-pencil" data, we consider it remiss of researchers of the social psychology of facial appearance that so very few studies have collected data of the psychophysiological variety. The most interesting hypothesis of Hansell, Sparacino, and Ronchi (1982) that "physical attractiveness is negatively related to the physiological stress generally experienced by people in social situations" is worthy of close examination. Hansell et al. found some support for their notion that unattractive people would have higher blood pressure, but they acknowledged that this "may represent a temporary accommodation to the measurement situations." However, even if this were the correct explanation of their findings it should still be of interest to social psychologists.

An even more important matter concerning the choice of dependent measure is brought into focus by findings that the notion of "what is beautiful is good" seems in need of some modification. Timmerman and Hewitt (1980) found increased facial attractiveness to heighten social attraction toward female stimuli, but not to affect trait ascriptions such as "sensitive" or "better mother." (Similar effects were observed by Kleck and Rubenstein [1975] and by Gallucci and Meyer [1984], who found physically attractive females to be rated as more egocentric.) Dermer and Thiel (1975) found that although physically attractive women were rated more positively on indices of social desirability (e.g., sociable, warm, exciting) they were also judged by other women to be more egotistical, snobbish, and materialistic. Unattractive female subjects rated the attractive women as less likely to be good parents. Bassili (1981) found evidence that the attractiveness stereotype may be more one of glamour than of goodness in that people assume that good looks are instrumental in leading to a socially and sexually exciting life, but that such a life-style may involve vanity and self-centeredness. His data suggested that physically attractive women are rated as having an active and exciting social orientation but are not judged as having greater personal integrity. In Chapter 2 we reviewed studies that noted that attractive women may be thought more likely to have extramarital affairs.

Kollar (1974) found that although males showed a strong preference for physically attractive females as dates, they (and females) rated beautiful women lower on expected marital happiness and adequacy as a wife and a mother. She also suggested that in certain circumstances people may be unwilling to approach highly attractive women. This is just what Dabbs and Stokes (1975) found in that on a sidewalk people passed closer to a female confederate when she looked unattractive rather than attractive. However, Powell and Dabbs (1976) found no such effect. Nevertheless, there seem to be good grounds for considering that the notion of "what is beautiful is good" is in large part the result of researchers' choices of dependent measures. Whether this criticism can be applied also to studies employing male stimuli is not yet known since the studies described above employed only female stimuli.

"What Is Good Is Beautiful"?

Another possible variation of the "what is beautiful is good" notion that future research should address is the extent to which individuals' other personal qualities can cause people to perceive their facial appearance to be different from that which it "objectively" is. That is, to what extent it is true that "what is good is beautiful"? Gross and Crofton (1977) were among the first to conduct a study specifically designed to find that reading a favorable personality description of a photographed person would lead male and female subjects to rate her as more physically attractive. Owens and Ford (1978) replicated this finding for female stimuli, but did not find an effect for male stimuli. However, as we noted in Chapter 4, although Efran (1974) made no comment on it, his female subjects who read of an (independently rated) attractive male's misdeeds did not find such a stimulus to be physically attractive. At the end of Chapter 6 we noted Felson and Bohrnstedt's (1979) finding that children's perceptions of their male and female classmates' physical attractiveness were more closely related to their judgments of their abilities than to "objective" indicators of the peers' physical attractiveness.

Some psychologists (e.g., Gross & Grofton, 1977) have suggested that it may be unpalatable for research to find that beautiful people do reap more of society's benefits. If future research were more closely to address the possibility that "what is good is beautiful" then the probable biases against the finding of research on the social psychology of facial appearance could be reduced. Whatever the final explanation of "what is good is beautiful" (and no adequate ones have yet been offered for this ascribing to/perceiving a target person in a way to justify one's feelings), this may turn out not only to be a more palatable notion, but also a more productive and useful one for future research to be concerned with, especially if it turns out to be of advantage to the facially unattractive/ugly/disfigured. In Chapter 8 we discussed some of the ways in which social psychology would be of use to those who suffer from facial prejudice. In 1981 Shaw (1981c) (a professor of orthdontics) made the point that, "As the dramatic progress in cosmetic surgery seen in recent decades now reaches a plateau, a search for better means of helping the disfigured individual to come to terms with his condition and more comfortably integrate with society, would seem appropriate." Our recent pilot study (Rumsey et al., 1986) suggesting social skills training seems to be one way forward.

Real-Life Social Interaction

If studies of the social psychology of facial appearance do come to be focused more on real-life social interaction rather than on laboratory-based reactions to photographs, then not only could the facial appearance of stimulus persons be examined within the context of their behavior, but the probable links between people's faces and their behavior could also be examined. In Chapter 2 we described the pioneering study by Snyder et al. (1977) that found stimulus facial appearance to have strong effects upon interpersonal behavioral dynamics. Even though Reingen et al. (1980) (see Chapter 3) did not find such strong dyadic effects, the notion of behavioral confirmation in social interaction merits close attention. The information from others that perceivers process in actual social interactions surely is in large part a product of their own actions toward those others (Snyder & Swann, 1978). This being so, then the defensive presentational style of the facially abnormal individual, rather than the face itself, may be the cause of fellow interactants' discomfort and/or avoidance behavior. Should this occur then such "an exacerbation cycle can become independent of the stimulus that originally gave rise to it" (Northcraft & Hastorf, 1986). This interactionist perspective is more likely to produce findings of benefit to society than has the majority of previous research. In his recent review of some of the literature on facial attractiveness Patzer (1985) stated that, "The findings reveal that physical attractiveness plays a dramatic but covert role in an individual's interpersonal interactions." We believe that sufficient research on real-life social interactions has not been conducted to support this contention, nor that "persons of different levels of physical attractiveness are perceived differently and are treated differently such that higher physical attractiveness is given overwhelmingly preferential treatment" (Patzer, 1985). In 1974 Berscheid and Walster pointed out that "there is no research directly addressed to the question of how the [physical attractiveness] stereotype stands up against contradictory information obtained in social interaction with another." Sadly, this remains the case today.

Although informing people (e.g., via this book) of research findings relating to the effects of facial appearance could possibly lead to a reduction where there is facial prejudice, since those involved in such reactions may well not have introspective access to their cognitive processing (Nisbett & Bellows, 1977), a more socially dynamic, rather than cognitive, approach would seem justified.

The "what is good is beautiful" notion is one that Lakoff and Scherr (1984) could have used when arguing that American society should replace its emphasis on the physical aspects of facial beauty by one in which "Beauty must be understood as something achieved through individual experience." They argued that this "is necessary if we believe in a world in which everyone has a choice for achievement, everyone can hope for autonomy, and everyone has the right to make choices." We take the weight of evidence cited in the present book to suggest that Lakoff and Scherr's hopes could be realized, and to support a statement made in the first published overview of psychologists' research on facial appearance, namely "it is not a forgone conclusion that attractive people should be happier than unattractive" (Berscheid & Walster, 1974).

References

Aamot, S. (1978). Reactions to facial deformities. *European Journal of Social Psychology, 8,* 315–334.

Abel, T. (1952). Personality characteristics of the facially disfigured. *Transactions of the New York Academy of Sciences, 4,* 325–329.

Adams, G. (1977a). Physical attractiveness research: Toward a developmental social psychology of beauty. *Human Development, 20,* 217–230.

Adams, G. (1977b). Physical attractiveness, personality, and social reactions to peer pressure. *Journal of Psychology, 96,* 287–296.

Adams, G. (1978). Racial membership and physical attractiveness effects on preschool teachers' expectations. *Child Study Journal, 8,* 29–41.

Adams, G. (1985). Attractiveness through the ages: Implications of facial attractiveness over the life cycle. In J. Graham & A. Kligman (Eds.), *The psychology of cosmetic treatments.* New York: Praeger.

Adams, G., and Cohen, A. (1974). Children's physical and interpersonal characteristics as they affect student-teacher interactions. *Journal of Experimental Education, 43,* 1–5.

Adams, G., and Cohen, A. (1976a). Characteristics of children and teacher expectancy: An extension to the child's social and family life. *Journal of Educational Research, 70,* 87–90.

Adams, G., and Cohen, A. (1976b). An examination of cumulative folder information used by teachers in making differential judgments of children's abilities. *Alberta Journal of Educational Research, 22,* 216–225.

Adams, G., and Crane, P. (1980). An assessment of parents' and teachers' expectations of preschool children's social preference for attractive or unattractive children and adults. *Child Development, 51,* 224–231.

Adams, G., and Crossman, S. (1978). *Physical attractiveness: A cultural imperative.* Rosslyn Heights, NY: Libra.

Adams, G., and LaVoie, J. (1974). The effect of student's sex, conduct and facial attractiveness on teacher expectancy. *Education, 95,* 76–85.

Adams, G., and LaVoie, J. (1975). Parental expectations of educational and personal-social performance and childrearing patterns as a function of attractiveness, sex and conduct of the child. *Child Study Journal, 5,* 125–142.

Adams, G., and Read, D. (1983). Personality and social influence styles of attractive and unattractive college women. *Journal of Psychology, 114,* 151–157.

Agarwal, P., and Prakash, N. (1977). Perceived physical attractiveness as related to attitudes towards women's liberation. *Indian Psychological Review, 15,* 31–34.

Agnew, R. (1984). Appearance and delinquency. *Criminology: An Interdisciplinary Journal, 22*, 421–440.

Albrecht, G., Walker, V., and Levy, J. (1982). Social distance from the stigmatized. *Social Science and Medicine, 16*, 1319–1327.

Alessi, D., and Anthony, W. (1969). The uniformity of children's attitudes toward physical disabilities. *Exceptional Children, 35*, 543–545.

Aloia, G. (1975). Effects of physical stigmata and labels on judgments of subnormality of preservice teachers. *Mental Retardation, 13*, 17–21.

Altemeyer, R., and Jones, K. (1974). Sexual identity, physical attractiveness and seating position. *Canadian Journal of Behavioral Science, 6*, 357–375.

Altman, I., and Haythorn, W. (1967). The ecology of isolated groups. *Behavioral Science, 12*, 169–182.

Andersen, S., and Bem, S. (1981). Sextyping and androgyny in dyadic interaction: Individual differences in responsiveness to physical attractiveness. *Journal of Personality and Social Psychology, 41*, 74–86.

Anderson, R., and Nida, S. (1978). Effect of physical attractiveness on opposite- and same-sex evaluations. *Journal of Personality, 46*, 401–413.

Andreasi, N., and Norris, A. (1972). Long-term adjustment and adaptation mechanisms in severely burned adults. *Journal of Nervous and Mental Disease, 154*, 352–362.

Archer, R., and Cash, T. (1985). Physical attractiveness and maladjustment among psychiatric inpatients. *Journal of Social and Clinical Psychology, 3*, 170–180.

Argyle, M. (1978). *The psychology of interpersonal behavior.* London: Penguin.

Argyle, M., and Dean, J. (1965). Eye contact, distance and affiliation. *Sociometry, 20*, 289–304.

Argyle, M., and McHenry, R. (1971). Do spectacles really affect judgments of intelligence? *British Journal of Social and Clinical Psychology, 4*, 27–29.

Argyle, M., Trower, P., and Bryant, B. (1974). Explorations in the treatment of personality disorders and neuroses by social skills training. *British Journal of Medical Psychology, 47*, 63–72.

Arkowitz, H., Lichtenstein, E., McGovern, K., & Hines, P. (1975). The behavioral assessment of social competence in males. *Behavior Therapy, 14*, 523–528.

Arndt, E., Lefebvre, A., Travis, F., and Munro, I. (1986). Fact and fantasy: Psychosocial consequences of facial surgery in 24 Down syndrome children. *British Journal of Plastic Surgery, 39*, 498–504.

Athanasiou, R., and Greene, P. (1973). Physical attractiveness and helping behavior. *Proceedings of the 81st Annual Convention of the American Psychological Association, 8*, 289–290.

Bailey, L., and Edwards, D. (1975) Psychological considerations in maxillofacial prosthetics. *Journal of Prosthetic Dentistry, 34*, 533–538.

Bailey, R., and Kelly, M. (1984). Perceived physical attractiveness in early, steady, and engaged daters. *Journal of Psychology, 116*, 39–43.

Bailey, R., and Price, J. (1978). Perceived physical attractiveness in married partners of long and short duration. *Journal of Psychology, 99*, 155–161.

Bailey, R., and Schreiber, T. (1981). Congruency of physical attractiveness perceptions and liking. *Journal of Social Psychology, 115*, 285–286.

Baker, M., and Churchill, G. (1977). The impact of physically attractive models on advertising evaluations. *Journal of Marketing Research, 14*, 538–555.

Baker, W., and Smith, L. (1939). Facial disfigurement and personality. *Journal of the American Medical Association, 112*, 301–304.

Baldwin, D., and Barnes, M. (1966). Patterns of motivation in families seeking orthodontic treatment. *International Association of Dental Research Abstracts, 44*, 412.

Banziger, G., and Hooker, L. (1979). The effects of attitudes toward feminism and perceived feminism on physical attractiveness ratings. *Sex Roles, 5*, 437–442.

Barker, R. (1948). The social psychology of physical disability. *Journal of Social Issues*, *4*, 28–38.

Barnes, M., and Rosenthal, R. (1985). Interpersonal effects of experimenter attractiveness, attire and gender. *Journal of Personality and Social Psychology*, *48*, 435–446.

Barocas, R., and Black, H. (1974). Referral rate and physical attractiveness in third-grade children. *Perceptual and Motor Skills*, *39*, 731–734.

Barocas, R., and Karoly, P. (1972). Effects of physical appearance on social responsiveness. *Psychological Reports*, *31*, 495–500.

Barocas, R., and Vance, F. (1974). Physical appearance and personal adjustment counseling. *Journal of Counseling Psychology*, *21*, 96–100.

Barrios, B., and Giesen, M. (1976). *Getting what you expect: Effects of expectation on intragroup attraction and interpersonal distance*. Paper presented at the meeting of the Southeastern Psychological Association, New Orleans.

Bar-Tal, D., and Saxe, L. (1976). Physical attractiveness and its relationship to sex role stereotyping. *Sex Roles*, *2*, 123–133.

Bassili, J. (1981). The attractiveness stereotype: Goodness or glamor? *Basic and Applied Psychology*, *2*, 235–252.

Baumeister, R., and Darley, J. (1982). Reducing the biasing effect of perpetrator attractiveness in jury simulation. *Personality and Social Psychology Bulletin*, *8*, 286–292.

Beaman, A., and Klentz, B. (1983). The supposed physical attractiveness bias against supporters of the women's movement: A meta-analysis. *Personality and Social Psychology Bulletin*, *9*, 544–550.

Beaman, A., Klentz, B., and Conrad, B. (1984). A direct test of and an alternative explanation for judgments of attractiveness of supporters of the women's movement. *Canadian Journal of Behavioral Science*, *16*, 191–195.

Beardsley, E. (1971). Privacy: Autonomy and selective disclosure. In J. Pennock & J. Chapman (Eds.), *Privacy*. New York: Atherton Press.

Beehr, T., and Gilmore, D. (1982). Applicant attractiveness as a perceived job-relevant variable in selection of management trainees. *Academy of Management Journal*, *25*, 607–617.

Belbin, E. (1979). Applicable psychology, and some national problems. *Bulletin of the British Psychological Society*, *32*, 241–244.

Bem, D. (1974). On predicting some of the people some of the time: The search for cross-situational consistencies in behavior. *Psychological Review*, *81*, 506–520.

Benassi, M. (1982). Effects of order of presentation, primacy, and physical attractiveness on attributions of ability. *Journal of Personality and Social Psychology*, *43*, 48–58.

Berkowitz, L., and Frodi, A. (1979). Reactions to a child's mistakes as affected by her/his looks or speech. *Social Psychology Quarterly*, *42*, 420–425.

Bernstein, I., Lin, T., and McClellan, P. (1982). Cross- vs. within-racial judgments of attractiveness. *Perception and Psychophysics*, *32*, 495–503.

Bernstein, N. (1976). *Emotional care of the facially burned and disfigured*. Boston: Little, Brown.

Bernstein, N. (1982). Psychosocial results of burns: The damaged self-esteem. *Clinics in Plastic Surgery*, *9*, 337–346.

Bernstein, W., Stephenson, B., Snyder, M., and Wicklund, R. (1983). Causal ambiguity and heterosexual affiliation. *Journal of Experimental Social Psychology*, *19*, 78–92.

Berry, D., and McArthur, L. (1985). Some components and consequences of a baby-face. *Journal of Personality and Social Psychology*, *48*, 312–323.

Berscheid, E. (1981). An overview of the psychological effects of physical attractiveness. In G. Lucker, K. Ribbens, & J. McNamara (Eds.), *Psychological aspects of facial form.* Ann Arbor: University of Michigan Press.

Berscheid, E. (1986). The question of the importance of physical attractiveness. In C. Herman, M. Zanna, & E. Higgins (Eds.), *Physical appearance, stigma and social behavior.* Hillsdale, NJ: Lawrence Erlbaum.

Berscheid, E., Dion, K., Walster, E., and Walster, G. (1971). Physical attractiveness and dating: A test of the matching hypothesis. *Journal of Experimental Social Psychology, 7,* 173–189.

Berscheid, E., and Gangestad, S. (1982). The social psychological implications of facial physical attractiveness. *Clinics in Plastic Surgery, 9,* 289–296.

Berscheid, E., Graziano, W., Monson, T., and Dermer, M. (1976). Outcome dependency: Attention, attribution, and attraction. *Journal of Personality and Social Psychology, 34,* 978–989.

Berscheid, E., and Walster, E. (1974). Physical attractiveness. *Advances in Experimental Social Psychology, 7,* 157–215.

Best, J., and Demmin, H. (1982). Victim's provocativeness and victim's attractiveness as determinants of blame in rape. *Psychological Reports, 51,* 255–258.

Bihm, E., Gaudet, I., and Sale, O. (1979). Altruistic responses under conditions of anonymity. *Journal of Social Psychology, 109,* 25–30.

Birdwhistell, R. (1952). *Introduction to kinesics: An annotation system for analysis of body motion and gesture.* Louisville, KY: University of Louisville Press.

Blass, T., Alperstein, L., and Block, S. (1974). Effects of communicators' race and beauty. *Personality and Social Psychology Bulletin, 1,* 132–134.

Boor, M. (1976). Beautiful is not dangerous, beauty is not talent: Two failures to replicate physical attractiveness effects. *Catalog of Selected Documents in Psychology, 6,* 109.

Boor, M., Wartman, S., and Reuben, D. (1983). Relationship of physical appearance and professional demeanor to interview evaluations and rankings of medical residency applicants. *Journal of Psychology, 113,* 61–65.

Boor, M., and Zeis, F. (1975). Effect of physical attractiveness and IQ estimation. A failure to extend results of prior research. *Catalog of Selected Documents in Psychology, 5,* 234–335.

Bordieri, J., Sotolongo, M., and Wilson, M. (1983). Physical attractiveness and attributions for disability. *Rehabilitation Psychology, 28,* 207–215.

Bradshaw, J., and McKenzie, B. (1971). Judging outline faces: A developmental study. *Child Development, 42,* 929–937.

Brantley, H., and Clifford, E. (1980). When my child was born: Maternal reactions to the birth of the child. *Journal of Personality Assessment, 44,* 620–623.

Bray, R., and Kerr, N. (1982). Methodological considerations in the study of the psychology of the courtroom. In N. Kerr & R. Bray (Eds.), *The psychology of the courtroom.* New York: Academic Press.

Brennan, T. (1982). Loneliness in adolescence. In L. Peplau & D. Perlman (Eds.), *Loneliness: A sourcebook of current theory, research and therapy.* New York: Wiley-Interscience.

Brigham, J. (1980). Limiting conditions of the "physical attractiveness stereotype". *Journal of Research in Personality, 14,* 365–375.

Brislin, R., and Lewis, S. (1968). Dating and physical attractiveness: Replication. *Psychological Reports, 22,* 976.

British Medical Journal. (1965). Physical disability and crime. *1,* 1448–1449.

Brooks, V., and Hochberg, J. (1960). A psychophysical study of "cuteness". *Perceptual and Motor Skills, 11,* 205.

Bryt, A. (1966). Psychiatric considerations in candidates for plastic surgery. *The Eye, Ear, Nose and Throat Monthly, 45,* 86–88, 102–105.

Bull, P. (1983). *Body Movement and Interpersonal Communication.* Chichester, England: Wiley.

Bull, R. (1979). The psychological significance of facial deformity. In M. Cook & G. Wilson (Eds.), *Love and attraction*. Oxford, England: Pergamon.

Bull, R. (1982). Can experimental psychology be applied psychology? In S. Canter & D. Canter (Eds.), *Psychology in practice*. Chichester, England: Wiley.

Bull, R. (1985). Society's reaction to facial deformity. In J. Graham & A. Kligman (Eds.), *The psychology of cosmetic treatments*. New York: Praeger.

Bull, R., and Brooking, J. (1985). Does marriage influence whether a facially disfigured person is judged to be physically unattractive? *Journal of Psychology, 119*, 163–167.

Bull, R., and Clifford, B. (1979). Eyewitness memory. In M. Gruneberg & P. Morris (Eds.), *Applied Problems in Memory*. London: Academic Press.

Bull, R., and David, I. (1986). Nigerian and English nurses' and office workers' ratings of normal and scarred faces. *Journal of Cross Cultural Psychology, 17*, 99–108.

Bull, R., and Green, J. (1980). The relationship between physical appearance and criminality. *Medicine, Science and the Law, 20*, 79–83.

Bull, R., and Hawkes, C. (1982). Judging politicians by their faces. *Political Studies, 30*, 95–191.

Bull, R., Jenkins, M., and Stevens, J. (1983). Evaluation of politicians' faces. *Political Psychology, 4*, 713–716.

Bull, R., and Shead, G. (1979). Pupil dilation, sex of stimulus, and age and sex of observer. *Perceptual and Motor Skills, 49*, 27–30.

Bull, R., and Stevens, J. (1979). The effects of attractiveness of writer and penmanship on essay grades. *Journal of Occupational Psychology, 52*, 53–59.

Bull, R., and Stevens, J. (1980). The effect of unsightly teeth on helping behaviour. *Perceptual and Motor Skills, 81*, 438.

Bull, R., and Stevens, J. (1981). The effects of facial deformity on helping behaviour. *Italian Journal of Psychology, 8*, 25–33.

Burns, M. (1972). Psychological aspects of orthodontics. In W. Cinotti., A. Grieder, & H. Springob (Eds.), *Applied psychology in dentistry*. St. Louis: Mosby.

Burns, R. (1979). *The self concept: Theory, measurement, development and behavior*. New York: Longman.

Burr, C. (1935). Personality and physiognomy. In *The human face: A symposium*. Philadelphia: The Dental Cosmos.

Busch-Rossnagel, N. (1981). Where is the handicap in disability?: The contextual impact of physical disability. In R. Lerner & N. Busch-Rossnagel (Eds.), *Individuals as producers of their development*. New York: Academic.

Buss, A. (1985). Self-consciousness and appearance. In J. Graham & A. Kligman (Eds.), *The psychology of cosmetic treatments*. New York: Praeger.

Byrne, D., Ervin, C., and Lamberth, J. (1970). Continuity between the experimental study of attraction and real-life computer dating. *Journal of Personality and Social Psychology, 16*, 157–165.

Byrne, D., London, O., and Reeves, K. (1968). The effects of physical attractiveness, sex and attitude similarity on interpersonal attraction. *Journal of Personality, 36*, 259–271.

Caballero, M., and Pride, W. (1984). Selected effects of salesperson sex and attractiveness in direct mail advertisements. *Journal of Marketing, 48*, 94–100.

Calhoun, L., Selby, J., Cann, A., and Keller, G. (1978). Effect of victim physical attractiveness and sex of respondent on social reactions. *British Journal of Social and Clinical Psychology, 17*, 191–192.

Cann, A., Siegfried, W., and Pearce, L. (1981). Forced attention to specific applicant qualifications: Impact on physical attractiveness and sex of applicant biases. *Personnel Psychology, 34*, 65–75.

Carducci, B., Cozby, P., and Ward, C. (1978). Sexual arousal and interpersonal evaluations. *Journal of Experimental Social Psychology, 14*, 449–457.

Carling, F. (1962). *And yet we are human*. London: Chatto & Windus.

Carlson, R., and Mayfield, E. (1967). Evaluating interview and employment application data. *Personnel Psychology, 20*, 441–460.

Carver, C., Glass, D., Snyder, M., and Katz, I. (1977). Favorable impressions of stigmatized others. *Personality and Social Psychology, 3*, 232–235.

Cash, T. (1985). Physical appearance and mental health. In J. Graham & A. Kligman (Eds.), *The psychology of cosmetic treatments*. New York: Praeger.

Cash, T., and Begley, P. (1976). Internal-external control, achievement orientation and physical attractiveness of college students. *Psychological Reports, 38*, 1205–1206.

Cash, T., Begley, P., McCown, D., and Weise, B. (1975). When counsellors are heard but not seen: Initial impact of physical attractiveness. *Journal of Counselling Psychology, 22*, 273–279.

Cash, T., and Burns, D. (1977). The occurrence of reinforcing activities in relation to locus of control, success-failure expectancies and physical attractiveness. *Journal of Personality Assessment, 41*, 387–391.

Cash, T., and Cash, D. (1982). Women's use of cosmetics: Psychosocial correlates and consequences. *International Journal of Cosmetic Science, 4*, 1–14.

Cash, T., and Derlega, V. (1978). The matching hypothesis: Physical attractiveness among same-sexed friends. *Personality and Social Psychology Bulletin, 4*, 240–243.

Cash, T., Gillen, B., and Burns, S. (1977). "Sexism" and "beautyism" in personnel consultant decision making. *Journal of Applied Psychology, 62*, 301–310.

Cash, T., and Horton, C. (1983). Aesthetic surgery: Effects of rhinoplasty on the social perception of patients by others. *Plastic and Reconstructive Surgery, 72*, 543–548.

Cash, T., and Kehr, J. (1978). Influence of non-professional counsellors' physical attractiveness and sex on perceptions of counsellor behavior. *Journal of Counselling Psychology, 25*, 336–342.

Cash, T., Kehr, J., Polyson, J., and Freeman, V. (1977). Role of physical attractiveness in peer attribution of psychological disturbance. *Journal of Consulting and Clinical Psychology, 45*, 987–993.

Cash, T., Rissi, J., and Chapman, R. (1985). Not just another pretty face: Sex roles, locus of control, and cosmetics use. *Personality and Social Psychology Bulletin, 11*, 246–257.

Cash, T., and Soloway, D. (1975). Self-disclosure correlates of physical attractiveness: An exploratory study. *Psychological Reports, 36*, 579–586.

Cash, T., and Trimer, C. (1984). Sexism and beautyism in women's evaluations of peer performance. *Sex Roles, 10*, 87–98.

Cavior, H., Hayes, S., and Cavior, N. (1974). Physical attractiveness of female offenders. *Criminal Justice and Behavior, 1*, 321–331.

Cavior, N., and Boblett, P. (1982). Physical attractiveness of dating versus married couples. *Proceedings of the 80th Annual Convention of the American Psychological Association, 7*, 175–176.

Cavior, N., and Dokecki, P. (1973). Physical attractiveness, perceived attitude similarity, and academic achievement as contributors to interpersonal attraction among adolescents. *Developmental Psychology, 9*, 44–54.

Cavior, N., and Howard, L. (1973). Facial attractiveness and juvenile delinquency. *Journal of Abnormal Child Psychology, 1*, 202–213.

Cavior, N., and Lombardi, D. (1973). Developmental aspects of judgment of physical attractiveness in children. *Developmental Psychology, 8*, 67–71.

Cavior, N., Miller, K., and Cohen, S. (1975). Physical attractiveness, attitude similarity and length of acquaintance as contributors to interpersonal attraction among adolescents. *Social Behavior and Personality, 3*, 133–141.

Centers, L., and Centers, R. (1963). Peer group attitudes toward the amputee child.

Journal of Social Psychology, *61*, 127–132.

Chaiken, S. (1979). Communicator physical attractiveness and persuasion. *Journal of Personality and Social Psychology*, *37*, 1387–1397.

Chaiken, S. (1980). Heuristic versus systematic information processing and the use of source versus message cues in persuasion. *Journal of Personality and Social Psychology*, *39*, 752–766.

Chaikin, A., Gillen, B., Derlega, V., Heinen, J., and Wilson, M. (1978). Students' reactions to teachers' physical attractiveness and nonverbal behavior: Two explanatory studies. *Psychology in the Schools*, *15*, 588–595.

Charon, S. (1979). *Symbolic interaction*. London: Prentice Hall.

Chelune, G., Sultan, F., and Williams, C. (1980). Loneliness, self-disclosure, and interpersonal effectiveness. *Journal of Counselling Psychology*, *27*, 462–468.

Chigier, E., and Chigier, M. (1968). Attitudes to disability of children in the multicultural society of Israel. *Journal of Health and Social Behavior*, *9*, 310–317.

Clifford, B., and Bull, R. (1978). *The psychology of person identification*. London: Routledge and Kegan Paul.

Clifford, E. (1973). Psychosocial aspects of orofacial anomalies: Speculations in search of data. In *Orofacial anomalies: Clinical and research implications*. Rockville, MD: American Speech and Hearing Association.

Clifford, E. (1974). Insights and speculations: Psychological explorations of the craniofacial experience. In *Proceedings of the Conference on evaluation of recent advances in craniofacial surgery*. Urbana: University of Illinois Medical Center.

Clifford, M. (1975). Physical attractiveness and academic performance. *Child Study Journal*, *5*, 201–209.

Clifford, M., and Walster, E. (1973). Research note: The effects of physical attractiveness on teacher expectations. *Sociology of Education*, *46*, 248–258.

Clingman, J., and Lushene, R. (1982). Perceptions of a woman's reasons for supporting feminism as a function of age, attractiveness and occupation. *Journal of Psychology*, *110*, 289–292.

Coleman, V., and Coleman, M. (1981). *Face values*. London: Pan.

Colligan, R., Sather, A., and Hollen, M. (1980). Psychological evaluation of the orthognathic surgical patient. In G. Lucker, K. Ribbens, & J. McNamara (Eds.), *Psychological aspects of facial form*. Ann Arbor: University of Michigan Press.

Comer, R., and Piliavin, J. (1972). The effects of physical deviance upon face-to-face interaction: The other side. *Journal of Personality and Social Psychology*, *23*, 33–39.

Cook, S. (1939). The judgment of intelligence from photographs. *Journal of Abnormal and Social Psychology*, *34*, 384–389.

Cooley, C. (1912). *Human nature and social order*. New York: Scribners.

Corrigan, J., Dell, D., Lewis, K., and Schmidt, L. (1980). Counselling as a social influence process: A review. *Journal of Counselling Psychology*, *27*, 395–441.

Corter, C., Trehub, S., Boukydis, C., Ford, L., Celhoffer, L., and Minde, K. (1978). Nurses' judgments of the attractiveness of premature infants. *Infant Behavior and Development*, *1*, 373–380.

Courtois, M., and Mueller, J. (1981). Target and distractor typicality in facial recognition. *Journal of Applied Psychology*, *66*, 639–645.

Cox, N., and van der Linden, F. (1971). Facial harmony. *American Journal of Orthodontics*, *60*, 175–183.

Craik, F., and Lockhart, R. (1972). Levels of processing: A framework for memory research. *Journal of Verbal Learning and Verbal Behavior*, *11*, 671–684.

Critelli, J., and Waid, L. (1980). Physical attractiveness, romantic love and equity restoration in dating relationships. *Journal of Personality Assessment*, *44*, 624–629.

Cross, J., and Cross, J. (1971). Age, sex, race and the perception of facial beauty. *Developmental Psychology*, *5*, 433–439.

Cross, J., Cross, J., and Daly, J. (1971). Sex, race, age and beauty as factors in recognition of faces. *Perception and Psychophysics, 10,* 393–396.

Crouse, B., and Mehrabian, A. (1977). Affiliation of opposite-sexed strangers. *Journal of Research in Personality, 11,* 38–47.

Cunningham, J. (1976). Boys meet girls. *Journal of Personality and Social Psychology, 34,* 334–343.

Cunningham, M. (1986). Measuring the physical in physical attractiveness: Quasi-experiments in the sociobiology of female facial beauty. *Journal of Personality and Social Psychology, 50,* 925–935.

Curran, J. (1973). Correlates of physical attractiveness, and interpersonal attraction in the dating situation. *Social Behavior and Personality, 1,* 153–157.

Curran, J. (1975). Convergence toward a single sexual standard. *Social Behavior and Personality, 3,* 189–195.

Curran, J., and Lippold, S. (1975). The effects of physical attractiveness and attitude similarity on attraction in dating dyads. *Journal of Personality, 43,* 528–539.

Curran, J., Neff, S., and Lippold, S. (1973). Correlates of sexual experience. *Journal of Sex Research, 9,* 124–131.

Dabbs, J., and Stokes, N. (1975). Beauty is power: The use of space on the sidewalk. *Sociometry, 38,* 551–557.

Dane, F., and Wrightsman, L. (1982). Effects of defendants' and victims' characteristics. In N. Kerr & R. Bray (Eds.), *The psychology of the courtroom.* New York: Academic.

Darwin, C. (1871). *The descent of man, and selection in relation to sex.* London: John Murray.

Davies, G., Ellis, H., and Shepherd, J. (Eds.). (1981). *Perceiving and remembering faces.* London: Academic.

Davis, F. (1961). Deviance disavowal: The management of strained interaction by the visibly handicapped. *Social Problems, 9,* 120–132.

Deitz, S., Littman, M., and Bentley, M. (1984). Attribution of responsibility for rape: The influence of observer empathy, victim resistance, and victim attractiveness. *Sex Roles, 10,* 261–280.

De Jong, W., and Kleck, R. (1986). The social psychological effects of overweight. In C. Herman, M. Zanna, & E. Higgins (Eds.), *Physical appearance, stigma and social behavior.* Hillsdale, NJ: Erlbaum.

Demeis, D., and Turner, R. (1978). Effects of students' race, physical attractiveness, and dialect on teachers' evaluations. *Contemporary Educational Psychology, 3,* 77–86.

Dermer, M., and Thiel, D. (1975). When beauty may fail. *Journal of Personality and Social Psychology, 31,* 1168–1176.

Dion, K. (1972). Physical attractiveness and evaluation of childrens' transgressions. *Journal of Personality and Social Psychology, 24,* 207–213.

Dion, K. (1973). Young children's stereotyping of facial attractiveness. *Developmental Psychology, 9,* 183–188.

Dion, K. (1974). Children's physical attractiveness and sex as determinants of adult punitiveness. *Developmental Psychology, 10,* 772–778.

Dion, K. (1977). The incentive value of physical attractiveness for young children. *Personality and Social Psychology Bulletin, 3,* 67–70.

Dion, K., and Berscheid, E. (1974). Physical attractiveness and peer perception among children. *Sociometry, 37,* 1–12.

Dion, K., Berscheid, E., and Walster, E. (1972). What is beautiful is good. *Journal of Personality and Social Psychology, 24,* 285–290.

Dion, K., and Stein, S. (1978). Physical attractiveness and interpersonal influence. *Journal of Experimental Social Psychology, 14,* 97–108.

Dipboye, R., Arvey, R., and Terpstra, D. (1977). Sex and physical attractiveness of raters and applicants as determinants of resume evaluations. *Journal of Applied Psychology, 62*, 288–294.

Dipboye, R., Fromkin, H., and Wiback, K. (1975). Relative importance of applicant sex attractiveness and scholastic standing in evaluation of job applicant resumes. *Journal of Applied Psychology, 60*, 39–43.

Dixon, J. (1977). Coping with prejudice: Attitudes of handicapped persons towards the handicapped. *Journal of Chronic Diseases, 30*, 307–322.

Dobo, P. (1982). Using literature to change attitudes towards the handicapped. *Reading Teacher, 36*, 290–292.

Donaldson, J. (1981). The visibility and image of handicapped people on television. *Exceptional Children, 47*, 413–416.

Donaldson, J., and Martinson, M. (1977). Modifying attitudes toward physically disabled persons. *Exceptional Children, 43*, 337–341.

Donley, B., and Allen, B. (1977). Influences of experimenter attractiveness and ego-involvement on paired-associates learning. *Journal of Social Psychology, 101*, 151–152.

Doob, A., and Ecker, B. (1970). Stigma and compliance. *Journal of Personality and Social Psychology, 14*, 302–304.

Dosey, M., and Meisels, M. (1969). Personal space and self-protection. *Journal of Personality and Social Personality, 11*, 93–97.

Dunn, M. (1982). *Social relationships and interpersonal skills: A guide for people with sensory and physical limitations.* Falls Church, VA: Institute for Informational Studies.

Dunn, M., and Herman, S. (1982). Social skills and physical disability. In D. Doleys, R. Meredity, & A. Ciminero (Eds.), *Behavioral medicine: Assessment and treatment strategies.* New York: Plenum.

Dunn, M., van Horn, E., and Herman, S. (1981). Social skills and spinal cord injury: A comparison of three training procedures. *Behavior Therapy, 12*, 153–164.

Dushenko, T., Perry, R., Schilling, J., and Smolarski, S. (1978). Generality of the physical attractiveness stereotype for age and sex. *Journal of Social Psychology, 105*, 303–304.

Dutton, D., and Aron, A. (1974). Some evidence for heightened sexual attraction under conditions of high anxiety. *Journal of Personality and Social Psychology, 30*, 510–517.

Dziurawiec, S., and Ellis, H. (1986). Neonates' attention to face-like stimuli: A replication of the study by Goren, Sarty and Wu (1975). *Bulletin of the British Psychological Society, 39*, A137.

Easson, W. (1966). Psychopathological environmental reaction to congenital defect. *Journal of Nervous and Mental Disease, 142*, 453–459.

Edgemon, C., and Clopton, C. (1978). The relationship between physical attractiveness, personal effectiveness and self concept. *Psychosocial Rehabilitation Journal, 2*, 21–25.

Edgerton, M., and Knorr, N. (1971). Motivational patterns of patients seeking cosmetic (esthetic) surgery. *Plastic and Reconstructive Surgery, 48*, 551–557.

Efran, M. (1974). The effect of physical appearance on the judgment of guilt, interpersonal attraction, and severity of recommended punishment in a simulated jury task. *Journal of Research in Personality, 8*, 45–54.

Efran, M., and Patterson, E. (1974). Voters vote beautiful: The effect of physical appearance on a national debate. *Canadian Journal of Behavioral Science, 6*, 352–356.

Ekman, P. (1965). Differential communication of affect by head and body cues. *Journal of Personality and Social Psychology, 2*, 726–735.

Elder, G. (1969). Appearance and education in marriage mobility. *American Sociological Review, 34*, 519–333.

Elliott, M., Bull, R., James, D., and Lansdown, R. (1986). Children's and adults' reactions to photographs taken before and after facial surgery. *Journal of Maxillofacial Surgery*, *14*, 18–21.

Elliott, T., and Byrd, E. (1982). Media and disability. *Rehabilitation Literature*, *43*, 348–355.

Ellis, H., Jeeves, M., Newcombe, F., and Young, A. (Eds.). (1986). *Aspects of face processing*. Dordrecht, Holland: Nijhoff.

Elms, A. (1975). The crisis of confidence in social psychology. *American Psychologist*, *30*, 967–976.

Elovitz, G., and Salvia, J. (1982). Attractiveness as a biasing factor in the judgments of school psychologists. *Journal of School Psychology*, *20*, 339–345.

Farina, A., Fischer, E., Sherman, S., Smith, W., Groh, T., and Mermin, P. (1977). Physical attractiveness and mental illness. *Journal of Abnormal Psychology*, *86*, 510–517.

Farina, A., Sherman, M., and Allen, J. (1968). Role of physical abnormalities in interpersonal perception and behavior. *Journal of Abnormal Psychology*, *73*, 590–593.

Feild, H. (1979). Rape trials and jurors' decisions. *Law and Human Behavior*, *3*, 261–284.

Feingold, A. (1981). Testing equity as an explanation for romantic couples "mismatched" on physical attractiveness. *Psychological Reports*, *49*, 247–250.

Feingold, A. (1982a). Do taller men have prettier girlfriends? *Psychological Reports*, *50*, 810.

Feingold, A. (1982b). Physical attractiveness and intelligence. *Journal of Social Psychology*, *118*, 283–284.

Feinman, S., and Gill, G. (1977). Females' responses to males' beardedness. *Perceptual and Motor Skills*, *44*, 533–534.

Feinman, S., and Gill, G. (1978). Sex differences in physical attractiveness preferences. *Journal of Social Psychology*, *105*, 43–52.

Felson, R. (1980). Physical attractiveness, grades and teachers' attributions. *Representative Research in Social Psychology*, *11*, 64–71.

Felson, R. (1981). Physical attractiveness and perceptions of deviance. *Journal of Social Psychology*, *114*, 85–89.

Felson, R., and Bohrnstedt, G. (1979). Are the good beautiful or the beautiful good? *Social Psychology Quarterly*, *42*, 386–392.

Fensterheim, H., and Tresselt, M. (1953). The influence of value systems on the perception of people. *Journal of Abnormal and Social Psychology*, *48*, 93–98.

Festinger, L. (1957). *A theory of cognitive dissonance*. London: Tavistock Publications.

Fleishman, J., Buckley, M., Klosinsky, M., Smith, N., and Tuck, B. (1976). Judged attractiveness in recognition memory of women's faces. *Perceptual and Motor Skills*, *43*, 709–710.

Folkes, V. (1982). Forming relationships and the matching hypothesis. *Personality and Social Psychology Bulletin*, *8*, 631–636.

Freedman, D. (1969). The survival value of the beard. *Psychology Today*, *3*, 36–39.

Friend, R., and Vinson, M. (1974). Learning over backwards: Jurors' responses to defendants' attractiveness. *Journal of Communication*, *24*, 124–129.

Frodi, A., Lamb, M., Leavitt, L., Donovan, W., Neff, L., and Sherry, D. (1978). Fathers' and mothers' responses to the faces and cries of normal and premature infants. *Developmental Psychology*, *14*, 490–498.

Fugita, S., Agle, T. Newman, I., and Walfish, N. (1977). Attractiveness, self concept and a methodological note about gaze behavior. *Personality and Social Psychology Bulletin*, *3*, 240–243.

Fugita, S., Panek, P., Balascoe, L., and Newman, I. (1977). Attractiveness, level of accomplishment, sex of rater, and the evaluation of feminine competence. *Representative Research in Social Psychology, 8*, 1–11.

Gallucci, N., and Meyer, R. (1984). People can be too perfect: Effect of subjects' and targets' attractiveness on interpersonal attraction. *Psychological Reports, 55*, 351–360.

Galton, F. (1907). *Inquiries into human faculty and its development* (2nd ed.). New York: Elsevier North Holland.

Geiselman, R., Haight, N., and Kimata, L. (1984). Context effects on the perceived physical attractiveness of faces. *Journal of Experimental Social Psychology, 20*, 409–424.

Gellman, W. (1974). Projections in the field of physical disability. *Rehabilitation Literature, 35*, 2–9.

Gerbasi, K., Zuckerman, M., and Reis, H. (1977). Justice needs a new blindfold: A review of mock jury research. *Psychological Bulletin, 84*, 323–345.

Gergen, K. (1975). *Experimental paradigm: Death and transfiguration.* Paper presented at the Annual Convention of the American Psychological Association, Chicago.

Gibbons, S., Stephan, W., Stephenson, B., and Petty, C. (1980). Reactions to stigmatized others: Response amplification vs. sympathy. *Journal of Experimental Social Psychology, 16*, 591–605.

Gillen, B. (1981). Physical attractiveness as a determinant of two types of goodness. *Personality and Social Psychology Bulletin, 7*, 277–281.

Glasgow, R., and Arkowitz, H. (1975). The behavioral assessment of male and female social competence in dyadic heterosexual interactions. *Behavior Therapy, 6*, 488–498.

Glenwick, D., Jason, L., and Elman, D. (1978). Physical attractiveness and social contact in singles bars. *Journal of Social Psychology, 105*, 311–312.

Goebel, B., and Cashen, V. (1979). Age, sex and attractiveness as factors in student ratings of teachers. *Journal of Educational Psychology, 71*, 646–653.

Goffman, E. (1963). *Stigma: Notes on the management of spoiled identity.* Englewood Cliffs, NJ: Prentice Hall.

Goffman, E. (1971). *Relations in public: Microstudies of the public order.* London: Allen Lane.

Going, M., and Read, J. (1974). Effects of uniqueness, sex of subject, and sex of photograph on facial recognition. *Perceptual and Motor Skills, 39*, 109–110.

Goldberg, P., Bernstein, N., and Crosby, R. (1975). Vocational development of adolescents with burn injury. *Rehabilitation Counseling Bulletin, 18*, 140–146.

Goldberg, P., Gottesdiener, M., and Abramson, P. (1975). Another put-down of women? Perceived attractiveness as a function of support for the feminist movement. *Journal of Personality and Social Psychology, 32*, 113–115.

Goldman, W., and Lewis, P. (1977). Beautiful is good: Evidence that the physically attractive are most socially skilful. *Journal of Experimental Social Psychology, 13*, 125–130.

Goldring, P. (1967). Role of distance and posture in the evaluation of interactions. In *Proceedings of the 75th Annual Convention of the American Psychological Association, 2*, 343–344.

Goldstein, A. (1983). Behavioral scientists' fascination with faces. *Journal of Nonverbal Behavior, 7*, 223–255.

Goldstein, A., Chance, J., and Gilbert, B. (1984). Facial stereotypes of good guys and bad guys: A replication and extension. *Bulletin of the Psychonomic Society, 22*, 549–552.

Goren, C., Sarty, M., and Wu, P. (1975). Visual following and pattern discrimination of face-like stimuli by newborn infants. *Pediatrics, 56*, 544–549.

Graber, L. (1980). Psychological considerations of orthodontic treatment. In G. Lucker, K. Ribbens, and J. McNamara (Eds.), *Psychological aspects of facial form*. Ann Arbor: University of Michigan Press.

Graham, J. (1985). Overview of the psychology of cosmetics. In J. Graham & A. Kligman (Eds.), *The psychology of cosmetic treatments*. New York: Praeger.

Graham, J., and Jouhar, A. (1980). Cosmetics considered in the context of physical attractiveness. *International Journal of Cosmetic Science, 2*, 77–101.

Graham, J., and Jouhar, A. (1981). The effects of cosmetics on person perception. *International Journal of Cosmetic Science, 3*, 199–210.

Greenwald, M. (1981). The effects of physical attractiveness, experience, and social performance on employer decision-making in job interviews. *Behavioral Counseling Quarterly, 1*, 275–287.

Greenwald, R. (1975). Consequences of prejudice against the null hypothesis. *Psychological Bulletin, 82*, 1–19.

Gresham, F. (1981). Social skills training with handicapped children: A review. *Review of Educational Research, 51*, 139–176.

Gross, A. (1975). Generosity and legitimacy of a model as determinants of helpful behavior. *Representative Research in Social Psychology, 6*, 45–50.

Gross, A., and Crofton, C. (1977). What is good is beautiful? *Sociometry, 40*, 85–90.

Haaf, R. (1974). Complexity and facial resemblance as determinants of response to facelike stimuli by 5- and 10-week old infants. *Journal of Experimental Child Psychology, 18*, 480–487.

Haaf, R. (1977). Visual response to complex facelike patterns by 15- and 20-week old infants. *Developmental Psychology, 13*, 77–78.

Haaf, R., and Bell, R. (1967). A facial dimension in visual discrimination by human infants. *Child Development, 38*, 893–899.

Haefner, J. (1976). Can TV advertising influence employers to hire or train disadvantaged persons? *Journalism Quarterly, 53*, 95–102.

Hafer, M., and Narcus, M. (1979). Information and attitudes toward disability. *Rehabilitation Counseling Bulletin, 23*, 95–102.

Hagiwara, S. (1975). Visual versus verbal information in impression formation. *Journal of Personality and Social Psychology, 32*, 692–698.

Hall, E. (1959). *The silent language*. Garden City, NY: Doubleday.

Halverson, C., and Waldrop, M. (1976). Relations between preschool activity and aspects of intellectual and social behavior at age 7. *Developmental Psychology, 12*, 107–112.

Handlers, A., and Austin, K. (1980). Improving attitudes of high school students toward their handicapped peers. *Exceptional Children, 47*, 228–229.

Hansell, S., Sparacino, J., and Ronchi, D. (1982). Physical attractiveness and blood pressure: Sex and age differences. *Personality and Social Psychology Bulletin, 8*, 113–121.

Harper, D., and Richman, L. (1978). Personality profiles of physically impaired adolescents. *Journal of Clinical Psychology, 34*, 636–642.

Harper, R., Wiens, A., and Matarazzo, J. (1978). *Nonverbal communication: The state of the art*. New York: Wiley.

Harrell, W. (1978). Physical attractiveness, self-disclosure and helping behavior. *Journal of Social Psychology, 104*, 15–18.

Harris, R., and Harris, A. (1977). A new perspective on the psychological effects of environmental barriers. *Rehabilitation Literature, 38*, 75–78.

Harrison, A., and Saeed, L. (1977). Let's make a deal: An analysis of revelations and stipulations in lonely hearts advertisements. *Journal of Personality and Social Psychology, 35*, 257–264.

Hartjen, C. (1972). Police-citizen encounters: Social order in interpersonal interaction. *Criminology, 10*, 61–84.

Hartnett, J., and Elder, D. (1973). The princess and the nice frog: Study in person perception. *Perceptual and Motor Skills*, *37*, 863–866.

Hartnett, J., Gottlieb, J., and Hayes, R. (1976). Social facilitation theory and experimenter attractiveness. *Journal of Social Psychology*, *99*, 293–294.

Hastorf, A., Northercraft, G., and Picciotto, S. (1979). Helping the handicapped. *Personality and Social Psychology Bulletin*, *5*, 373–376.

Hastorf, A., Wildfogel, J., and Cassman, T. (1979). Acknowledgment of handicap as a tactic in social interaction. *Journal of Personality and Social Psychology*, *37*, 1790–1797.

Hatfield, E., and Sprecher, S. (1986). *Mirror, mirror. . . : The importance of looks in everyday life*. Albany: State University of New York.

Hay, G. (1970). Psychiatric aspects of cosmetic nasal operations. *British Journal of Psychiatry*, *116*, 85–97.

Hebb, D. (1974). What psychology is about. *American Psychologist*, *29*, 71–79.

Heese, G. (1975). The handicapped in literature. *Heilpadagogik*, *44*, 204–209.

Heider, F. (1958). *The psychology of interpersonal relationships*. New York: Wiley.

Heilman, M., and Saruwatari, L. (1979). When beauty is beastly. *Organizational Behavior and Human Performance*, *23*, 360–372.

Heilman, M., and Stopeck, M. (1985a). Being attractive, advantage or disadvantage? Performance-based evaluations and recommended personnel actions as a function of appearance, sex and job type. *Organizational Behavior and Human Decision Processes*, *35*, 202–215.

Heilman, M., and Stopeck, M. (1985b). Attractiveness and corporate success: Different causal attributions for males and females. *Journal of Applied Psychology*, *70*, 379–388.

Heimberg, R., Montgomery, D., Madsen, C., and Heimberg, J. (1977). Assertion training: A review of the literature. *Behavior Therapy*, *8*, 953–971.

Heinemann, W., Pellander, F., Vogelbusch, A., and Wojtek, B. (1981). Meeting a deviant person: Subjective norms and affective reactions. *European Journal of Social Psychology*, *11*, 1–25.

Helm, S., Kreiborg, S., and Solow, B. (1985). Psychological implications of malocclusion: A 15-year follow-up study in 30-year-old Danes. *American Journal of Orthodontics*, *78*, 110–118.

Herman, C., Zanna, M., and Higgins, E. (1986). *Physical appearance, stigma, and social behavior*. Hillsdale, NJ: Lawrence Erlbaum.

Hess, E. (1975). The role of pupil size in communication. *Scientific American*, *233*, 110–119.

Hewett, S. (1970). *The family and the handicapped child*. London: Allen & Unwin.

Hicks, R., Evans, E., Martin, R., and Moore, J. (1978). Test anxiety and pupil size. *Polygraph*, *7*, 101–105.

Hicks, R., McNicholas, G., and Armogida, R. (1981). Iride pigmentation, sex and type A behavior. *Psychological Record*, *31*, 43–46.

Hicks, R., Pellegrini, R., and Tomlinson, N. (1978). Attributions of female college students to male photographs as a function of attractiveness and pupil size. *Perceptual and Motor Skills*, *47*, 1265–1266.

Hicks, R., Reaney, H., and Hill, L. (1967). Effects of pupil size and facial angle on preference for photographs of a young woman. *Perceptual and Motor Skills*, *24*, 388–390.

Hicks, R., Williams, S., and Ferrante, F. (1979a). Pupillary attributions of college students to happy and angry faces. *Perceptual and Motor Skills*, *48*, 401–402.

Hicks, R., Williams, S., and Ferrante, F. (1979b). Eye color and the pupillary attributions of college students to happy and angry faces. *Bulletin of the Psychonomic Society*, *13*, 55–56.

Hildebrandt, K. (1982). The role of physical appearance in infant and child development. In H. Fitzgerald, B. Lester, & M. Yogman (Eds.), *Theory and research in behavioral pediatrics* (Vol. 1). New York: Plenum.

Hildebrandt, K. (1983). Effects of facial expression variations on ratings of infants' physical attractiveness. *Developmental Psychology, 19,* 414–417.

Hildebrandt, K., and Fitzgerald, H. (1978). Adults' responses to infants varying in perceived cuteness. *Behavioral Processes, 3,* 159–172.

Hildebrandt, K., and Fitzgerald, H. (1979). Facial feature determinants of perceived infant attractiveness. *Infant Behavior and Development, 2,* 329–339.

Hildebrandt, K., and Fitzgerald, H. (1983). The infant's physical attractiveness: Its effect on bonding and attachment. *Infant Mental Health Journal, 4,* 3–12.

Hill, C., Rubin, Z., and Peplau, L. (1976). Breakups before marriage: The end of 103 affairs. *Journal of Social Issues, 32,* 147–168.

Hill, M., and Lando, H. (1976). Physical attractiveness and sex-role stereotypes in impression formation. *Perceptual and Motor Skills, 43,* 1251–1255.

Himmelfarb, S., and Fishbein, M. (1971). Studies in the perception of ethnic group members: II. Attractiveness, response bias, and anti-semitism. *Journal of Social Psychology, 83,* 289–298.

Hirschenfang, M., Goldberg, M., and Benton, J. (1969). Psychological aspects of patients with facial paralysis. *Diseases of the Nervous System, 30,* 257–261.

Hobfoil, S., and Penner, L. (1978). Effect of physical attractiveness on therapists' initial judgments of a person's self-concept. *Journal of Consulting and Clinical Psychology, 46,* 200–201.

Hocking, J., Walker, B., and Fink, E. (1982). Physical attractiveness and judgments of morality following an "immoral" act. *Psychological Reports, 51,* 111–116.

Hoffman, S. (1968). An empirical study of representational hand movements. *Dissertation Abstracts International, 28,* 4379B.

Holahan, C., and Stephan, C. (1981). When beauty isn't talent: The influence of physical attractiveness, attitudes towards women, and competence on impression formation. *Sex Roles, 7,* 867–876.

Holmes, S., and Hatch, C. (1938). Personal appearance as related to scholastic records and marriage selection in college women. *Human Biology, 10,* 65–76.

Horai, J., Naccari, N., and Fatoullah, E. (1974). The effects of experience and physical attractiveness upon opinion agreement and liking. *Sociometry, 36,* 601–606.

Hore, T. (1971). Assessment of teaching practice: An "attractive" hypothesis. *British Journal of Educational Psychology, 41,* 327–328.

Hornstein, H., Fisch, E., and Holmes, M. (1968). Influence of a model's feeling about his behavior and his relevance as a comparison other on observers' helping behavior. *Journal of Personality and Social Psychology, 10,* 222–226.

Horowitz, L., and French, R. (1979). Interpersonal problems of people who describe themselves as lonely, *Journal and Counseling and Clinical Psychology, 47,* 462–464.

Howard, C., Cohen, S., and Cavior, N. (1974). More results on increasing the persuasiveness of a low prestige communicator: The effects of the communicator's physical attractiveness and sex of the receiver. *Personality and Social Psychology Bulletin, 1,* 393–395.

Hoyt, J. (1978). Feeling free. *American Education, 14,* 24–28.

Husain, A., and Kureshi, A. (1983). Opposite-sex attraction as a function of perceiver's self-evaluation and physical attractiveness of the perceiver and perceived. *Personality Study and Group Behavior, 3,* 35–42.

Husband, R. (1934). The photograph on the application blank. *Personnel Journal, 13,* 69–72.

Huston, T. (1973). Ambiguity of acceptance, social desirability, and dating choice. *Journal of Experimental Social Psychology, 9,* 32–42.

Huston, T., and Levinger, G. (1978). Interpersonal attraction and relationships. *Annual Review of Psychology, 29,* 115–156.

Ibrahim, F., and Herr, E. (1982). Modification of attitudes toward disability: Differential effect of two educational models. *Rehabilitation Counselling Bulletin*, *26*, 29–36.

Iliffe, A. (1960). A study of preferences in feminine beauty. *British Journal of Psychology*, *51*, 267–273.

Innes, J., and Gilroy, S. (1980). The semantics of asking a favor: Asking for help in three countries. *Journal of Social Psychology*, *110*, 3–7.

Irilli, J. (1978). *Students' expectations: Ratings of teacher performance as biased by teachers' physical attractiveness*. Paper presented at the Annual Meeting of the American Educational Research Association, Toronto.

Izzett, R., and Fishman, L. (1976). Defendant sentences as a function of attractiveness and justifications for actions. *Journal of Social Psychology*, *100*, 285–290.

Izzett, R., and Sales, B. (1979). Person perception and jurors' reactions to defendants: An equity theory explanation. In B. Sales (Ed.), *Perspectives in law and psychology. Vol. 2: The jury, judicial and trial processes*. New York: Plenum.

Jackson, D., and Huston, T. (1975). Physical attractiveness and assertiveness. *Journal of Social Psychology*, *96*, 79–84.

Jackson, L. (1983a). The influence of sex, physical attractiveness, sex role, and occupational sex-linkage on perceptions of occupational suitability. *Journal of Applied Social Psychology*, *13*, 31–44.

Jackson, L. (1983b). Gender, physical attractiveness, and sex role in occupational treatment discrimination: The influence of trait and role assumptions. *Journal of Applied Social Psychology*, *13*, 443–458.

Jacobson, M., and Koch, W. (1978). Attributed reasons for support of the feminist movement as a function of attractiveness. *Sex Roles*, *4*, 169–174.

Jacobson, S., and Berger, C. (1974). Communication and justice: Defendant attributes and their effects on the severity of his sentence. *Speech Monographs*, *41*, 282–286.

Jacobson, W., Edgerton, M., Meyer, E., Canter, A., and Slaughter, R. (1961). Psychiatric evaluation of male patients seeking cosmetic surgery. *Plastic and Reconstructive Surgery*, *26*, 356–372.

Jahoda, G. (1954). Political attitudes and judgments of other people. *Journal of Abnormal and Social Psychology*, *49*, 331–334.

Jenny, J. (1975). A social perspective on need and demand for orthodontic treatment. *International Dental Journal*, *25*, 248–256.

Jensen, S. (1978). The psychosocial dimensions of oral and maxillofacial surgery: A critical review of the literature. *Journal of Oral Surgery*, *36*, 447–453.

Johnson, D. (1985). Appearance and the elderly. In J. Graham & A. Kligman (Eds.), *The psychology of cosmetic treatments*. New York: Praeger.

Johnson, R. (1981). Perceived physical attractiveness of supporters of Canada's political parties. Stereotype or in-group bias? *Canadian Journal of Behavioral Science*, *13*, 320–325.

Johnson, R., Dannenbring, G., Anderson, N., and Villa, R. (1983). How different cultural and geographic groups perceive the attractiveness of active and inactive feminists. *Journal of Social Psychology*, *119*, 111–117.

Johnson, R., Doiron, D., Brooks, G., and Dickinson, J. (1978). Perceived attractiveness as a function of support for the feminist movement. *Canadian Journal of Behavioral Science*, *10*, 214–221.

Johnson, R., Holborn, S., and Turcotte, S. (1979). Perceived attractiveness as a function of active vs. passive support for the feminist movement. *Personality and Social Psychology Bulletin*, *5*, 227–230.

Jones, Q., and Moyel, I. (1971). The influence of iris color and pupil size on experienced affect. *Psychonomic Science*, *23*, 126–127.

Jones, R. (1982). Perceiving other people: Stereotyping as a process of social cognition. In A. Miller (Ed.), *In the eye of the beholder: Contemporary issues in stereotyping*. New York: Praeger.

Jones, R., and Adams, G. (1982). Assessing the importance of physical attractiveness across the life-span. *Journal of Social Psychology*, *118*, 131–132.

Jones, T., Sorrell, V., Jones, J., and Butler, L. (1981). Changing children's perceptions of handicapped people. *Exceptional Children*, *47*, 365–368.

Jones, W., Hansson, R., and Phillips, A. (1978). Physical attractiveness and judgments of psychopathology. *Journal of Social Psychology*, *105*, 79–84.

Jones, W., Hobbs, S., and Hockenbury, D. (1982). Loneliness and social skill deficits. *Journal of Personality and Social Psychology*, *42*, 682–689.

Jones-Molfese, V. (1975). Preferences of infants for regular and distorted facial stimuli. *Child Development*, *46*, 1005–1009.

Joseph, W. (1982). The credibility of physically attractive communicators: A review. *Journal of Advertising*, *11*, 15–24.

Kaats, C., and Davis, K. (1970). The dynamics of sexual behavior of college students. *Journal of Marriage and the Family*, *32*, 390–399.

Kagan, J., Henker, B., Hen-Tov, A., Levine, J., and Lewis, M. (1966). Infants' differential reactions to familiar and distorted faces. *Child Development*, *3*, 519–532.

Kahle, L., and Homer, P. (1985). Physical attractiveness of the celebrity endorser: A social adaptation perspective. *Journal of Consumer Research*, *11*, 954–961.

Kahneman, D., and Tversky, A. (1973). On the psychology of prediction. *Psychological Review*, *80*, 237–251.

Kalick, S. (1977). *Plastic surgery, physical appearance and person perception*. Doctoral dissertation, Harvard University, Cambridge, MA.

Kalick, S. (1982). Clinician, social scientist and body image: Collaboration and future prospects. *Clinics In Plastic Surgery*, *9*, 379–385.

Kalick, S., and Hamilton, T. (1986). The matching hypothesis re-examined. *Journal Personality and Social Psychology*, *51*, 673–682.

Kanekar, S., and Kolsawalla, M. (1980). Responsibility of a rape victim in relation to her respectibility, attractiveness, and provocativeness. *Journal of Social Psychology*, *112*, 153–154.

Kanfer, F. (1960). Verbal rate, eyeblink and content in structured psychiatric interviews. *Journal of Abnormal and Social Psychology*, *61*, 341–347.

Kaplan, R. (1978). Is beauty talent? Sex interaction in the attractiveness halo effect. *Sex Roles*, *4*, 195–204.

Kapp, K. (1979). Self concept of the child with cleft lip and/or palate. *Cleft Palate Journal*, *16*, 171–176.

Kapp-Simon, K. (1980). Psychological adaptation of patients with craniofacial malformations. In G. Lucker, K. Ribbens, & J. McNamara (Eds.), *Psychological aspects of facial form*. Ann Arbor: University of Michigan Press.

Kassarjian, H. (1963). Voting intention and political perception. *Journal of Psychology*, *56*, 85–88.

Katz, I. (1981). *Stigma: A social psychological analysis*. Hillsdale, NJ: Lawrence Erlbaum.

Katz, S., and Shurka, M. (1977). The influence of contextual variables on evaluation of the physically disabled by the nondisabled. *Rehabilitation Literature*, *38*, 369–373.

Katz, S., Shurka, E., and Florian, V. (1978). The relationship between physical disability, social perception and psychological stress. *Scandinavian Journal of Rehabilitation Medicine*, *10*, 109–113.

Kehle, T., Bramble, W., and Mason, E. (1974). Teachers' expectations: Ratings of student performance. *Journal of Experimental Education*, *43*, 54–60.

Kellerman, J., and Laird, J. (1982). The effect of appearance on self-perceptions. *Journal of Personality*, *50*, 296–315.

Kelley, H. (1971). *Attribution in social psychology*. Morristown, NJ: General Learning Press.

Kemp, A. (1982, March 24). *The Guardian*.

Kendon, A. (1967). Some functions of gaze-direction in social interaction. *Acta Psychologica, 26*, 22–63.

Kenny, C., and Fletcher, D. (1973). Effects of beardedness on person perception. *Perceptual and Motor Skills, 37*, 413–414.

Kenrick, D., and Gutierres, S. (1980). Contrast effects and judgments of physical attractiveness: When beauty becomes a social problem. *Journal of Personality and Social Psychology, 38*, 131–140.

Kerber, K., and Coles, M. (1978). The role of perceived physiological activity in affective judgments. *Journal of Experimental Social Psychology, 14*, 419–433.

Kernis, M., and Wheeler, L. (1981). Beautiful friends and ugly strangers: Radiation and contrast effects in perception of same-sex pairs. *Personality and Social Psychology Bulletin, 7*, 617–620.

Kerr, N. (1978). Beautiful and blameless: Effects of victim attractiveness and responsibility on mock jurors' verdicts. *Personality and Social Psychology Bulletin, 4*, 479–482.

Kerr, N. (1982). Trial participants' behaviors and jury verdicts: An exploratory field study. In V. Konecni & E. Ebbesen (Eds.), *The criminal justice system: A social-psychological analysis*. San Francisco: Freeman.

Kerr, N., Bull, R., MacCoun, R., and Rathborn, H. (1985). Effects of victim attractiveness, care and disfigurement on the judgements of American and British mock jurors. *British Journal of Social Psychology, 24*, 47–58.

Kiesler, S., and Baral, R. (1970). The search for a romantic partner: The effects of self-esteem and physical attractiveness on romantic behavior. In K. Kergen & D. Marlowe (Eds.), *Personality and social behavior*. New York: Addison-Wesley.

King, M. (1986). *Psychology in and out of court*. Oxford, England: Pergamon.

Kirkland, J., and Smith, J. (1978). Preferences for infant pictures with modified eye-pupils. *Journal of Biological Psychology, 20*, 33–34.

Kirkpatrick, C., and Cotton, J. (1951). Physical attractiveness, age and marital adjustment. *American Sociological Review, 16*, 81–86.

Klatzky, R., Martin, G., and Kane, R. (1982). Semantic interpretation effects on memory for faces. *Memory and Cognition, 10*, 195–206.

Kleck, R. (1969). Physical stigma and task oriented interactions. *Human Relations, 22*, 53–60.

Kleck, R. (1970). Interaction distance and nonverbal agreeing responses. *British Journal of Social and Clinical Psychology, 9*, 180–182.

Kleck, R., Buck, P., Goller, W., London, R., Pfeiffer, J., and Vukcevic, D. (1968). Effect of stigmatizing conditions on the use of personal space. *Psychological Reports, 23*, 111–118.

Kleck, R., and Nuessle, W. (1968). Congruence between the indicative and communicative functions of eye contact in interpersonal relations. *British Journal of Social and Clinical Psychology, 7*, 241–246.

Kleck, R., Ono, H., and Hastorf, A. (1966). The effects of physical deviance upon face-to-face interaction. *Human Relations, 19*, 425–436.

Kleck, R., and Rubenstein, C. (1975). Physical attractiveness, perceived attitude similarity, and interpersonal attraction in an opposite-sex encounter. *Journal of Personality and Social Psychology, 31*, 107–114.

Kleck, R., and Strenta, A. (1980). Perceptions of the impact of negatively valued physical characteristics on social interaction. *Journal of Personality and Social Psychology, 39*, 861–873.

Kleck, R., and Strenta, A. (1985a). Physical deviance and the perception of social outcomes. In J. Graham & A. Kligman (Eds.), *The psychology of cosmetic treatments*. New York: Praeger.

Kleck, R., and Strenta, A. (1985b). Gender and responses to disfigurement in self and others. *Journal of Social and Clinical Psychology, 3*, 257–267.

Kleinke, C. (1974). *First impressions: The psychology of encountering others*. Englewood Cliffs, NJ: Prentice Hall.

Kleinke, C., Staneski, R., and Pipp, S. (1975). Effects of gaze, distance, and attractiveness on males' first impressions of females. *Representative Research in Social Psychology*, 6, 7–12.

Kligman, A. (1985). Medical aspects of skin and its appearance. In J. Graham & A. Kligman (Eds.). *The psychology of cosmetic treatments*. New York: Prager.

Knapp, M. (1985). The study of physical appearance and cosmetics in western culture. In J. Graham and A. Kligman (Eds.), *The psychology of cosmetic treatments*. New York: Praeger.

Knorr, N., Edgerton, M., and Hoopes, J. (1967). The "insatiable" cosmetic surgery patient. *Plastic and Reconstructive Surgery*, 40, 285–289.

Kollar, M. (1974). The beautiful is rotten phenomenon: A negative stereotype of physical attraction. *Dissertation Abstracts International*, 34, 4632.

Korabik, K. (1981). Changes in physical attractiveness and interpersonal attraction. *Basic and Applied Social Psychology*, 2, 59–65.

Kozeny, E. (1962). Experimental investigation of physiognomy utilizing a photographic-statistical method. *Archiv fur die Gesamte Psychologie*, 114, 55–71.

Krebs, D., and Adinolfi, A. (1975). Physical attractiveness, social relations, and personality style. *Journal of Personality and Social Psychology*, 31, 245–253.

Kulka, R., and Kessler, J. (1978). Is justice really blind? *Journal of Applied Social Psychology*, 8, 366–381.

Kupke, T., Calhoun, K., and Hobbs, S. (1979). Selection of heterosocial skills, II: Experimental validity. *Behavior Therapy*, 10, 336–346.

Kupke, T., Hobbs, S., and Cheney, T. (1979). Selection of heterosexual skills, I: Criteria related validity. *Behavior Therapy*, 10, 327–335.

Kurtzberg, R., Lewin, M., Cavior, N., and Lipton, D. (1967). Psychologic screening of inmates requesting cosmetic operations: A preliminary report. *Plastic and Reconstructive Surgery*, 39, 387–396.

Kurtzberg, R., Safar, H., and Cavior, N. (1968). Surgical and social rehabilitation of adult offenders. *Proceedings of the 76th Annual Convention of the American Psychological Association*, 3, 649–650.

Lakoff, R., and Scherr, R. (1984). *Face value: The politics of beauty*. Boston: Routledge and Kegan Paul.

Lampel A., and Anderson, N. (1968). Combining visual and verbal information in an impression-formation task. *Journal of Personality and Social Psychology*, 9, 1–6.

Landy, D., and Aronson, E. (1969). The influence of the character of the criminal and his victim on the decisions of simulated jurors. *Journal of Experimental Social Psychology*, 5, 141–152.

Landy, D., and Sigall, H. (1974). Beauty is talent: Task evaluation as a function of the performer's physical attractiveness. *Journal of Personality and Social Psychology*, 29, 299–304.

Lange, A., and Jakubowski, P. (1976). *Responsible assertive behavior*. Champaign, IL: Research Press.

Langer, E., Fiske, S., Taylor, S., and Chanowitz, B. (1976). Stigma, staring and discomfort: A novel-stimulus hypothesis. *Journal of Experimental Social Psychology*, 12, 451–463.

Langlois, J. (1986). From the eye of the beholder to behavioral reality: Development of social behaviors and social relations as a function of physical attractiveness. In C. Herman, M. Zanna, & E. Higgins (Eds.), *Physical appearance, stigma, and social behavior*. Hillsdale, NJ: Lawrence Erlbaum.

Langlois, J., and Casey, R. (1984). *Baby beautiful: The relationship between infant physical attractiveness and maternal behavior*. Paper presented at the fourth biennial International Conference on Infant Studies, New York.

Langlois, J., and Downs, A. (1979). Peer relations as a function of physical attractiveness. *Child Development*, 50, 409–418.

Langlois, J., and Stephan, C. (1977). The effects of physical attractiveness and ethnicity on children's behavioral attributions and peer preferences. *Child Development*, *48*, 1694–1698.

Langlois, J., and Stephan, C. (1981). Beauty and the beast: The role of physical attractiveness in the development of peer relations and social behavior. In S. Brehm, S. Kassin, & F. Gibbons (Eds.), *Developmental social psychology: Theory and research*. New York: Oxford University Press.

Langlois, J., and Styczynski, L. (1979). The effects of physical attractiveness on the behavioral attributions and peer preferences of acquainted children. *International Journal of Behavioral Development*, *2*, 325–341.

Lansdown, R. (1976). *The psychological management of children with a facial deformity*. (Available from the author, The Hospital for Sick Children, Great Ormond Street, London, U.K.).

Lansdown, R. (1981). Cleft lip and palate: A prediction of psychological disfigurement. *British Journal of Orthodontics*, *8*, 83–88.

Larrance, D., and Zuckerman, M. (1981). Facial attractiveness and vocal likeability as determinants of nonverbal sending skills. *Journal of Personality*, *49*, 349–362.

La Voie, J., and Adams, G. (1974). Teaching expectancy and its relation to physical and interpersonal characteristics of the child. *Alberta Journal of Educational Research*, *20*, 122–132.

La Voie, J., and Adams, G. (1978). Physical and interpersonal attractiveness of model and imitation in adults. *Journal of Social Psychology*, *106*, 191–202.

Lawson, E. (1971). Hair color, personality and the observer. *Psychological Reports*, *28*, 311–322.

Lee, L., Adams, G., and Dobson, W. (1984). Male and female attributions and social influence behavior towards a physically attractive female. *Journal of Psychology*, *117*, 97–103.

Lefebvre, A., and Munro, I. (1978). The role of psychiatry in a cranio facial team. *Plastic and Reconstructive Surgery*, *61*, 564.

Lefebvre, A., Travis, F., Arndt, E., and Munro, I. (1986). A psychiatric profile before and after reconstructive surgery in children with Apert's syndrome. *British Journal of Plastic Surgery*, *39*, 510–513.

Leonard, B. (1978). *Impaired view: Television portrayal of handicapped people*. Unpublished doctoral dissertation, Boston University, Boston, MA.

Lerner, M. (1970). The desire for justice and reactions to victims. In J. Macaulay & L. Berkowitz (Eds.), *Altruism and helping behavior*. New York: Academic Press.

Lerner, R., and Lerner, J. (1977). Effects of age, sex and physical attractiveness on child-peer relations, academic performance, and elementary school adjustment. *Developmental Psychology*, *13*, 585–590.

Leventhal, G., and Krate, R. (1977). Physical attractiveness and severity of sentencing. *Psychological Reports*, *40*, 315–318.

Levitt, L., and Kornhaber, R. (1977). Stigma and compliance: A re-examination. *Journal of Social Psychology*, *103*, 13–18.

Lewis, K., and Walsh, W. (1978). Physical attractiveness: Its impact on the perception of a female counselor. *Journal of Counseling Psychology*, *25*, 210–216.

Lewis, M. (1969). Infants' responses to facial stimuli during the first year of life. *Developmental Psychology*, *1*, 75–86.

Lewison, E. (1974). Twenty years of prison surgery: An evaluation. *Canadian Journal of Otolaryngology*, *3*, 42–50.

Lewit, D., and Virolainen, K. (1968). Conformity and independence in adolescents' motivation for orthodontic treatment. *Child Development*, *39*, 1189–1200.

Libet, J., and Lewinsohn, P. (1973). Concept of social skill with special reference to the behavior of depressed persons. *Journal of Consulting and Clinical Psychology*, *40*, 304–312.

Liebert, R. (1975). *Television and attitudes toward the handicapped.* Albany, NY: New York State Education Department.

Liggett, J. (1974). *The human face.* London: Constable.

Light, L., Hollander, S., and Kayra-Stuart, F. (1981). Why attractive people are harder to remember. *Personality and Social Psychology Bulletin, 7,* 269–276.

Linn, E. (1966). Social meanings of dental appearance. *Journal of Health and Social Behavior, 7,* 289–295.

Lipson, A., Przybyla, D., and Byrne, D. (1983). Physical attractiveness, self-awareness and mirror gazing behavior. *Bulletin of the Psychonomic Society, 21,* 115–116.

Livneh, H. (1982). On the origins of negative attitudes toward people with disabilities. *Rehabilitation Literature, 43,* 338–347.

Lombardi, J., and Tocci, M. (1979). Attribution of positive and negative characteristics of instructors as a function of attractiveness and sex of instructor and sex of subject. *Perceptual and Motor Skills, 48,* 491–494.

Longacre, J. (1973). *Rehabilitation of the facially disfigured.* Springfield, IL: Charles C. Thomas.

Lowenstein, L. (1978). The bullied and non-bullied child. *Bulletin of the British Psychological Society, 31,* 316–318.

Lown, C. (1977). Legal approaches to juror stereotyping by physical characteristics. *Law and Human Behavior, 1,* 87–100.

Lucker, G. (1976). Physical attractiveness, individual differences and personality stereotyping. *Dissertation Abstracts International, 36,* 4219B.

Lucker, G. (1981). Esthetics and a quantitative analysis of facial appearance. In G. Lucker, K. Ribbens, & J. McNamara (Eds.), *Psychological aspects of facial form.* Ann Arbor: University of Michigan Press.

Lucker, G., and Graber, L. (1980). Physiognomic features and facial appearance judgments in children. *Journal of Psychology, 104,* 261–268.

Lucker, G., Ribbens, K., and McNamara, J. (Eds.). (1981). *Psychological aspects of facial form.* Ann Arbor: University of Michigan Press.

Lyman, B., Hatlelid, D., and Macurdy, C. (1981). Stimulus-person cues in first-impression attraction. *Perceptual and Motor Skills, 52,* 59–66.

Macgregor, F. (1951). Some psycho-social problems associated with facial deformities. *American Sociological Review, 16,* 629–638.

Macgregor, F. (1974). *Transformation and identity: The face and plastic surgery.* New York: Quadrangle/New York Times Books.

Macgregor, F. (1981). Patient dissatisfaction with results of technically satisfactory surgery. *Aesthetic Plastic Surgery, 5,* 27–32.

Macgregor, F. (1982). Social and psychological considerations in plastic surgery. *Clinics in Plastic Surgery, 9,* 283–288.

Madan, R. (1962). Facial disfigurement. In J. Garrett & E. Levine (Eds.), *Psychological practices with the physically disabled.* New York: Columbia University Press.

Maddi, S. (1968). *Personality theories: A comparative analysis.* Homewood, IL: Dorsey Press.

Maddux, J., and Rogers, R. (1980). Effects of source expertness, physical attractiveness, and supporting arguments on persuasion: A case of brains over beauty. *Journal of Personality and Social Psychology, 39,* 235–244.

Manstead, A., and McCulloch, C. (1981). Sex-role stereotyping in British television advertisements. *British Journal of Social Psychology, 20,* 171–180.

Manz, W., and Lueck, H. (1968). Influences of wearing glasses upon judgment of personality traits: Cross-cultural validation of an old experiment. *Perceptual and Motor Skills, 27,* 704.

Marinelli, R. (1974). State anxiety in interactions with visibly disabled persons. *Rehabilitation Counseling Bulletin, 18,* 72–77.

Markle, A., Rinn, R., and Bell, C. (1984). Eye color as a predictor of outcomes in behavior therapy. *Journal of Clinical Psychology, 40*, 489–495.

Marks, G., Miller, N., and Maruyama, G. (1981). Effects of targets' physical attractiveness on assumptions of similarity. *Journal of Personality and Social Psychology, 41*, 198–206.

Marks-Greenfield, P. (1984). *Mind and media: The effects of television, computers and video games*. London: Fontana.

Martinek, T. (1981) Physical attractiveness: Effects on teacher expectations and dyadic interactions in elementary age children. *Journal of Sport Psychology, 3*, 196–205.

Maruyama, G., and Miller, N. (1980). Physical attractiveness, race and essay evaluation. *Personality and Social Psychology Bulletin, 6*, 384–390.

Maruyama, G., and Miller, N. (1981). Physical attractiveness and personality. In B. Mahrer (Ed.), *Progress in experimental research in personality* (Vol. 10). New York: Academic Press.

Marwit, S. (1982). Students' race, physical attractiveness and teachers' judgments of transgressions: Follow-up and clarification. *Psychological Reports, 50*, 242.

Marwit, K., Marwit, S., and Walker, E. (1978). Effects of student race and physical attractiveness on teachers' judgments of transgressions. *Journal of Educational Psychology, 70*, 911–915.

Marzillier, J. (1978). Outcome studies of social skills training: A review. In P. Trower, P. Bryant, & M. Argyle (Eds.), *Social skills and mental health*. London: Methuen.

Mashman, R. (1978). Effect of physical attractiveness on perception of attitude similarity. *Journal of Social Psychology, 106*, 103–110.

Massimo, M. (1978). Development of the concept of physical attractiveness in children and the operation of the matching hypothesis. *Dissertation Abstracts International, 38*, 6245B–6246B.

Masters, F., and Greaves, D. (1967). The Quasimodo complex. *British Journal of Plastic Surgery, 20*, 204–210.

Matarazzo, J., and Wiens, A. (1972). *The interview: Research on its anatomy and structure*. Chicago: Aidine-Atherton.

Mathes, E. (1974). The effects of physical attractiveness on behavior: A test of the self-fulfilling prophecy theory. *Dissertation Abstracts International, 34*, 5226B.

Mathes, E. (1975). The effects of physical attractiveness and anxiety on heterosexual attraction. *Journal of Marriage and the Family, 37*, 769–773.

Mathes, E., and Edwards, L. (1978). Physical attractiveness as an input in social exchanges. *Journal of Psychology, 98*, 267–275.

Matthews, V., and Westie, C. (1966). A preferred method for obtaining rankings: Reactions to physical handicaps. *American Sociological Review, 31*, 851–854.

Maurer, D., and Barrera, M. (1981). Infants' perception of natural and distorted arrangement of a schematic face. *Child Development, 52*, 196–202.

Maxwell, E., and Maxwell, R. (1979). *Evaluations for contempt expressed toward old people*. Paper presented at the 32nd Annual Scientific Meeting of the Gerontological Society, Washington, DC.

May, J., and Hamilton, P. (1980). Effects of musically evoked affect on women's interpersonal attraction toward and perceptual judgments of physical attractiveness in men. *Motivation and Emotion, 4*, 217–228.

McAfee, L., Fox, R., and Hicks, R. (1982). Attributions of male college students to variations in facial features in the line drawing of a woman's face. *Bulletin of the Psychonomic Society, 19*, 143–144.

McArthur, L. (1982). Judging a book by its cover: A cognitive analysis of the relationship between physical appearance and stereotyping. In A. Hastorf & A. Isen (Eds.), *Cognitive social psychology*. New York: Elsevier.

McArthur, L., and Baron, R. (1983). Toward an ecological theory of social perception. *Psychological Review*, *90*, 215–238.

McCabe, V. (1984). Abstract perceptual information for age level: A risk factor for maltreatment? *Child Development*, *55*, 267–276.

McDaniel, J. (1969). *Physical disability and human behavior*. New York: Pergamon Press.

McDonald, P., and Eilenfield, V. (1980). Physical attractiveness and the approach/avoidance of self-awareness. *Personality and Social Psychology Bulletin*, *6*, 391–395.

McFatter, R. (1978). Effects of punishment philosophy on sentencing decisions. *Journal of Personality and Social Psychology*, *36*, 1490–1500.

McGill, P. (1984, February 19). East faces up to West. *The Observer*.

McGinnis, J. (1976). *The selling of the president*. New York: Andre Deutsch.

McKeachie, W. (1952). Lipstick as a determiner of first impressions of personality: An experiment for the general psychology course. *Journal of Social Psychology*, *36*, 241–244.

McKelvie, S., and Matthews, S. (1976). Effects of physical attractiveness and favorableness of character on liking. *Psychological Reports*, *38*, 1223–1230.

McKillip, J., and Riedel, S. (1983). External validity of matching on physical attractiveness for same and opposite sex couples. *Journal Applied Social Psychology*, *13*, 328–337.

McLean, J. (1974). *The social significance of the pupil*. Unpublished doctoral dissertation, University of Chicago.

McWilliams, B. (1982). Social and psychological problems associated with cleft palate. *Clinics in Plastic Surgery*, *9*, 317–326.

Mead, G. (1934). *Mind, self and society*. University of Chicago Press.

Mehrabian, A. (1968). Inference of attitudes from the posture, orientation, and distance of a communicator. *Journal of Consulting and Clinical Psychology*, *32*, 296–308.

Mehrabian, A. (1972). *Nonverbal communication*. Chicago: Aldine Atherton.

Mehrabian, A., and Friar, P. (1969). Encoding of attitude by a seated communicator via posture and seating cues. *Journal of Consulting and Clinical Psychology*, *33*, 330–336.

Meiners, M., and Sheposh, J. (1977). Beauty or brains. *Personality and Social Psychology Bulletin*, *3*, 262–265.

Melamed, L., and Moss, M. (1975). The effect of context on ratings of attractiveness of photographs. *Journal of Psychology*, *90*, 129–136.

Meyer, J., Hoopes, J., Jabaley, M., and Allan, R. (1973). Is plastic surgery effective in the rehabilitation of deformed delinquent adolescents? *Plastic and Reconstructive Surgery*, *51*, 53–58.

Michelini, R., and Snodgrass, S. (1980). Defendant characteristics and juridic decisions. *Journal of Research in Personality*, *14*, 340–350.

Middleton, D., and Edwards, D. (1985). Pure and applied psychology: Re-examining the relationship. *Bulletin of the British Psychological Society*, *38*, 146–150.

Milgram, S. (1963). Behavioral study of obedience. *Journal of Abnormal and Social Psychology*, *67*, 371–378.

Miller, A. (1970a). The role of physical attractiveness in impression formation. *Psychonomic Science*, *19*, 241–243.

Miller, A. (1970b). Social perception of internal-external control. *Perceptual and Motor Skills*, *30*, 103–109.

Miller, A. (1982). *In the eye of the beholder: Contemporary issues in stereotyping*. New York: Praeger.

Miller, A., Gillen, B., Schenker, C., and Radlove, S. (1974). The prediction and perception of obedience to authority. *Journal of Personality*, *42*, 23–42.

Miller, H., and Rivenbark, W. (1970). Sexual differences in physical attractiveness as a determinant of heterosexual liking. *Psychological Reports, 27,* 701–702.

Miller, L., and Cox, C. (1982). For appearance's sake: Public self-consciousness and make-up use. *Personality and Social Psychology Bulletin, 8,* 748–751.

Miller, M., Armstrong, S., and Hagan, M. (1981). Effects of teaching on elementary students' attitudes towards handicaps. *Educational Training of the Mentally Retarded, 16,* 110–113.

Mills, J., and Aronson, E. (1965). Opinion change as a function of the communicator's attractiveness and desire to influence. *Journal of Personality and Social Psychology, 1,* 173–177.

Mills, J., and Harvey, J. (1972). Opinion change as a function of when information about the communicator is received and whether he is attractive or expert. *Journal of Personality and Social Psychology, 21,* 52–55.

Mishler, W. (1978). Nominating attractive candidates for Parliament: Recruitment to the Canadian House of Commons. *Legislative Studies Quarterly, 3,* 581.

Mitchell, K., and Orr, F. (1976). Heterosexual social competence, anxiety, avoidance and self-judged physical attractiveness. *Perceptual and Motor Skills, 43,* 533–554.

Monson, D., and Shurtleff, C. (1979). Altering attitudes toward the physically handicapped through print and nonprint media. *Language Art, 56,* 163–170.

Morgan, E., Hohmann, G., and Davis, J. (1974). Psychological rehabilitation in Veterans Administration spinal cord injury centers. *Rehabilitation Psychology, 21,* 3–33.

Morgan, B., and Leung, P. (1980). Effects of assertion training on the acceptance of disability by physically disabled university students. *Journal of Counseling Psychology, 27,* 209–212.

Morrison, R., and Bellack, A. (1981). The role of social perception in social skill. *Behavior Therapy, 12,* 69–79.

Morrow, P., and McElroy, J. (1984). The impact of physical attractiveness in evaluative contexts. *Basic and Applied Social Psychology, 5,* 171–182.

Morse, S., Gruzen, J., and Reis, H. (1976). The "eye of the beholder": A neglected variable in the study of physical attractiveness. *Journal of Personality, 44,* 209–225.

Morse, S., Reis, H., Gruzen, J., and Wolff, E. (1974). The "eye of the beholder": Determinants of physical attractiveness judgments in the U.S. and South Africa. *Journal of Personality, 42,* 528–542.

Moss, M., Miller, R., and Page, R. (1975). The effects of racial context on the perception of physical attractiveness. *Sociometry, 38,* 525–535.

Mueller, J., Heesacker, M., and Ross, M. (1984). Likability of targets and distractors in facial recognition. *American Journal of Psychology, 97,* 235–247.

Mueller, J., Thompson, W., and Vogel, J. (1988). Perceived honesty and face memory. *Personality and Social Psychology Bulletin, 14,* (in press).

Mueser, K., Grau, B., Sussman, S., and Rosen, A. (1984). You're only as pretty as you feel: Facial expression as a determinant of physical attractiveness. *Journal of Personality and Social Psychology, 43,* 469–478.

Munro, I. (1981). The psychological effects of surgical treatment of facial deformity. In G. Lucker, K. Ribbens, & J. McNamara (Eds.), *Psychological aspects of facial form.* Ann Arbor: University of Michigan Press.

Murphy, M., and Hellkamp, D. (1976). Attractiveness and personality warmth: Evaluations of paintings rated by college men and women. *Perceptual and Motor Skills, 43,* 1163–1166.

Murphy, M., Nelson, D., and Cheap, T. (1981). Rated and actual performance of high school students as a function of sex and attractiveness. *Psychological Reports, 48,* 103–106.

Murray, J., Rubenstein, E., and Comstock, G. (1972). *Television and social behavior volume 2: Television and social learning.* Washington, DC: U.S. Government Printing Office.

Murstein, B. (1972). Physical attractiveness and marital choice. *Journal of Personality and Social Psychology*, 22, 8–12.

Murstein, B., and Christy, P. (1976). Physical attractiveness and marriage adjustment in middle-aged couples. *Journal of Personality and Social Psychology*, 34, 537–542.

Napoleon, T., Chassin, L., and Young, R. (1980). A replication and extension of "physical attractiveness and mental illness". *Journal of Abnormal Psychology*, 89, 250–253.

Nida, S., and Williams, J. (1977). Sex-stereotyped traits, physical attractiveness, and interpersonal attraction. *Psychological Reports*, 41, 1311.

Nisbett, R., and Bellows, N. (1977). Verbal reports about causal influences on social judgments: Private versus public theories. *Journal of Personality and Social Psychology*, 35, 613–624.

Nisbett, R., and Wilson, T. (1977). The halo effect: Evidence for unconscious alteration of judgments. *Journal of Personality and Social Psychology*, 35, 250–256.

Noles, S. (1983). *Body image and depression in a college student sample.* Unpublished doctoral dissertation. Virginia Consortium of Professional Psychology. Dominion University, Norfolk, Virginia.

Nordholm, (1980). Physical attractiveness and attributions for disability. *Rehabilitation Psychology*, 28, 207–215.

Norman, R. (1976). When what is said is important: A comparison of expert and attractive sources. *Journal of Experimental Psychology*, 12, 294–300.

Northcraft, G., and Hastorf, A. (1986). Maturation and social behavior: A framework for the analysis of deviance. In C. Herman, M. Zanna, & E. Higgins (Eds.), *Physical appearance, stigma and social behavior.* Hillsdale, NJ: Lawrence Erlbaum.

Novak, P., and Lerner, M. (1968). Rejection as a consequence of perceived similarity. *Journal of Personality and Social Psychology*, 9, 147–152.

Owens, G., and Ford, J. (1978). Further consideration of the "what is good is beautiful" findings. *Social Psychology Quarterly*, 41, 73–75.

Pallak, S. (1983). Salience of a communicator's physical attractiveness and persuasion: A heuristic versus systematic processing interpretation. *Social Cognition*, 2, 158–170.

Pallak, S., Murroni, E., and Koch, J. (1983). Communicator attractiveness and expertise, emotional versus rational appeals, and persuasion: A heuristic versus systematic processing interpretation. *Social Cognition*, 2, 122–141.

Pancer, S., and Meindl, J. (1978). Length of hair and beardedness. *Perceptual and Motor Skills*, 46, 1328–1330.

Paschall, N. (1974). The effects of targets' clothing, raters' attractiveness, and type of photograph on rating of physical attractiveness. *Dissertation Abstracts International*, 35, 3071B.

Patzer, G. (1983). Source credibility as a function of communicator physical attractiveness. *Journal of Business Research*, 11, 229–241.

Patzer, G. (1985). *The physical attractiveness phenomena.* New York: Plenum.

Pavlos, A., and Newcomb, J. (1974). Effects of physical attractiveness on attempted suicide. *Personality and Social Psychology Bulletin*, 1, 36–38.

Pellegrini, R., Hicks, S., and Meyers-Winton, B. (1979). Situational affective arousal and heterosexual attraction: Some effects of success, failure, and physical attractiveness. *Psychological Record*, 29, 453–462.

Pellegrini, R., Hicks, R., and Meyers-Winton, S. (1980). Self-evaluations of attractiveness and perceptions of mate-attraction in the interpersonal marketplace. *Perceptual and Motor Skills*, 50, 812–814.

Pellegrini, R., Hicks, R., Meyers-Winton, S., and Antal, B. (1978). Physical attractiveness and self-disclosure in mixed-sex dyads. *Psychological Record*, 28, 509–516.

Pennebaker, J., Dyer, M., Caulkins, R., Litowitz, D., Ackreman, P., Anderson, D., and McGraw, K. (1979). Don't girls get prettier at closing time: A country and western application to psychology. *Personality and Social Psychology Bulletin*, *5*, 122–125.

Pennock, J. (1971). Introduction. In J. Pennock & J. Chapman (Eds.), *Privacy*. New York: Atherton Press.

Peplau, L., and Perlman, D. (1979). Blueprint for a social psychological theory of loneliness. In M. Cook & G. Wilson (Eds.), *Love and attraction: An international conference*. Oxford: Pergamon Press.

Perkins, B., and Karniski, M. (1978). The effect of increased knowledge of body systems and functions on attitudes toward the disabled. *Rehabilitation Counseling Bulletin*, *22*, 16–20.

Perrin, F. (1921). Physical attractiveness and repulsiveness. *Journal of Experimental Psychology*, *4*, 203–217.

Pertschuk, M. (1985). Appearance in psychiatric disorder. In J. Graham & A. Kligman (Eds.), *The psychology of cosmetic treatments*. New York: Praeger.

Pertschuk, M., and Whitaker, L. (1982). Social and psychological effects of craniofacial deformity and surgical reconstruction. *Clinics in Plastic Surgery*, *9*, 297–306.

Peter, J., Chinsky, R., and Fisher, M. (1975). Sociological aspects of cleft palate adults in social integration. *Cleft Palate Journal*, *12*, 304–310.

Peterson, J., and Miller, C. (1980). Physical attractiveness and marriage adjustment in older American couples. *Journal of Psychology*, *105*, 247–252.

Peterson, K., and Curran, J. (1976). Trait attribution as a function of hair length and correlates of subjects' preferences for hair style. *Journal of Psychology*, *93*, 331–339.

Peterson, N. (1982). Social integration of handicap and nonhandicap preschoolers: A study of playmate preferences. *Topics in Early Childhood Special Education*, *2*, 56–69.

Pheterson, M., and Horai, J. (1976). The effects of sensation seeking, physical attractiveness of stimuli, and exposure frequency on liking. *Social Behavior and Personality*, *4*, 241–247.

Pick, J. (1948). Ten years of plastic surgery in a penal institution: Preliminary report. *Journal of the International College of Surgeons*, *11*, 315–319.

Piehl, J. (1977). Integration of information in the "courts": Influence of physical attractiveness on amount of punishment for a traffic offender. *Psychological Reports*, *41*, 551–556.

Piff, C. (1985). *Let's face it*. London: Gollancz.

Piliavin, I., and Briar, S. (1964). Police encounters with juveniles. *American Journal of Sociology*, *70*, 206–214.

Piliavin, I., Piliavin, J., and Rodin, J. (1975). Costs, diffusion, and stigmatized victim. *Journal of Personality and Social Psychology*, *32*, 429–438.

Piliavin, I., Rodin, J., and Piliavin, J. (1969). Good samaritanism: An underground phenomenon? *Journal of Personality and Social Psychology*, *13*, 289–299.

Pilkonis, P., Heape, C., and Klein, R. (1980). Treating shyness and other relationship difficulties in psychiatric outpatients. *Communication Education*, *29*, 250–255.

Pilkonis, P., Lewis, P., Calpin, J., Senatore, V., and Hersen, M. (1980). Training complex social skills for use in a psychotherapy group: A case study. *International Journal of Group Psychotherapy*, *30*, 3.

Pittenger, J., Johnson, D., and Mark, L. (1983). Aesthetic equivalence of three representations of the face. *Bulletin of the Psychonomic Society*, *21*, 111–114.

Porter, J., Beuf, A., Nordlund, J., and Lerner, A. (1978). Personal responses of patients to vitiligo. *Archives of Dermatology*, *2*, 114.

Potter, R. (1978). Understanding exceptionality through TV. *Teacher*, *96*, 42–48.

Powell, P., and Dabbs, J. (1976). Physical attractiveness and personal space. *Journal of Social Psychology*, *100*, 59–64.

Price, R., and Vandenberg, S. (1979). Matching for physical attractiveness in married couples. *Personal and Social Psychology Bulletin*, *5*, 398–400.

Priestley, P., McGuire, J., Flegg, D., Hemsley, V., and Welham, D. (1978). *Social skills and personal problem solving*. London: Tavistock Publications.

Quay, H. (1972). Patterns of aggression, withdrawal and immaturity. In H. Quay & J. Werry (Eds.), *Psychopathological disorders of childhood*. New York: Wiley.

Rand, C., and Hall, J. (1983). Sex differences in the accuracy of self-perceived attractiveness. *Social Psychology Quarterly*, *46*, 359–363.

Raskin, N. (1956). *The attitude of sighted people toward blindness*. Paper presented at the National Psychological Research Council on Blindness.

Reece, M., and Whitman, R. (1962). Expressive movements, warmth and verbal reinforcement. *Journal of Abnormal and Social Psychology*, *64*, 234–236.

Reich, J. (1975). Factors influencing patients satisfaction with the results of aesthetic plastic surgery. *Plastic and Reconstructive Surgery*, *55*, 5–13.

Reich, J. (1982). The interface of plastic surgery and psychiatry. *Clinics in Plastic Surgery*, *9*, 367–377.

Reingen, P., Gresham, L., and Kernan, J. (1980). Behavioral consequences of the physical attractiveness stereotype in personal selling. In R. Bagozzi, K. Bernhardt, P. Busch, D. Cravens, J. Hair, & C. Scott (Eds.), *Marketing in the '80's*. Chicago: American Marketing Association.

Reis, H., Nezlek, J., and Wheeler, L. (1980). Physical attractiveness in social interaction. *Journal of Personality and Social Psychology*, *38*, 604–617.

Reis, H., Wheeler, L., Spiegel, N., Kernis, M., Nezlek, J., and Perri, M. (1982). Physical attractiveness in social interaction II: Why does appearance affect social experience? *Journal of Personality and Social Psychology*, *43*, 979–996.

Rich, A., and Schroeder, H. E. (1976). Research issues in assertive training. *Psychological Bulletin*, *88*, 1081–1096.

Rich, J. (1975). Effects of children's physical attractiveness on teachers' evaluations. *Journal of Educational Psychology*, *67*, 599–609.

Richardson, S. (1963). Some social psychological consequences of handicapping. *Pediatrics*, *32*, 291–297.

Richardson, S. (1970). Age and sex differences in values toward physical handicaps. *Journal of Health and Social Behavior*, *11*, 207–214.

Richardson, S. (1971). Handicap, appearance and stigma. *Social Science and Medicine*, *5*, 621–628.

Richardson, S., Goodman, N., Hastorf, A., and Dornbusch, S. (1961). Cultural uniformity in reaction to physical disabilities. *American Sociological Review*, *26*, 241–247.

Richman, L. (1976). Behavior and achievement of cleft palate children. *Cleft Palate Journal*, *13*, 4–10.

Richman, L. (1978). The effects of facial disfigurement on teachers' perceptions of ability in cleft palate children. *Cleft Palate Journal*, *15*, 155–160.

Richman, L., and Harper, D. (1978). School adjustment of children with observable disabilities. *Journal of Abnormal Child Psychology*, *6*, 11–18.

Riggio, R., and Woll, S. (1984). The role of nonverbal cues and physical attractiveness in the selection of dating partners. *Journal of Social and Personal Relationships*, *1*, 347–357.

Robertiello, R. (1976). The myth of physical attractiveness. *Psychotherapy: Theory, Research and Practice*, *13*, 54–55.

Robinson, J. (1978). *Catching criminals: Some basic skills*. London: Police Review Publications.

Robinson, T. (1981). Eye-color, sex, and personality: A case of negative findings for Worthy's sociability hypothesis. *Perceptual and Motor Skills*, *52*, 855–863.

Roll, S., and Verinis, J. (1971). Stereotypes of scalp and facial hair as measured by the semantic differential. *Psychological Reports*, *28*, 975–980.

Rosenberg, M. (1975). Self esteem and anxiety. In S. Dragastin & G. Eider (Eds.), *Adolescence in the life cycle: Psychological change and social context*. Washington, DC: Hemisphere.

Rosenfeld, H. (1966). Instrumental affiliative functions of facial and gestural expressions. *Journal of Personality and Social Psychology*, *4*, 65–72.

Rosenthal, R., and Jacobson, L. (1968). *Pygmalion in the classroom*. New York: Holt, Rinehart and Winston.

Ross, J., and Ferris, K. (1981). Interpersonal attraction and organizational outcomes: A field examination. *Administrative Science Quarterly*, *26*, 617–632.

Ross, M., and Salvia, J. (1975). Attractiveness as a biasing factor in teacher judgments. *American Journal of Mental Deficiency*, *80*, 96–98.

Rumsey, N. (1983). *Psychological problems associated with facial disfigurement*. Unpublished doctoral thesis, North East London Polytechnic, London, England.

Rumsey, N., and Bull, R. (1986). The effects of facial disfigurement on social interaction. *Human Learning*, *5*, 203–208.

Rumsey, N., Bull, R., and Gahagan, D. (1982). The effect of facial disfigurement on the proxemic behavior of the general public. *Journal of Applied Social Psychology*, *12*, 137–150.

Rumsey, N., Bull, R., and Gahagan, D. (1986). A preliminary study of the potential of social skills training for improving the quality of social interaction for the facially disfigured. *Social Behaviour*, *1*, 143–145.

Rusalem, H. (1973). The homebound. In J. Garrett & E. Levine (Eds.), *Rehabilitation practices with the disabled*. New York: Columbia University Press.

Rutter, D., and Stephenson, G. (1972). Visual interaction in a group of schizophrenic and depressive patients. *British Journal of Social and Clinical Psychology*, *11*, 57–65.

Rutzen, S. (1973). The social importance of orthodontic rehabilitation: Report of a five year follow-up study. *Journal of Health and Social Behavior*, *14*, 233–240.

Sadlick, M., and Penta, F. (1975). Changing nurse attitudes towards quadraplegics through use of television. *Rehabilitation Literature*, *36*, 274–283.

Salvia, J., Algozzine, R., and Sheare, J. (1977). Attractiveness and school achievement. *Journal of School Psychology*, *15*, 60–67.

Samerotte, G., and Harris, M. (1976). Some factors influencing helping: The effects of a handicap on responsibility and requesting help. *Journal of Social Psychology*, *98*, 39–45.

Samuels, C., and Ewy, R. (1985). Aesthetic perception of faces during infancy. *British Journal of Developmental Psychology*, *3*, 221–228.

Sandler, A. (1975). *The effects of patients' physical attractiveness on therapists' clinical judgment*. Unpublished doctoral dissertation. University of Texas.

Saxe, L., and Bar-Tal, D. (1977). *The effect of a teacher's physical attractiveness on students' evaluations*. Unpublished manuscript.

Schlenker, B. (1974). Social psychology and science. *Journal of Personality and Social Science*, *29*, 1–15.

Schneider, W., and Shiffrin, R. (1977). Controlled and automatic human information processing: 1. Detection, search and attention. *Psychological Review*, *84*, 1–66.

Schoedel, J., Frederickson, W., and Knight, J. (1975). An explanation of the physical attractiveness and sex variables within the Byrne attraction paradigm. *Memory and Cognition*, *3*, 527–530.

Schofield, W. (1964). *Psychotherapy: The purchase of friendship*. Englewood Cliffs, NJ: Prentice Hall.

Schulz, R. (1976). The effects of control and predictability on the psychological and physical well-being of the institutionalized aged. *Journal of Personality and Social Psychology*, *33*, 563–573.

Schuring, A., and Dodge, R. (1967). The role of cosmetic surgery in criminal rehabilitation. *Plastic and Reconstructive Surgery, 40*, 268–270.

Schwartz, J., and Abramowitz, S. (1978). Effects of female client physical attractiveness. *Psychotherapy: Theory, Research and Practice, 15*, 251–257.

Schwibbe, G., and Schwibbe, M. (1981). Judgment and treatment of people of varied attractiveness. *Psychological Reports, 48*, 11–14.

Sears, D. (1968). Political behavior. In G. Lindzey & E. Aronson (Eds.), *Handbook of Social Psychology* (Vol. 2). New York: Academic Press.

Secord, P. (1958). Facial features and inference processes in interpersonal attraction. In R. Tagiuri & L. Petrullo (Eds.), *Person perception and interpersonal behavior*. Stanford, CA: Stanford University Press.

Secord, P., and Backman, C. (1959). Malocclusion and psychological factors. *Journal of the American Dental Association, 59*, 931–938.

Secord, P., and Backman, C. (1964). *Social psychology*. New York: McGraw Hill.

Secord, P., and Bevan, W. (1956). Personalities in faces: III, across-cultural comparison of impressions of physiognomy and personality in faces. *Journal of Social Psychology, 43*, 283–288.

Secord, P., and Muthard, J. (1955). Personalities in faces: IV, A descriptive analysis of the perception of women's faces and the identification of some physiognomic determinants. *Journal of Psychology, 29*, 269–278.

Seligman, C., Brickman, J., and Koulack, D. (1977). Rape and physical attractiveness: Assigning responsibility to victims. *Journal of Personality, 45*, 554–563.

Seligman, C., Paschall, N., and Takata, G. (1974). Effects of physical attractiveness on attribution of responsibility. *Canadian Journal of Behavioral Science, 6*, 290–296.

Sergl, H., and Stodt, W. (1970). Experimental investigation of the aesthetic effect of various tooth positions after loss of an incisor tooth. *Transactions of the European Orthodontic Society, 2*, 497–507.

Shakespeare, R. (1975). *The psychology of handicap*. London: Methuen.

Shanteau, J., and Nagy, G. (1979). Probability of acceptance in dating choice. *Journal of Personality and Social Psychology, 37*, 522–533.

Shaw, J. (1972). Reactions to victims and defendants of varying degrees of attractiveness. *Psychonomic Science, 27*, 329–330.

Shaw, W. (1981a). The influence of children's dentofacial appearance on their social attractiveness as judged by peers and lay adults. *American Journal of Orthodontics, 79*, 399–415.

Shaw, W. (1981b). Factors influencing the desire for orthodontic treatment. *European Journal of Orthodontics, 3*, 151–162.

Shaw, W. (1981c). Folklore surrounding facial deformity and the origins of facial prejudice. *British Journal of Plastic Surgery, 34*, 237–246.

Shaw, W., and Humphreys, S. (1982). Influence of children's dentofacial appearance on teacher expectations. *Community Dental and Oral Epidemiology, 10*, 313–319.

Shaw, W., Lewis, H., and Robertson, N. (1975). Perception of malocclusion. *British Dental Journal, 138*, 211–217.

Shaw, W., Rees, G., Dawe, M., and Charles, C. (1985). The influence of dentofacial appearance on the social attractiveness of young adults. *American Journal of Orthodontics, 87*, 21–26.

Shea, J., Crossman, S., and Adams, G. (1978). Physical attractiveness and personality development. *Journal of Psychology, 99*, 59–62.

Sheed, W. (1980, August 25). On being handicapped. *Newsweek*.

Shepherd, J., and Ellis, H. (1972). Physical attractiveness and selection of marriage partners. *Psychological Reports, 30*, 1004.

Shepherd, J., and Ellis, H. (1973). The effect of attractiveness on recognition memory for faces. *American Journal of Psychology, 86*, 627–633.

Shepherd, J., Ellis, H., McMurran, M., and Davies, G. (1978). Effect of character attribution on photofit construction of a face. *European Journal of Social Psychology*, *8*, 263–268.

Shoemaker, D., and South, D. (1978). Nonverbal images of criminality and deviance: Existence and consequence. *Criminal Justice Review*, *3*, 65–80.

Shoemaker, D., South, D., and Lowe, J. (1973). Facial stereotypes of deviants and judgments of guilt or innocence. *Social Forces*, *51*, 427–433.

Shortridge, S. (1982). Facilitating attitude change toward the handicapped. *American Journal of Occupational Therapy*, *36*, 456–460.

Sigal, J., Braden, J., and Aylward, G. (1978). The effects of attractiveness of defendant, number of witnesses, and personal motivation of defendant on jury decision making behavior. *Psychology*, *15*, 4–10.

Sigall, H., and Aronson, E. (1969). Liking for an evaluator as a function of her physical attractiveness and nature of the evaluation. *Journal of Experimental Social Psychology*, *5*, 93–100.

Sigall, H., and Landy, D. (1973). Radiating beauty: Effects of having a physically attractive partner on person perception. *Journal of Personality and Social Psychology*, *28*, 218–224.

Sigall, H., and Ostrove, N. (1975). Beautiful but dangerous: Effects of offender attractiveness and nature of crime on juridic judgment. *Journal of Personality and Social Psychology*, *31*, 410–414.

Sigall, H., and Page, R. (1972). Reducing attenuation in the expression of interpersonal affect via the bogus pipeline. *Sociometry*, *35*, 629–642.

Siller, J. (1976). Attitudes toward disability. In H. Rusalem & D. Maliken (Eds.), *Contemporary vocational rehabilitation*. New York: New York University Press.

Simms, T. (1967). Pupillary response of male and female subjects to pupillary difference in male and female picture stimuli. *Perception and Psychophysics*, *2*, 553–555.

Singer, J. (1964). The use of manipulative strategies: Machiavellianism and attractiveness. *Sociometry*, *27*, 128–150.

Singleton, R., and Hofacre, S. (1976). Effects of victim's physical attractiveness on juridic judgments. *Psychological Reports*, *39*, 73–74.

Siperstein, G., and Gottlieb, J. (1977). Physical stigma and academic performance as factors affecting children's first impressions of handicapped peers. *American Journal of Mental Deficiency*, *81*, 455–462.

Smith, D., and Williamson, L. (1977). *Interpersonal communication*. Dubuque, IA: Brown.

Smith, E., and Hed, A. (1979). Effects of offenders' age and attractiveness on sentencing by mock juries. *Psychological Reports*, *44*, 691–694.

Smith, R., Sprecher, S., and De Lamater, J. (1983a). *The impact of physical attractiveness and gender on perceptions of sexuality*. Department of Sociology, University of Wisconsin-Madison. Photocopy.

Smith, R., Sprecher, S., and De Lamater, J. (1983b). *Perceptions of the intimacy of matched vs. mismatched couples*. Department of Sociology, University of Wisconsin-Madison. Photocopy.

Smits, G., and Cherhoniak, I. (1976). Physical attractiveness and friendliness in interpersonal attraction. *Psychological Reports*, *39*, 171–174.

Snyder, M. (1981). On the self-perpetuating nature of social stereotypes. In D. Hamilton (Ed.), *Cognitive processes in stereotyping and intergroup behavior*. Hillsdale, NJ: Lawrence Erlbaum.

Snyder, M., and Rothbart, M. (1971). Communicator attractiveness and opinion change. *Canadian Journal of Behavioral Science*, *3*, 377–387.

Snyder, M., and Swann, W. (1978). Behavioral confirmation in social interaction: From social perception to social reality. *Journal of Experimental Social Psychology*, *14*, 148–162.

Snyder, M., Tanke, E., and Berscheid, E. (1977). Social perception and interpersonal behavior: On the self-fulfilling nature of social stereotypes. *Journal of Personality and Social Psychology, 35*, 656–666.

Soble, S., and Strickland, L. (1974). Physical stigma, interaction and compliance. *Bulletin of the Psychonomic Society, 4*, 130–132.

Solender, E., and Solender, E. (1976). Minimizing the effects of the unattractive client on the jury. *Human Rights, 5*, 201–214.

Solomon, M., and Schopler, J. (1978). The relationship of physical attractiveness and punitiveness: Is the linearity assumption out of line? *Personality and Social Psychology Bulletin, 4*, 483–486.

Sommer, R. (1969). *Personal space: The behavioral basis of design.* Englewood Cliffs, NJ: Prentice Hall.

Sorell, G., and Nowak, C. (1981). The role of physical attractiveness as a contributor to individual development. In R. Lerner & N. Busch-Rossnagel (Eds.), *Individuals as producers of their development.* New York: Academic Press.

Sparacino, J. (1980). Physical attractiveness and occupational prestige among male college graduates. *Psychological Reports, 47*, 1275–1280.

Sparacino, J., and Hansell, S. (1979). Physical attractiveness and academic performance. *Journal of Personality, 47*, 449–469.

Spira, M., Chizen, J., Gerow, F., and Hardy, S. (1966). Plastic surgery in the Texas prison system. *British Journal of Plastic Surgery, 19*, 364–371.

Spreadbury, C., and Reeves, J. (1979). Physical attractiveness, dating behavior and implications for women. *Personnel and Guidance Journal, 57*, 338–340.

Sprecher, S., De Lamater, J., Neuman, N., Neuman, M., Kahn, P., Orbuch, D., and McKinney, K. (1984). Asking questions in bars: The girls (and boys) may not be getting prettier at closing time and other interesting results. *Personality and Social Psychology Bulletin, 10*, 482–488.

Spricstersbach, D. (1963). Psychosocial factors of cleft lip and palate rehabilitation. In B. Rogers (Ed.), *Facial disfigurement: A rehabilitation problem.* Washington, DC: Vocational Rehabilitation Administration.

Springbett, B. (1958). Factors affecting the final decision in the employment interview. *Canadian Journal of Psychology, 12*, 13–22.

Spuhler, J. (1968). Assortative mating with respect to physical characteristics. *Eugenics Quarterly, 15*, 128–140.

Sroufe, R., Chaiken, A., Cook, R., and Freeman, V. (1977). The effects of physical attractiveness on honesty: A socially desirable response. *Personality and Social Psychology Bulletin, 3*, 59–62.

Staffieri, R., and Klappersack, B. (1960). An attempt to change attitudes toward the cerebral palsied. *Rehabilitation Counseling Bulletin, 3*, 5–6.

Starr, P. (1978). Self esteem and behavioral functioning of teenagers with oral-facial clefts. *Rehabilitation Literature, 39*, 233–235.

Starr, P. (1980). Facial attractiveness and behavior of patients with cleft lip and/or palate. *Psychological Reports, 46*, 579–582.

Stass, J., and Willis, F. (1967). Eye contact, pupil dilation and personal preference. *Psychonomic Science, 7*, 375–376.

Steffen, J., and Redden, J. (1977). Assessment of social competence in an evaluation-interaction analog. *Human Communication Research, 4*, 30–37.

Stephan, C., Berscheid, E., and Walster, E. (1971). Sexual arousal and heterosexual perception. *Journal of Personality and Social Psychology, 20*, 93–101.

Stephan, C., and Langois, J. (1984). Baby beautiful: Adult attributions of infant competence as a function of infant attractiveness. *Child Development, 55*, 576–585.

Stephan, C., and Tully, J. (1977). The influence of physical attractiveness of a plaintiff on the decisions of simulated jurors. *Journal of Social Psychology, 101*, 149–150.

Sternglatz, S., Gray, J., and Murakami, M. (1977). Adult preferences for infantile facial features: An ethological approach. *Animal Behavior*, *25*, 108–115.

Stewart, J. (1980). Defendant's attractiveness as a factor in the outcome of criminal trials: An observational study. *Journal of Applied Social Psychology*, *10*, 348–361.

Stone, M. (1984). *Proof of fact in criminal trials*. Edinburgh, Scotland: Green.

Storck, J., and Sigall, H. (1979). Effect of harm-doer's attractiveness and the victim's history of prior victimization on punishment of the harm-doer. *Personality and Social Psychology Bulletin*, *5*, 344–347.

Straith, C., and De Kleine, E. (1938). Plastic surgery in children. *Journal of American Medical Association*, *111*, 2364–2370.

Strane, K., and Watts, C. (1977). Females judged by attractiveness of partner. *Perceptual and Motor Skills*, *45*, 225–226.

Strauss, R. (1980). Surgery, activism and aesthetics: A sociological perspective on treating facial disfigurement. In G. Lucker, K. Ribbens, & J. McNamara (Eds.), *Psychological aspects of facial form*. Ann Arbor: University of Michigan Press.

Strenta, A., and Kleck, R. (1985). Physical disability and the attribution dilemma: Perceiving the causes of social behavior. *Journal of Social and Clinical Psychology*, *3*, 129–142.

Stretch, R., and Figley, C. (1980). Beauty and the boast: Predictors of interpersonal attraction in a dating experiment. *Psychology*, *17*, 35–43.

Stricker, G. (1970). Psychological issues pertaining to malocclusion. *American Journal of Orthodontics*, *58*, 276–283.

Stritch, T., and Secord, P. (1956). Interaction effects in the perception of faces. *Journal of Personality*, *24*, 272–284.

Stroebe, W., Insko, C., Thompson, V., and Layton, B. (1971). Effects of physical attractiveness, attitude similarity, and sex on various aspects of interpersonal attraction. *Journal of Personality and Social Psychology*, *18*, 79–91.

Strohmer, D., and Biggs, D. (1983). Effects of counselor disability status on disabled subjects' perceptions of counselor attractiveness and expertness. *Journal of Counseling Psychology*, *30*, 202–208.

Strong, S. (1968). Counseling: An interpersonal influence process. *Journal of Counseling Psychology*, *15*, 215–224.

Styczynski, L., & Langlois, J. (1977). The effects of familiarity on behavioral stereotypes associated with physical attractiveness in young children. *Child Development*, *48*, 1137–1141.

Suben, M., and McKeever, W. (1977). Differential right hemisphere memory storage of emotional and nonemotional faces. *Neuropsychologica*, *15*, 757–768.

Sussman, S., Mueser, K., Grau, B., and Yarnold, P. (1983). Stability of females' facial attractiveness during childhood. *Journal of Personality and Social Psychology*, *44*, 1231–1233.

Tan, A. (1979). TV beauty advertisements and the role expectations of adolescent female viewers. *Journalism Quarterly*, *56*, 283–288.

Tanke, E. (1982). Dimensions of the physical attractiveness stereotype: A factoranalytic study. *Journal of Psychology*, *110*, 63–73.

Tarrahian, G., and Hicks, R. (1979). Attribution of pupil size as a function of facial valence and age in American and Persian children. *Journal of Cross-cultural Psychology*, *10*, 243–250.

Taylor, J. (1981). Portrayal of persons with disabilities by the media. *Mental Retardation Bulletin*, *9*, 38–53.

Taylor, P., and Glenn, N. (1976). The utility of education and attractiveness for females' status. *American Sociological Review*, *41*, 484–498.

Tennis, G., and Dabbs, J. (1975). Judging physical attractiveness. *Personality and Social Psychology Bulletin*, *1*, 513–516.

Terry, R. (1977). Further evidence on components of facial attractiveness. *Perceptual and Motor Skills*, *45*, 130.

Terry, R. (1982). The psychology of visual correctives: Social and psychological effects of eyeglasses and contact lenses. *Optometric Monthly, 73*, 137–142.

Terry, R., and Brady, C. (1976). Effects of framed spectacles and contact lenses on self ratings of facial attractiveness. *Perceptual and Motor Skills, 42*, 789–790.

Terry, R., and Davis, J. (1976). Components of facial attractiveness. *Perceptual and Motor Skills, 42*, 918.

Terry, R., and Kroger, D. (1976). Effects of eye correctives on ratings of attractiveness. *Perceptual and Motor Skills, 42*, 562.

Terry, R., and Macklin, E. (1977). Accuracy of identifying married couples on the basis of similarity of attractiveness. *Journal of Psychology, 97*, 15–20.

Terry, R., and Zimmerman, D. (1970). Anxiety induced by contact lenses and framed spectacles. *Journal of the American Optometric Association, 41*, 257–259.

Thomas, S., and Wolfensberger, W. (1982). The importance of social imagery in interpreting societally devalued people to the public. *Rehabilitation Literature, 43*, 356–358.

Thoreson, R., and Kerr, B. (1978). The stigmatising aspects of severe disability: Strategies for change. *Journal of Applied Rehabilitation Counseling, 9*, 21–26.

Thornton, B. (1977). Effect of rape victim's attractiveness in a jury simulation. *Personality and Social Psychology Bulletin, 3*, 666–669.

Thornton, B., and Linnstaedter, L. (1980). The influence of physical attractiveness and sex-role congruence on interpersonal attraction. *Representative Research in Social Psychology, 11*, 55–63.

Thornton, G. (1939). The ability to judge crimes from photographs of criminals. *Journal of Abnormal and Social Psychology, 34*, 378–383.

Thornton, G. (1943). The effect upon judgments of personality traits of varying a single factor in a photograph. *Journal of Social Psychology, 18*, 127–148.

Thornton, G. (1944). The effect of wearing glasses upon judgments of personality traits of persons seen briefly. *Journal of Applied Psychology, 28*, 203–207.

Thredkeld, R., and DeJong, W. (1982). Changing behavior toward the handicapped: An evaluation of the film "First Encounters". *Rehabilitation Counseling Bulletin, 25*, 282–285.

Timmerman, K., and Hewitt, J. (1980). Examining the halo effect of physical attractiveness. *Perceptual and Motor Skills, 51*, 607–612.

Tolor, A., and Salafia, W. (1971). The social schemata technique as a projective device. *Psychological Reports, 28*, 423–429.

Tomlinson, N., Hicks, R., and Pellegrini, R. (1978). Attributions of female college students to variations in pupil size. *Bulletin of the Psychonomic Society, 12*, 477–478.

Tompkins, R., and Boor, M. (1980). Effects of students' physical attractiveness and name popularity on student teachers' perceptions of social and academic attributes. *Journal of Psychology, 106*, 37–42.

Touhey, J. (1979). Sex-role stereotyping and individual differences in liking for the physically attractive. *Social Psychology Quarterly, 42*, 285–289.

Triandis, H. (1975). Social psychology and cultural analysis. *Journal for the Theory of Social Behavior, 5*, 81–106.

Trower, P., Bryant, B., and Argyle, M. (1978). *Social skills and mental health*. London: Methuen.

Trust, D. (1977). *Skin deep: An introduction to skin camouflage and disfigurement therapy*. Edinburgh, Scotland: Harris.

Turkat, D., and Dawson, J. (1976). Attributions of responsibility for a chance event as a function of sex and physical attractiveness of target individual. *Psychological Reports, 39*, 275–279.

Tversky, A., and Kahneman, D. (1977). Causal schemata in judgments under uncertainty. In M. Fishbein (Ed.), *Progress in social psychology*. Hillsdale, NJ: Lawrence Erlbaum.

Udry, J. (1977). The importance of being beautiful. *American Journal of Sociology*, *83*, 154–160.

Udry, J. (1965). Structural correlates of feminine beauty preferences in Britain and the U.S.: A comparison. *Sociology and Social Research*, *49*, 330–342.

Udry, R., and Eckland, B. (1984). Benefits of being attractive: Differential payoffs for men and women. *Psychological Reports*, *54*, 47–56.

Ungar, S. (1979). The effects of effort and stigma on helping. *Journal of Social Psychology*, *107*, 23–28.

Unger, R., Hilderbrand, M., and Madar, T. (1982). Physical attractiveness and assumptions about social deviance: Some sex-by-sex comparisons. *Personality and Social Psychology Bulletin*, *8*, 293–301.

Valins, S. (1966). Cognitive effects of false heart rate feedback. *Journal of Personality and Social Psychology*, *4*, 400–408.

Vandenberg, S. (1972). Assortative mating, or who marries whom. *Behavior Genetics*, *2*, 127–157.

Van Denmark, D., and Van Denmark, A. (1970). Speech and socio-vocational aspects of individuals with cleft palate. *Cleft Palate Journal*, *7*, 284–299.

Vaughn, B., and Langlois, J. (1983). Physical attractiveness as a correlate of peer status and social competence in preschool children. *Developmental Psychology*, *19*, 561–567.

Villemur, N., and Hyde, J. (1983). Effects of sex of defence attorney, sex of juror and attractiveness of the victim on mock juror decision making in a rape case. *Sex Roles*, *9*, 879–889.

Waldrop, M., Bell, R., and Goering, J. (1976). Minor physical anomalies and inhibited behavior in elementary school girls. *Journal of Child Psychology and Psychiatry*, *17*, 113–122.

Waldrop, M., and Goering, J. (1971). Hyperactivity and minor physical anomalies in elementary school children. *American Journal of Orthopsychiatry*, *41*, 602–607.

Waldrop, M., and Halverson, C. (1971). Minor physical anomalies and hyperactive behavior in young children. In J. Hellmuth, (Ed.), *The exceptional infant: Studies in abnormalities* (Vol. 2). London: Butterworths.

Waldrop, M., Pederson, F., and Bell, R. (1968). Minor physical anomalies and behavior in preschool children. *Child Development*, *39*, 391–400.

Walker, M., Harriman, S., and Costello, S. (1980). The influence of appearance on compliance with a request. *Journal of Social Psychology*, *112*, 159–160.

Walster, E., Aronson, E., Abrahams, D., and Rottman, L. (1966). The importance of physical attractiveness in dating behavior. *Journal of Personality and Social Psychology*, *4*, 508–516.

Warford, J. (1973). An analysis of the factors motivating children to seek orthodontic treatment. Unpublished Master's thesis, Northwestern University, Chicago.

Warr, P., and Knapper, C. (1968). *The perception of people and events*. Chichester, England: Wiley.

Washburn, P., and Hakel, M. (1973). Visual cues and verbal content as influences on impressions formed after simulated employment interviews. *Journal of Applied Psychology*, *58*, 137–141.

Waters, J. (1985). Cosmetics and the job market. In J. Graham & A. Kligman (Eds.), *The psychology of cosmetic treatments*. New York: Praeger.

Weinberg, N. (1976). Social stereotyping of the physically handicapped. *Rehabilitation Psychology*, *23*, 115–124.

Weinberg, N. (1978). Preschool children's perceptions of orthopaedic disability. *Rehabilitation Counseling Bulletin*, *21*, 183–189.

Weinberg, N., and Santana, R. (1978). Comic books: Champions of the disabled stereotype. *Rehabilitation Literature*, *39*, 327–331.

Weinberger, H., and Cash, T. (1982). The relationship of attributional style to learned helplessness in an interpersonal context. *Basic and Applied Psychology*, *3*, 141–154.

Weiss, J., and Eiser, H. (1977). Psychological timing of orthodontic treatment. *American Journal of Orthodontics*, *72*, 198–204.

Weiss, R. (1973). *Loneliness: The experience of emotional and social isolation*. Cambridge, MA: MIT Press.

Wells, B. (1983). *Body and personality*. London: Longman.

West, S., and Brown, J. (1975). Physical attractiveness, the severity of the emergency and helping: A field experiment and interpersonal simulation. *Journal of Experimental Social Psychology*, *11*, 531–538.

Westervelt, V., and McKinney, J. (1980). Effects of a film on nonhandicapped children's attitude toward handicapped children. *Exceptional Children*, *46*, 294–296.

Westin, A. (1970). *Privacy and freedom*. New York: Atheneum.

White, G. (1980). Physical attractiveness and courtship progress. *Journal of Personality and Social Psychology*, *39*, 660–668.

Wiemann, J. (1974). *An experimental study of visual attention in dyads: The effect of four gaze conditions on evaluation of applicants in employment interviews*. Paper presented at the meeting of the Speech Communication Association, Chicago.

Wilcox, B. (1969). Visual preferences of human infants for representations of the human face. *Journal of Experimental Child Psychology*, *7*, 10–20.

Wilkinson, J., and Canter, S. (1982). *Social skills training manual*. Chichester, England: Wiley.

Williams, S., and Hicks, R. (1980). Sex, iride pigmentation and the pupillary attributions of college students to happy and angry faces. *Bulletin of the Psychonomic Society*, *16*, 67–68.

Wilson, D., and Donnerstein, E. (1977). Guilty or not guilty? A look at the "simulated" jury paradigm. *Journal of Applied Psychology*, *7*, 175–190.

Wilson, G., and Brazendale, A. (1974). Psychological correlates of sexual attractiveness: An empirical demonstration of denial and fantasy gratification phenomena. *Social Behavior and Personality*, *2*, 30–34.

Wolfgang, J., and Wolfgang, A. (1968). Personal space—an unobtrusive measure of attitudes toward the physically handicapped. *Proceedings of the 76th Annual Convention of the American Psychological Association*, *3*, 121–128.

Woll, S., and McFall, M. (1979). The effects of false feedback on attributed arousal and rated attractiveness in female subjects. *Journal of Personality*, *47*, 214–229.

Worthington, M. (1974). Personal space as a function of the stigma effect. *Environmental Behavior*, *6*, 289–294.

Worthy, M. (1974). *Eye color, sex and race*. Anderson, SC: Droke House/Hallux.

Wright, B. (1960). *Physical disability—a psychological approach*. New York: Harper & Row.

Wright, B. (1974, March). An analysis of attitudes—dynamics and effects. *The New Outlook*, 108–118.

Wrightsman, L. (1977). *Social psychology*. Monterey, CA: Brooks Cole.

Yardley, K. (1979). Social skills training—a critique. *British Journal of Medical Psychology*, *52*, 55–62.

Yarmey, A. (1977). *The effects of attractiveness, feature sailency, and liking on memory for faces*. Paper presented at the International Conference on Love and Attraction, Swansea, Wales.

Yarmey, A. (1982). Eyewitness identification and stereotypes of criminals. In A. Trankell (Ed.) *Reconstructing the past: The role of psychologists in criminal trials*. Stockholm: Norstedt.

Young, J. (1979). Symptom disclosure to male and female physicians. *Journal of Behavioral Medicine*, *2*, 157–169.

Young, L., and Cooper, D. (1944). Some factors associated with popularity. *Journal of Educational Psychology*, *25*, 513–535.

Zakariya, S. (1978). Helping children understand disabilities. *National Elementary Principal*, *58*, 46–47.

Zakin, D. (1983). Physical attractiveness, sociability, athletic ability, and children's preference for their peers. *Journal of Psychology*, *115*, 117–122.

Ziller, R. (1973). *The social self*. New York: Pergamon.

Zimbardo, P. (1981). *Shyness*. New York: Pan.

Zlotlow, S., and Allen, G. (1981). Comparison of analogue strategies for investigating the influence of counselor's physical attractiveness. *Journal of Counseling Psychology*, *28*, 194–202.

Author Index

A

Aamot, S.   194
Abel, T.   193
Abrahams, D.   9, 10, 11, 14, 15, 20, 30, 293
Abramowitz, S.   249
Abramson, P.   57, 58, 59, 60
Ackreman, P.   24
Adams, G.   4, 48, 124, 125, 126, 127, 130, 131, 161, 173, 177, 178, 181, 189, 254, 257, 258, 269, 290, 295
Adinolfi, A.   18, 19, 20, 259
Agarwal, P.   59
Agle, T.   255
Agnew, R.   93, 94
Albrecht, G.   195
Alessi, D.   165
Algozzine, R.   143, 144
Allan, G.   248
Allan, R.   99
Allen, B.   285
Allen, J.   195
Aloia, G.   131
Alperstein, L.   48
Altemeyer, R.   44
Altman, I.   199
Andersen, S.   21, 22
Anderson, D.   24
Anderson, N.   11, 60

Anderson, R.   136, 137
Andreasa, N.   193
Antal, B.   257
Anthony, W.   165
Archer, R.   251
Argyle, M.   196, 198, 200, 259, 275, 295
Arkowitz, H.   257, 258
Armogida, R.   274
Armstrong, S.   225
Arndt, E.   239, 240
Aron, A.   284
Aronson, E.   9, 10, 11, 14, 15, 20, 30, 41, 42, 43, 106, 107, 109, 293
Arvey, R.   64, 65
Athanasiou, R.   203
Austin, K.   236
Aylward, G.   108, 111

B

Backman, C.   272, 292
Bailey, L.   247
Bailey, R.   12, 31, 38
Baker, M.   75, 76, 78
Baker, W.   239
Balascoe, L.   139
Baldwin, D.   244, 271
Banziger, G.   59
Baral, R.   16

Barker, R. 187
Barnes, M. 244, 271, 295
Barocas, R. 143, 249, 286
Baron, R. 293
Barrera, M. 163
Barrios, B. 170
Bar-Tal, D. 32, 36, 37, 148
Bassili, J. 296
Baumeister, R. 119
Beaman, A. 61
Beardsley, E. 199
Beehr, T. 67, 68, 72
Begley, P. 66, 247
Belbin, E. 217
Bell, C. 274
Bell, R. 155, 162
Bellack, A. 267
Bellows, N. 77, 299
Bem, D. 138
Bem, S. 21, 22
Benassi, M. 295
Bentley, M. 105
Benton, J. 187, 194
Berger, C. 108
Berkowitz, L. 154
Bernstein, I. 296
Bernstein, N. 146, 181, 183, 184,
    188, 194, 197, 199, 200, 201,
    210, 245, 259, 267
Bernstein, W. 16
Berry, D. 280, 281
Berscheid, E. 2, 3, 9, 10, 15, 18, 19,
    21, 22, 23, 46, 47, 172, 174, 177,
    207, 211, 227, 253, 254, 281, 284,
    287, 288, 289, 293, 298, 299
Best, J. 105
Beuf, A. 245
Bevan, W. 296
Biggs, D. 248
Bihm, E. 205
Birdwhistell, R. 195
Black, H. 143
Blass, T. 48
Block, S. 48
Boblett, P. 30
Bohrnstedt, G. 176, 177, 297

Boor, M. 11, 69, 130
Bordieri, J. 66
Boukydis, C. 159
Braden, J. 108, 111
Bradshaw, J. 161, 165, 166
Brady, C. 274, 279
Bramble, W. 123
Brantley, H. 180
Bray, R. 120
Brazendale, A. 25
Brennan, T. 261
Briar, S. 84
Brickman, J. 37, 102, 103, 104, 108
Brislin, R. 9, 30
Brooking, J. 35
Brooks, G. 58
Brooks, V. 158
Brown, J. 203
Bryant, B. 259
Bryt, A. 193, 213
Buck, P. 196, 197
Buckley, M. 87, 89
Bull, P. 273
Bull, R. 3, 35, 52, 53, 55, 81, 83,
    84, 85, 106, 111, 125, 135, 136,
    139, 153, 166, 170, 171, 189,
    190, 195, 196, 197, 203, 204,
    205, 206, 207, 210, 211, 217,
    224, 242, 253, 260, 264, 270,
    273, 287, 295, 296, 298
Burns, D. 27
Burns, M. 270
Burns, R. 181
Burns, S. 65, 66, 72
Burr, C. 185
Busch-Rossnagel, N. 238
Buss, A. 277
Butler, L. 225
Byrd, E. 228, 229, 230, 231, 233,
    235, 237
Byrne, D. 10, 12, 255, 289, 290

C
Caballero, M. 78
Calhoun, K. 255

Calhoun, L.   103, 105
Calpin, J.   264
Cann, A.   69, 70, 71, 103, 105
Canter, A.   193
Canter, S.   265
Carducci, B.   284
Carling, F.   188
Carlson, R.   63
Carver, C.   225
Casey,   159
Cash, D.   1, 277
Cash, T.   1, 17, 27, 30, 65, 66, 72,
    138, 239, 241, 247, 248, 249,
    250, 251, 260, 277
Cashen, V.   147, 148, 149
Cassman, T.   202
Caulkins, R.   24
Cavior, H.   91, 92, 93
Cavior, N.   8, 13, 30, 44, 92, 98,
    161, 166, 167, 224, 286
Celhoffer, L.   159
Centers, L.   188
Centers, R.   188
Chaiken, A.   203
Chaiken, S.   44, 47, 49, 76, 149, 256
Chance, J.   83
Chanowitz, B.   201
Chapman, R.   277
Charles, C.   270
Charon, S.   200, 291
Chassin, L.   251
Cheap, T.   146
Chelune, G.   261
Cheney, T.   10, 11, 255
Cherhoniak, I.   10
Chigier, E.   165
Chigier, M.   165
Chinsky, R.   184, 193, 194
Chizen, J.   95, 96
Christy, P.   30, 38, 286
Churchill, G.   75, 76, 78
Clifford, B.   3, 81, 84, 287
Clifford, E.   180, 181, 184, 186, 187,
    213, 237
Clifford, M.   122, 124, 125, 140, 141
Clingman, J.   58

Clopton, C.   255
Cohen, A.   126, 127
Cohen, S.   13, 44
Coleman, M.   1
Coleman, V.   1
Coles, M.   285
Colligan, R.   191, 243, 244
Comer, R.   197
Comstock, G.   229
Conrad, B.   61
Cook, R.   203
Cook, S.   141
Cooley, C.   291
Cooper, D.   172
Corrigan, J.   248
Corter, C.   159
Costello, S.   203
Cotton, J.   37, 38
Courtois, M.   89
Cox, C.   277
Cox, N.   279
Cozby, P.   284
Craig, F.   49
Crane, P.   173, 177
Critelli, J.   29
Crofton, C.   15, 24, 31, 38, 73, 94,
    162, 176, 297
Crosby, R.   194
Cross, J.   85, 88, 89, 161, 166
Crossman, S.   4, 161, 189, 258, 269
Crouse, B.   22
Cunningham, J.   20
Cunningham, M.   281, 282
Curran, J.   13, 15, 25, 276

D

Dabbs, J.   283, 297
Daly, J.   86, 88, 89
Dane, F.   119, 120
Dannenbring, G.   60
Darley, J.   119
Darwin, C.   15
David, I.   296
Davies, G.   84, 85
Davis, F.   194

Davis, J.   233, 279
Davis, K.   24
Dawe, M.   270
Dawson, J.   102
Dean, J.   196
Deitz, S.   105
De Jong, W.   1, 235
De Kleine, E.   99, 100, 101
De Lamater, J.   24
Dell, D.   248
De Meis, D.   130
Demmin, H.   105
Derlega, V.   30, 149
Dermer, M.   37, 104, 287, 296
Dickinson, J.   58
Dion, K.   9, 10, 15, 18, 23, 124, 128,
     151, 152, 153, 154, 163, 164,
     166, 167, 169, 172, 174, 177,
     254, 256, 281
Dipboye, R.   63, 64, 65
Dixon, J.   225
Dobo, P.   235
Dobson, W.   48
Dodge, R.   99
Doiron, D.   58
Dokecki, P.   8, 286
Donaldson, J.   228, 235
Donley, B.   285
Donnerstein, E.   116, 117
Donovan, W.   180
Doob, A.   203, 206, 207
Dornbusch, S.   202
Dosey, M.   199
Downs, A.   155, 156, 157, 283
Dunn, M.   205, 220, 263, 264, 265,
     266
Dushenko, T.   295
Dutton, D.   284
Dyer, M.   24
Dzuirawiec, S.   163

E
Easson, W.   180, 192, 213
Ecker, B.   203, 206, 207

Eckland, B.   34
Edgemon, C.   255
Edgerton, M.   193, 244
Edwards, D.   217, 247
Edwards, L.   12
Efran, M.   15, 51, 52, 107, 108, 297
Eilenfield, V.   255
Eiser, H.   238
Ekman, P.   85, 196
Elder, D.   35
Elder, G.   32, 286
Elliott, M.   166, 170, 171, 190
Elliott, T.   228, 229, 230, 231, 233,
     235, 237
Ellis, H.   30, 84, 85, 86, 87, 88, 89
Ellis, H.   163
Elman, D.   24
Elms, A.   286
Elovitz, G.   128, 129
Evans, E.   274
Ewy, R.   164

F
Farina, A.   195, 251
Fatoullah, E.   42, 43
Feild, H.   103, 104, 108
Feingold, A.   32, 34, 146
Feinman, S.   274, 275, 276
Felson, R.   145, 146, 154, 155, 176,
     177, 297
Fensterheim, H.   282
Ferrante, F.   273, 274
Ferris, K.   71, 72, 73, 74
Festinger, L.   200
Figley, C.   15
Fink, E.   25
Fisch, E.   205
Fischer, E.   251
Fishbein, M.   296
Fisher, M.   184, 193, 194
Fishman, L.   115, 116
Fiske, S.   201
Fitzgerald, H.   158, 159, 160, 279
Flegg, D.   258, 266

Fleishman, J.   87, 89
Fletcher, D.   275
Florian, V.   223
Folkes, V.   23
Ford, J.   297
Ford, L.   159
Fox, R.   279
Frederickson, W.   13, 14
Freedman, D.   275
Freeman, V.   203, 249
French, R.   261
Friar, P.   196
Friend, R.   108
Frodi, A.   154, 180
Fromkin, H.   63, 64, 65
Fugita, S.   139, 255

G

Gahagan, D.   166, 170, 171, 189,
    196, 197, 211, 242, 253, 264,
    295, 298
Gallucci, N.   296
Galton, F.   88
Gangestad, S.   3, 227
Gaudet, I.   205
Geiselman, R.   36, 284
Gellman, W.   218
Gerbasi, K.   113
Gergen, K.   285
Gerow, F.   95, 96
Gibbons, S.   226
Giesen, M.   170
Gilbert, B.   83
Gill, G.   274, 275, 276
Gillen, B.   65, 66, 67, 72, 75, 93,
    149, 281
Gilmore, D.   67, 68, 72
Gilroy, S.   206
Glasgow, R.   258
Glenn, N.   33, 34
Glenwick, D.   24
Goebel, B.   147, 148, 149
Goering, J.   155

Goffman, E.   187, 194, 195, 198,
    199, 207, 208, 292
Going, M.   86, 87, 88
Goldberg, M.   187, 194
Goldberg, P.   57, 58, 59, 60, 194
Goldman, W.   260
Goldring, P.   196
Goldstein, A.   2, 83
Goller, W.   196, 197
Goodman, N.   202
Goren, C.   163
Gottesdiener, M.   57, 58, 59, 60
Gottlieb, J.   189, 285
Graber, L.   242, 244, 279, 280
Graham, J.   277
Grau, B.   4, 295
Gray, J.   158
Graziano, W.   287
Greaves, D.   96, 97
Green, J.   83, 84
Greene, P.   203
Greenwald, M.   65
Greenwald, R.   111
Gresham, F.   262
Gresham, L.   46, 289, 298
Groh, T.   251
Gross, A.   15, 24, 31, 38, 73, 94,
    162, 176, 205, 297
Gruzen, J.   18, 282
Gutierres, S.   36, 283, 284

H

Haaf, R.   162
Haefner, J.   233
Hafer, M.   236
Hagan, M.   225
Hagiwara, S.   18
Haight, N.   36, 284
Hakel, M.   211, 252
Hall, E.   197
Hall, J.   282
Halverson, C.   100, 101, 155, 157,
    160
Hamilton, P.   285

Hamilton, T.   31
Handlers, A.   236
Hansell, S.   144, 145, 296
Hansson, R.   249
Hardy, S.   95, 96
Harper, D.   182, 183, 184
Harper, R.   212
Harrell, W.   203
Harriman, S.   203
Harris, A.   231
Harris, M.   204, 206
Harris, R.   231
Harrison, A.   23
Hartjen, C.   84
Hartnett, J.   35, 285
Harvey, J.   43, 44
Hastorf, A.   202, 203, 204, 206, 207,
    298
Hatch, C.   29, 141, 145
Hatfield, E.   1, 3, 9, 24, 72, 285,
    293, 294
Hatlelid, D.   295
Hawkes, C.   52, 53, 55
Hay, G.   239
Hayes, R.   285
Hayes, S.   91, 92, 93
Haythorn, W.   199
Heape, C.   263
Hebb, D.   286
Hed, A.   114
Heesacker, M.   89, 90
Heese, G.   231
Heider, F.   202
Heilman, M.   62, 66, 67, 72, 73, 74
Heimberg, J.   262
Heimberg, R.   262
Heinemann, W.   191
Heinen, J.   149
Hellkamp, D.   75
Helm, S.   271
Hemsley, V.   258, 266
Henker, B.   161, 162
Hen-Tov, A.   161, 162
Herman, C.   294
Herman, S.   205, 220, 263, 265

Herr, E.   235
Hersen, M.   264
Hess, E.   272, 273, 274
Hewett, S.   183
Hewitt, J.   296
Hicks, R.   18, 257, 272, 273, 274,
    279
Hicks, S.   284
Higgins, E.   294
Hildebrandt, K.   158, 159, 160, 279
Hilderbrand, M.   58, 93
Hill, C.   28
Hill, L.   272
Hill, M.   66
Himmelfarb, S.   296
Hines, P.   257
Hirschenfang, M.   187, 194
Hobbs, S.   10, 11, 255, 261
Hobfoil, S.   249
Hochberg, J.   158
Hockenbury, D.   261
Hocking, J.   25
Hofacre, S.   106
Hoffman, S.   195
Hohmann, G.   233
Holahan, C.   137, 138
Holborn, S.   59
Hollander, S.   88, 89, 90
Hollen, M.   191, 243, 244
Holmes, M.   205
Holmes, S.   29, 141, 145
Homer, P.   77
Hooker, L.   59
Hoopes, J.   99
Hoopes, J.   193
Horai, J.   12, 42, 43
Hore, T.   148, 149
Hornstein, H.   205
Horowitz, L.   261
Horton, C.   239, 241
Howard, C.   44
Howard, L.   91, 92
Hoyt, J.   233
Humphreys, S.   131, 132, 270
Husain, A.   12

Husband, R. 34
Huston, T. 16, 17, 23, 259, 282
Hyde, J. 105

I

Ibrahim, F. 235
Iliffe, A. 278
Innes, J. 206
Insko, C. 10, 13, 38
Irilli, J. 147
Izzett, R. 115, 116

J

Jabaley, M. 99
Jackson, D. 259
Jackson, L. 67, 68, 72, 73, 121
Jacobson, M. 57, 58
Jacobson, S. 108
Jacobson, W. 193
Jahoda, G. 52
Jakubowski, P. 262
James, D. 166, 170, 171, 190
Jason, L. 24
Jeeves, M. 85
Jenkins, M. 52, 55
Jenny, J. 271
Jensen, S. 243
Johnson, D. 280, 295
Johnson, R. 54, 58, 59, 60
Jones, J. 225
Jones, K. 44
Jones, Q. 274
Jones, R. 3, 7, 288, 295
Jones, T. 225
Jones, W. 249, 261
Jones-Molfese, V. 162, 163
Joseph, W. 75, 76
Jouhar, A. 277

K

Kaats, C. 24
Kagan, J. 161, 162

Kahle, L. 77
Kahn, P. 24
Kahneman, D. 68, 207
Kalick, S. 31, 239, 243, 253, 267
Kane, R. 90
Kanekar, S. 105
Kanfer, F. 212
Kaplan, R. 136, 137
Kapp, K. 180, 182
Kapp-Simon, K. 242, 253
Karniski, M. 225
Karoly, P. 286
Kassarjian, H. 54
Katz, I. 188, 190, 191, 218, 220
Katz, S. 222, 223
Kayra-Stuart, F. 88, 89, 90
Kehle, T. 123
Kehr, J. 248, 249
Keller, G. 275
Kelley, H. 291
Kelly, M. 31, 38
Kemp, A. 229, 232
Kendon, A. 211, 252
Kenny, C. 275
Kenrick, D. 36, 283, 284
Kerber, K. 285
Kernan, J. 46, 289, 298
Kernes, M. 25, 26, 27, 36, 254, 284
Kerr, B. 225
Kerr, N. 106, 119, 120
Kessler, J. 103, 105, 113, 114
Kiesler, S. 16
Kimata, L. 36, 284
King, M. 286
Kirkland, J. 273
Kirkpatrick, C. 37, 38
Klappersack, B. 236
Klatzky, R. 90
Kleck, R. 1, 189, 190, 194, 195,
   196, 197, 202, 203, 206, 207,
   208, 209, 210, 260, 296
Klein, R. 263
Kleinke, C. 2, 10, 256
Klentz, B. 61
Kligman, A. 219, 245

Klosinsky, M. 87, 89
Knapp, M. 213, 295
Knapper, C. 151, 282
Knight, J. 13, 14
Knorr, N. 193, 244
Koch, J. 76, 77
Koch, W. 57, 58
Kollar, M. 296
Kolsawalla, M. 105
Korabik, K. 271, 272
Kornhaber, R. 204
Koulack, D. 102, 103, 104, 108
Kozeny, E. 82
Krate, R. 112
Krebs, D. 18, 19, 20, 259
Kreiborg, S. 271
Kroger, D. 275
Kulka, R. 113, 114
Kupke, T. 10, 11, 255
Kureshi, A. 12
Kurtzberg, R. 92, 98, 224

L

Laird, J. 275
Lakoff, R. 282, 299
Lamb, M. 180
Lamberth, J. 12
Lampel, A. 11
Lando, H. 66
Landy, D. 34, 36, 106, 107, 109,
    134, 135, 136, 137, 138, 139
Lange, A. 262
Langer, E. 201
Langlois, J. 151, 155, 156, 157, 159,
    160, 166, 167, 168, 169, 172, 173,
    174, 175, 176, 177, 283, 286
Lansdown, R. 170, 171, 180, 183,
    184, 190, 207
Larrance, D. 255
La Voie, J. 124, 125, 126, 127, 131,
    295
Lawson, E. 276
Layton, B. 10, 13, 38
Leavitt, L. 180

Lee, L. 48
Lefebvre, A. 193, 239, 240
Leonard, B. 228
Lerner, A. 245
Lerner, J. 142, 146
Lerner, M. 201
Lerner, M. 290
Lerner, R. 142, 146
Leung, P. 262
Leventhal, G. 112
Levine, J. 161, 162
Levinger, G. 282
Levitt, L. 204
Levy, J. 195
Lewin, M. 98, 224
Lewinsohn, P. 259
Lewis, H. 271
Lewis, K. 248
Lewis, M. 161, 162
Lewis, P. 260, 264
Lewis, S. 9, 30
Lewison, E. 97, 98
Lewit, D. 270
Libet, J. 259
Lichtenstein, E. 257
Liebert, R. 237
Liggett, J. 81
Light, L. 88, 89, 90
Lin, T. 296
Linn, E. 244, 271
Linnstaedter, L. 10
Lippold, S. 13, 25
Lipson, A. 255
Lipton, D. 98, 224
Litowitz, D. 24
Littman, M. 105
Livneh, H. 218, 219, 220, 221, 222,
    223, 224
Lockhart, R. 49
Lombardi, D. 161, 166, 167
Lombardi, J. 147
London, O. 10, 12, 289, 290
London, R. 196, 197
Longacre, J. 95, 181
Lowe, J. 81, 82

Lowenstein, L. 101
Lown, C. 112, 113
Lucker, G. 3, 279, 280, 282
Lueck, H. 275
Lushene, R. 58
Lyman, B. 295

M

MacCoun, R. 106
Macgregor, F. 179, 181, 185, 186, 187, 188, 198, 200, 209, 222, 240, 241
Macklin, E. 31
Macurdy, C. 295
Madan, R. 201
Madar, T. 58, 93
Maddi, S. 258
Maddux, J. 47, 48, 49, 76
Madsen, C. 262
Manstead, A. 229
Manz, W. 275
Marinelli, R. 194
Mark, L. 280
Markle, A. 274
Marks, G. 14
Marks-Greenfield, P. 228, 229
Martin, G. 90
Martin, R. 274
Martinek, T. 133, 134
Martinson, M. 235
Maruyama, G. 1, 14, 138, 146, 295
Marwit, S. 153, 154
Marzillier, J. 265, 266
Mashman, R. 14
Mason, E. 123
Massimo, M. 167
Masters, F. 96, 97
Matarazzo, J. 195, 212
Mathes, E. 12, 20, 289
Matthews, S. 11
Matthews, V. 165
Maurer, D. 163
Maxwell, R. 219
Maxwell, E. 219

May, J. 285
Mayfield, E. 63
McAfee, L. 279
McArthur, L. 3, 280, 281, 293
McCabe, V. 157, 158
McClellan, P. 296
McCown, D. 247
McCulloch, C. 229
McDaniel, J. 219
McDonald, P. 255
McElroy, J. 132, 133
McFall, M. 285
McFatter, R. 117, 118
McGhee, J. 195
McGill, P. 192
McGinnis, J. 50
McGovern, K. 257
McGraw, K. 24
McGuire, J. 258, 266
McHenry, R. 275, 295
McKeachie, W. 276
McKeever, W. 214
McKelvie, S. 11
McKenzie, B. 161, 165, 166
McKillip, J. 30
McKinney, J. 236
McKinney, K. 24
McLean, J. 273
McMurran, M. 84
McNamara, J. 3
McNicholas, G. 274
McWilliams, B. 180
Mead, G. 291
Mehrabian, A. 22, 196, 195, 211
Meindl, J. 275, 276
Meiners, M. 35
Meisels, M. 199
Melamed, L. 283, 284
Mermin, P. 251
Meyer, E. 193
Meyer, J. 99
Meyer, R. 296
Meyers-Winton, B. 284
Meyers-Winton, S. 18, 257
Michelini, R. 116

Middleton, D. 217
Milgram, S. 93
Miller, A. 9, 10, 19, 66, 93, 287, 288
Miller, C. 28, 37
Miller, H. 10
Miller, K. 13
Miller, L. 277
Miller, M. 225
Miller, N. 1, 14, 138, 146, 295
Miller, R. 296
Mills, J. 41, 42, 43, 44
Minde, K. 159
Mishler, W. 51
Mitchell, K. 258
Monson, D. 236
Monson, T. 287
Montgomery, D. 262
Moore, J. 274
Morgan, B. 262
Morgan, E. 223
Morrison, R. 267
Morrow, P. 132, 133
Morse, S. 18, 282
Moss, M. 283, 284, 296
Moyel, I. 274
Mueller, J. 81, 89, 90, 91
Mueser, K. 4, 295
Munro, I. 185, 193, 238, 239, 240, 241, 242
Murakami, M. 158
Murroni, E. 76, 77
Murphy, M. 75, 146
Murray, J. 229
Murstein, B. 30, 38, 286
Muthard, J. 282

N
Naccari, N. 42, 43
Nagy, G. 17, 23
Napoleon, T. 251
Narcus, M. 236
Neff, L. 180

Neff, S. 25
Nelson, D. 146
Newcomb, J. 66, 102
Newcombe, F. 85
Newman, I. 139, 255
Neuman, M. 24
Neuman, N. 24
Nezlek, J. 25, 26, 27, 254
Nida, S. 29, 36, 136, 137
Nisbett, R. 3, 77, 299
Noles, S. 250
Nordholm 249
Nordlund, J. 245
Norman, R. 43, 48
Norris, A. 193
Northcraft, G. 298
Northercraft, G. 204
Novak, P. 201
Nowak, C. 121, 178, 285, 286
Nudler, S. 195
Nuessle, R. 195

O
Ono, H. 202, 203, 206, 207
Orbuch, D. 24
Orr, F. 258
Orvin, C. 12
Ostrove, N. 108, 109, 110, 111, 114, 116
Owens, G. 297

P
Page, R. 296
Pallak, S. 49, 76, 77
Pancer, S. 275, 276
Panek, P. 139
Paschall, N. 66, 101, 102, 283
Patterson, E. 51, 52
Patzer, G. 78, 79, 278, 283, 298
Pavlos, A. 66, 102
Pearce, L. 69, 70, 71
Pederson, F. 155

Pellander, F. 191
Pellegrini, R. 18, 257, 272, 273, 284
Pennebaker, J. 24
Penner, L. 249
Pennock, J. 199
Penta, F. 236
Peplau, L. 28, 261, 264
Perkins, B. 225
Perlman, D. 261, 264
Perri, M. 25, 26, 27, 254
Perrin, F. 2
Perry, R. 295
Pertschuk, M. 238, 251
Peter, J. 184, 193, 194
Peterson, J. 28, 37
Peterson, K. 276
Peterson, N. 181
Petty, C. 226
Pfeiffer, J. 196, 197
Pheterson, M. 12
Phillips, A. 249
Piciotto, S. 204
Pick, J. 99
Piehl, J. 112
Piff, C. 251
Piliavin, J. 84, 197, 204, 207, 290
Pilkonis, P. 263, 264
Pipp, S. 10, 256
Pittenger, J. 280
Polyson, J. 249
Pope, B. 195
Porter, J. 245
Potter, R. 233
Powell, P. 297
Prakash, N. 59
Price, J. 31, 38
Price, R. 30
Pride, W. 78
Priestley, P. 258, 266
Przybla, D. 255

Q
Quay, H. 92

R
Radlove, S. 93
Rand, C. 282
Raskin, N. 218
Rathborn, H. 106
Read, D. 257
Read, J. 86, 87, 88
Reaney, H. 272
Redden, J. 256
Reece, M. 265
Rees, G. 270
Reeves, J. 18
Reeves, K. 10, 12, 289, 290
Reich, J. 239, 241, 243, 244
Reingen, P. 46, 289, 298
Reis, H. 18, 25, 26, 27, 113, 254, 282
Reuben, D. 69
Ribbens, K. 3
Rich, A. 262
Rich, J. 101, 104, 127, 128, 152, 153, 154
Richardson, S. 164, 165, 189, 202, 220, 223
Richman, L. 132, 182, 183, 184
Riedel, S. 30
Riggio, R. 23
Rinn, R. 274
Rissi, J. 277
Rivenbark, W. 10
Robertiello, R. 15
Robertson, N. 271
Robinson, J. 84
Robinson, T. 274
Rodin, J. 204, 207, 290
Rogers, R. 47, 48, 49, 76
Roll, S. 275, 276
Ronchi, D. 296
Rosen, A. 4
Rosenberg, M. 226
Rosenfeld, H. 196
Rosenthal, R. 121, 295
Ross, J. 71, 72, 73, 74
Ross, M. 128

Rothbart, M.   43
Rottman, L.   9, 10, 11, 14, 15, 20,
    30, 293
Rubenstein, C.   1, 296
Rubenstein, E.   229
Rubin, Z.   28
Rumsey, N.   166, 170, 171, 186, 187,
    188, 189, 192, 193, 195, 196,
    197, 198, 199, 203, 205, 206,
    207, 209, 210, 211, 214, 222,
    228, 232, 234, 238, 242, 243,
    245, 246, 251, 253, 260, 264,
    265, 266, 295, 298
Rusalem, H.   262
Rutter, D.   259
Rutzen, S.   271

S

Sadlick, M.   236
Saeed, L.   23
Safar, H.   92, 98
Salafia, W.   197
Sale, O.   205
Sales, B.   115, 116
Salvia, J.   128, 129, 143, 144
Samarotte, G.   204, 206
Samuels, C.   164
Sandler, A.   250
Santana, R.   230
Sarty, M.   163
Saruwatari, L.   66, 67, 72
Sather, A.   191, 243, 244
Saxe, L.   32, 36, 37, 148
Schenker, C.   93
Scherr, R.   282, 299
Schilling, J.   295
Schlenker, B.   286
Schmidt, L.   248
Schneider, W.   49
Schoedel, J.   13, 14
Schofield, W.   248
Schopler, J.   114, 115
Schreiber, T.   12
Schroeder, H.E.   262

Schulz, R.   264
Schuring, A.   99
Schwartz, J.   249
Schwibbe, G.   108
Schwibbe, M.   108
Sears, D.   50
Secord, P.   158, 190, 272, 281, 282,
    292, 296
Selby, J.   103, 105
Seligman, C.   66, 101, 102, 103, 104,
    108
Senatore, V.   264
Sergl, H.   270
Shakespeare, R.   180, 183, 186, 191,
    192, 221, 231
Shanteau, J.   17, 23
Shaw, J.   104
Shaw, W.   131, 132, 185, 188, 192,
    219, 270, 271, 298
Shea, J.   258
Shead, G.   273
Sheare, J.   143, 144
Sheed, W.   229
Shepherd, J.   30, 35, 84, 85, 86, 87,
    88, 89
Sheposh, J.   *35*
Sherman, M.   195
Sherman, S.   251
Sherry, D.   180
Shiffrin, R.   49
Shoemaker, D.   81, 82
Shortridge, S.   235
Shurka, E.   223
Shurka, M.   222, 223
Shurtleff, C.   236
Siegfried, W.   69, 70, 71
Sigal, J.   108, 111
Sigall, H.   34, 36, 42, 106, 108, 109,
    110, 111, 114, 116, 134, 135,
    136, 137, 138, 139, 296
Siller, J.   220
Simms, T.   274
Singer, J.   41, 141, 142, 146
Singleton, R.   106
Siperstein, G.   189

Slaughter, R.   193
Smith, J.   273
Smith, L.   239
Smith, N.   87, 89
Smith, R.   24
Smith, W.   251
Smits, G.   10
Smolarski, S.   295
Snodgrass, S.   116
Snyder, M.   16, 21, 22, 43, 46, 47,
    207, 211, 253, 288, 289, 298
Soble, S.   203, 206
Solender, E.   110
Solomon, M.   114, 115
Solow, B.   271
Soloway, D.   260
Sommer, R.   200
Sorell, G.   121, 178, 285, 286
Sorrell, V.   225
Sotolongo, M.   66
South, D.   81, 82
Sparacino, J.   71, 72, 73, 74, 144,
    145, 296
Spiegel, N.   25, 26, 27, 254
Spira, M.   95, 96
Spreadbury, C.   18
Sprecher, S.   1, 3, 9, 24, 72, 285,
    293, 294
Spriestersbach, D.   180
Springbett, B.   62
Spuhler, J.   30
Sroufe, R.   203
Staffieri, R.   236
Staneski, R.   10, 256
Starr, P.   182
Stass, J.   273
Steffen, J.   256
Stein, S.   256
Stephan, C.   112, 137, 138, 151, 160,
    172, 173, 177, 284, 286
Stephen, W.   226
Stephenson, B.   16, 226
Stephenson, G.   259
Sternglatz, S.   158
Stewart, J.   118, 120

Stevens, J.   52, 55, 125, 135, 136,
    139, 153, 203, 204, 206, 260, 270
Stodt, W.   270
Stokes, N.   297
Stone, M.   118
Stopeck, M.   62, 73, 74
Storck, J.   106
Straith, C.   99, 100, 101
Strane, K.   35
Strauss, R.   187, 191, 244
Strenta, A.   189, 194, 207, 208, 209,
    210, 260
Stretch, R.   15
Stricker, G.   213, 272
Strickland, L.   203, 206
Stritch, T.   281
Stroebe, W.   10, 13, 38
Strohmer, D.   248
Strong, S.   247
Stycznski, L.   167, 168, 169, 174,
    175, 176, 177
Suben, M.   214
Sultan, F.   261
Sussman, S.   4, 295
Swann, W.   298

T
Takata, G.   66, 101, 102
Tan, A.   230
Tanke, E.   21, 22, 46, 47, 207, 211,
    253, 281, 288, 289, 298
Tarrahian, G.   273
Taylor, J.   231
Taylor, P.   33, 34
Taylor, S.   201
Tennis, G.   283
Terpstra, D.   64, 65
Terry, R.   31, 274, 275, 279
Thiel, D.   37, 104, 296
Thomas, S.   232
Thompson, V.   10, 13, 38
Thompson, W.   81, 90, 91
Thoreson, R.   225
Thornton, B.   10, 104

Thornton, G.   82, 83, 275
Thredkeld, R.   235
Timmerman, K.   296
Tocci, M.   147
Tolor, A.   197
Tomlinson, N.   272, 273
Tompkins, R.   130
Touhey, J.   12
Travis, F.   239, 240
Tresselt, M.   282
Trehub, S.   159
Triandis, H.   286
Trimer, C.   138
Trower, P.   259
Trust, D.   187, 199
Tuck, B.   87, 89
Tully, J.   112
Turcotte, S.   59
Turkat, D.   102
Turner, R.   130
Tversky, A.   68, 207

U
Udry, J.   33, 278
Udry, R.   34
Ungar, S.   203
Unger, R.   58, 93

V
Valins, S.   284, 285
Vance, F.   249
Vandenberg, S.   29, 30
Van Denmark, A.   185
Van Denmark, D.   185
van der Linden, F.   279
van Horn, E.   175, 177, 263, 265
Verinis, J.   275, 276
Vilemur, N.   105
Villa, R.   60
Vinson, M.   108
Virolainen, K.   270
Vogel, J.   81, 90, 91
Vogelbusch, A.   191

Vonkorff, M.   195
Vukcevic, D.   196, 197

W
Waid, L.   29
Waldrop, M.   100, 101, 155, 157, 160
Walfish, N.   255
Walker, B.   25
Walker, E.   153, 154
Walker, M.   203
Walker, V.   195
Walsh, W.   248
Walster, E.   9, 10, 11, 14, 15, 18, 19,
      20, 23, 30, 122, 124, 125, 140,
      141, 254, 281, 284, 293, 298, 299
Ward, C.   284
Warford, J.   245
Warr, P.   151, 282
Wartman, S.   69
Washburn, P.   211, 252
Waters, J.   69
Watts, C.   35
Weinberg, N.   189, 213, 230
Weinberger, H.   17
Weise, B.   247
Weiss, J.   238
Weiss, R.   261
Welham, D.   258, 266
Wells, B.   4, 11
West, S.   203
Westervelt, V.   236
Westie, C.   165
Westin, A.   198
Wheeler, L.   25, 26, 27, 36, 254, 284
Whitaker, L.   238
White, G.   28
Whitman, R.   265
Wiback, K.   63, 64, 65
Wicklund, R.   16
Wiemann, J.   195
Wiens, A.   195, 212
Wilcox, B.   164
Wildfogel, J.   202
Wilkinson, J.   265

Williams, C.   261
Williams, J.   29, 36
Williams, S.   273, 274
Williamson, L.   200
Willis, F.   273
Wilson, D.   116, 117
Wilson, G.   25
Wilson, M.   66
Wilson, M.   149
Wilson, T.   3, 77
Wolfensberger, W.   232
Wolff, E.   18
Wolfgang, A.   198
Wolfgang, J.   198
Woll, S.   23, 285
Worthington, M.   197
Worthy, M.   274
Wojtek, B.   191
Wright, B.   187, 191, 213, 218, 223, 232
Wrightsman, L.   119, 120, 286
Wu, P.   163

Y
Yardley, K.   265, 267
Yarmey, A.   87, 88, 89
Yarmey, A.   84, 85
Yarnold, P.   295
Young, A.   85
Young, J.   257
Young, L.   172
Young, R.   251

Z
Zakariya, S.   235
Zakin, D.   11
Zanna, M.   294
Zeis, F.   130
Ziller, R.   200, 201
Zimbardo, P.   208, 225, 260, 263
Zimmerman, D.   274
Zlotlow, S.   248
Zuckerman, M.   113, 255

Subject Index

A

Abnormality 95–101
Abuse 157–161
Academic performance 134–147
Acceptance 16
Acquaintance 167–169, 172–175
Adults 190
Advertising 75–79, 229–230
Age 161–177
Applicant selection 62–71
Arousal 284
Attitudes 12–14, 218–226, 236
Attractiveness 10, 12, 14–15, 63, 67,
    85, 90, 92, 122, 142, 155, 161,
    163, 166, 170, 214, 254–255,
    278–283, 297
Attribution theory 287–288
Avoidance 201–203

B

Babies 158–161
Beards 275–276
Beauty 281, 297
Behavior 10, 127, 207–209,
    223–227
Bias 129
Body image 220
Bullying 101

C

Care 244–247
Character 11
Childhood 219
Children 11, 151–177, 179–185,
    235–256
Chin 281
Cleft lip/palate 182
Clients 248–251
Cognitive explanations 287–288
Communication 123
Competence 168
Computer dating 22–24
Conduct 126
Cosmetics 1, 191–192, 276–277
Cosmetic surgery 240–241
Counseling 247–251
Credibility 43
Criminality 81–85, 91–101
Cultural effects 192, 219

D

Dating 14–29
Defendants 106–108, 116–118
Deformity 170, 179–267
Delinquency 91–94
Dental appearance 132, 270–272
Dependent variables 296–297

Developmental effects   121, 181–182, 184–185, 188–190
Deviancy   91–93
Disability   218–223
Disadvantage   217–267
Discipline   151–154
Discrimination   3
Disfigurement   95–101, 170, 179–267
Distinctiveness   89
Dynamics of encounters   20–22

E
Ecological validity   5, 11, 18, 78–79, 113–115, 154–157, 293
Education   121–149, 225
Employment   62–75
Equity theory   290
Evidence   119–120
Expectations   123
Experience   130
Expertise   44–47
Eyes   272–275, 281

H
Hair   276
Handicap   165, 203
Health   237–247
Help   203–207, 212–213, 247–267
History   185, 218–219
Hyperactivity   100

I
Impartiality   108–109
Individual differences   11–12, 17–18, 282–283
Infants   158–164
Information processing   49–50, 76
In-group bias   60
In-post evaluation   71–75
Interjudge agreement   278
IQ   121, 124–125, 130, 140
Isolation   199–200

J
Job status   69
Jurors   104
Justice   81–120

L
Law   3, 81–120
Liking   9–14, 87, 90, 164
Loneliness   199–200, 260–264
Long-term interactions   25–29

M
Marital adjustment   36–38
Marriage   29–39
Media   227–237
Meeting   14–19
Mental health   250–251
Meta-analysis   61
MMPI   182
Motivation   243

N
Nonfacial information   69, 124–132, 144–146
Nose   281
Null effects   111
Number of arguments   47–48
Nursing   159–160

O
Objectivity   48
Occupation   90

P
Personality   10–11, 221
Persuasion   41–50, 256
Police   84–85
Political inclination   52–56
Politics   50–62

Preoccupation with appearance
     209–210
Prison   95–101
Privacy   198–199

R
Race   138–139
Rape   102–103, 104–106
Real-life   118–119
Recognizability   85–91
Reinforcement theory   14, 289–290
Research quality   2, 132–134
Responsibility   102–104
Role theory   292

S
School   129, 143
Self
     -definition   200–201
     -disclosure   257
     -esteem   240
     -evaluation   258
     -fulfilling prophecy   3, 288–289
     -help   251
     -ratings   17–18
Sexual experience   24
Shyness   260–264
Similarity of partners   29–36
Social
     interaction   193–198, 210–212,
          254, 257, 298

     skills   252–267
Societal values   186
Spectacles   274–275
Stereotypes   3, 90, 176, 187–190
Subnormality   131
Success   74
Surgery   95–101, 239–244
Symbolic interaction   291

T
Teachers   121–134, 142, 147–149,
     183
Teeth   132, 270–272
Television   227
Theories   115–116, 285–292
Type of job   65–67, 73–74
Typicality   88

U
Ugliness   63, 175
Unconscious processing   3
Uniqueness   86, 88
University   141

V
Votes   51, 56

W
Women's movement   56–62

Springer Series in Social Psychology

Attention and Self-Regulation: A Control-Theory Approach to Human Behavior
Charles S. Carver/Michael F. Scheier

Gender and Nonverbal Behavior
Clara Mayo/Nancy M. Henley (Editors)

Personality, Roles, and Social Behavior
William Ickes/Eric S. Knowles (Editors)

Toward Transformation in Social Knowledge
Kenneth J. Gergen

The Ethics of Social Research: Surveys and Experiments
Joan E. Sieber (Editor)

The Ethics of Social Research: Fieldwork, Regulation, and Publication
Joan E. Sieber (Editor)

Anger and Aggression: An Essay of Emotion
James R. Averill

The Social Psychology of Creativity
Teresa M. Amabile

Sports Violence
Jeffrey H. Goldstein (Editor)

Nonverbal Behavior: A Functional Perspective
Miles L. Patterson

Basic Group Processes
Paul B. Paulus (Editor)

Attitudinal Judgment
J. Richard Eiser (Editor)

Social Psychology of Aggression: From Individual Behavior to Social Interaction
Amélie Mummendey (Editor)

Directions in Soviet Social Psychology
Lloyd H. Strickland (Editor)

Sociophysiology
William M. Waid (Editor)

Compatible and Incompatible Relationships
William Ickes (Editor)

Facet Theory: Approaches to Social Research
David Canter (Editor)

Action Control: From Cognition to Behavior
Julius Kuhl/Jürgen Beckmann (Editors)

Springer Series in Social Psychology

The Social Construction of the Person
Kenneth J. Gergen/Keith E. Davis (Editors)

Entrapment in Escalating Conflicts: A Social Psychological Analysis
Joel Brockner/Jeffrey Z. Rubin

The Attribution of Blame: Causality, Responsibility, and Blameworthiness
Kelly G. Shaver

Language and Social Situations
Joseph P. Forgas (Editor)

Power, Dominance, and Nonverbal Behavior
Steve L. Ellyson/John F. Dovidio (Editors)

Changing Conceptions of Crowd Mind and Behavior
Carl F. Graumann/Serge Moscovici (Editors)

Changing Conceptions of Leadership
Carl F. Graumann/Serge Moscovici (Editors)

Friendship and Social Interaction
Valerian J. Derlega/Barbara A. Winstead (Editors)

An Attributional Theory of Motivation and Emotion
Bernard Weiner

Public Self and Private Self
Roy F. Baumeister (Editor)

Social Psychology and Dysfunctional Behavior: Origins, Diagnosis, and Treatment
Mark R. Leary/Rowland S. Miller

Communication and Persuasion: Central and Peripheral Routes to Attitude Change
Richard E. Petty/John T. Cacioppo

Theories of Group Behavior
Brian Mullen/George R. Goethals (Editors)

Changing Conceptions of Conspiracy
Carl F. Graumann/Serge Moscovici (Editors)

Controversial Issues in Social Research Methods
Jerald Greenberg/Robert G. Folger

The Social Psychology of Facial Appearance
Ray Bull/Nichola Rumsey